BRAIN TRAINING for RUNNERS

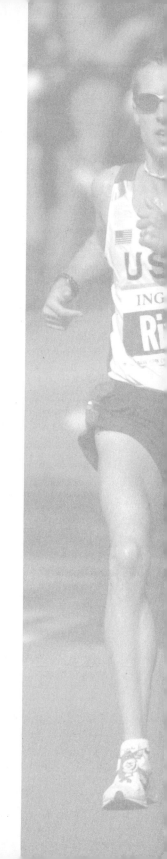

BRAIN
TRAINING
for RUNNERS

A Revolutionary New

Training System

to Improve

Endurance,

Speed,

Health,

and **Results**

Matt Fitzgerald

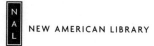

NEW AMERICAN LIBRARY

New American Library

Published by New American Library, a division of
Penguin Group (USA) Inc., 375 Hudson Street,
New York, New York 10014, USA
Penguin Group (Canada), 90 Eglinton Avenue East, Suite 700, Toronto,
Ontario M4P 2Y3, Canada (a division of Pearson Penguin Canada Inc.)
Penguin Books Ltd., 80 Strand, London WC2R 0RL, England
Penguin Ireland, 25 St. Stephen's Green, Dublin 2,
Ireland (a division of Penguin Books Ltd.)
Penguin Group (Australia), 250 Camberwell Road, Camberwell, Victoria 3124,
Australia (a division of Pearson Australia Group Pty. Ltd.)
Penguin Books India Pvt. Ltd., 11 Community Centre, Panchsheel Park,
New Delhi - 110 017, India
Penguin Group (NZ), 67 Apollo Drive, Rosedale, North Shore 0745,
Auckland, New Zealand (a division of Pearson New Zealand Ltd.)
Penguin Books (South Africa) (Pty.) Ltd., 24 Sturdee Avenue,
Rosebank, Johannesburg 2196, South Africa

Penguin Books Ltd., Registered Offices:
80 Strand, London WC2R 0RL, England

First published by New American Library,
a division of Penguin Group (USA) Inc.

First Printing, September 2007
10 9 8 7 6 5 4 3

(*For art credits and permissions see page 563.*)

 REGISTERED TRADEMARK—MARCA REGISTRADA

LIBRARY OF CONGRESS CATALOGING-IN-PUBLICATION DATA

Fitzgerald, Matt.
    Brain training for runners: a revolutionary new training system to improve endurance, speed,
health, and results/Matt Fitzgerald.
        p. cm.
    ISBN: 978-0-451-22232-9
1. Running—Training.   2. Running—Physiological aspects.   I. Title.
    GV1061.5.F57   2007
    613.7'172—dc22   2007004618

Set in 10 pt Goudy
Designed by Patrice Sheridan

Printed in the United States of America

CONTENTS

FOREWORD

There was a time, not so long ago, when we really did know everything about human exercise physiology. After all, it was all so very simple. The heart, you see, is the reason why we become tired during exercise. For the heart was designed so that it does not have quite enough capacity to supply our hungry muscles with all the oxygen they require when running at very fast speeds.

For when we attempt to run as fast as we can for as long as possible, the heart is unable to keep up. So the blood and oxygen supply to the muscles is too little; as a result the muscles develop an oxygen deficit, becoming "anaerobic." In this state, instead of producing energy only from oxygen-requiring (aerobic) sources, the exercising muscles must turn to their short-term savior, lactic acid, which can be produced in the absence of oxygen, that is, anaerobically. But according to a theory first proposed between 1907 and 1924, this can only ever be a short-term solution. For the lactic acid so produced is the ultimate cellular poison. So as the muscle cells become increasingly anaerobic, their lactic acid concentrations increase, leading ultimately to exhaustion. Since the basis for this fatigue is centered in the muscles rather than the brain, it has been called peripheral fatigue.

But there are two additional components crucial to this explanation. First, the end result is always a catastrophic failure of muscle function. Second, this outcome occurs in the absence of any intervention by the brain. Thus the brain has no capacity to "anticipate" what will happen in the future and so to act in a timely manner to forestall that catastrophe.

This model of catastrophic peripheral fatigue is also used to explain why we tire when we run for more than an hour or two. Then our exhaustion is not caused by an excess of lactic acid in the exercising muscles but by the opposite: by a lack of sufficient stores of the crucial muscle fuel, glycogen, to supply the muscles' energy requirements. Emptied of their most important fuel, the muscles refuse to work, terminating the exercise bout.

According to this model, the outcome of the changes we produce in our bodies with training must be to lessen the impact of these limiting processes. So the heart becomes stronger and better able to pump more blood to the muscles; the network of blood vessels in the muscles expands to hasten the delivery of oxygen from the blood to the muscle cells. And the intracellular engines, the mitochondria, which produce the energy to power the function of the cells, improve their capacity. As a result, the muscles become less "anaerobic" during exercise and better able to function at a higher capacity and for a longer time.

The prediction of this explanation, as so clearly identified in this book, is that the only way to improve our running performance is forever to be training at the limit. Only in this way can we maximize these adaptations in our muscles and heart and so lessen the barriers to performance that they pose. For how can we train our hearts and muscles to the maximum other than by always working them to the limit of their capacities?

The first problem with this catastrophic model is that it runs contrary to some fundamental principles in human physiology. For example, in the early 1940s, Dr. Walter Cannon from Harvard University published his seminal work showing that the reason why earthly creatures survive in a variety of different environmental niches is because all have the capacity to sustain internal homeostasis. He described homeostasis as a state of relative constancy of the chemical composition of all the bodily organs. The point, of course, is that the catastrophic model of exercise predicts that whereas human functioning is designed to maintain homeostasis at rest, that control is completely lost during exercise. Indeed the basis for this theory is that fatigue represents a state of homeostatic failure.

In time it was realized that this state of internal homeostasis (at rest) is achieved by the interaction of feed-forward and feedback controls within the body so that all the bodily organs act as a unified whole. The feed-forward component of this control is most usually regulated by the brain, which initiates each response to a new challenge on the basis of what it "knows" will be required to complete the biological task, whatever that task might be. But once the action is begun, the brain no longer works in isolation. Rather, on a second-by-second basis, the brain received sensory feedback from every organ in the body, each telling the brain how it is faring and what support it might need from the brain and other organs to keep it in homeostasis. On the basis of this feedback, the brain continually modifies its original response to ensure that every part of the body remains in homeostasis.

When it comes to exercise, the principal component of this feed-forward control is the number of muscle fibers that the brain chooses to activate in the exercising muscles. For the speed that the athlete can achieve is principally the result of the number of muscle fibers that the brain chooses to activate for any exercise bout. When fewer fibers are active, the speed is slower; when more are recruited, the athlete speeds up. In the words of Matt Fitzgerald, "only the brain can hold the muscles back." Or as might be added: Only the brain can speed up the muscles. But the crucial point is that the more fibers that are activated, the greater will be the risk to homeostasis.

For the more muscle fibers become active, the more blood flow they require; the more oxygen that must be delivered; the faster the rate at which energy must be produced; and the quicker the body produces heat. So the quickest way to quell any of these threats to homeostasis is simply to reduce the number of muscle fibers that are recruited by the brain. This represents a simple and elegant solution that would have been forged in the error-reducing crucible of evolution.

But the more compelling challenge for the traditional model is that it simply cannot explain the obvious. For instance, why do athletes run at different paces during races of different distances? For the lactic-acid-as-poison model predicts that there can only ever be one running pace. So each athlete must begin every race at the same very fast pace until his muscles produce enough lactic acid to poison their function, causing the runner to slow down to a more sustainable pace, just below that at which this poisoning effect becomes marked.

The result is that once this poisoning effect is fully activated, the athlete will have reached his steady state pace, which will be maintained presumably until the muscles encounter their next limiting factor when they become depleted of their crucial glycogen stores. So this explanation predicts that every athlete will only ever have one pace for all races regardless of distance. That pace may indeed be different among different runners, yet for each individual there is only ever one running pace.

It does not require a degree in advanced mathematics to appreciate that all athletes begin races of different distances at different running speeds, such that the longer the racing distance, the slower will be the starting speed. As a result, the much beloved lactic acid model fails to explain that which is the most obvious. Yet there is more.

Perhaps even more compelling is the observation that athletes speed up near the end of races at distances beyond about 1500 meters. This invites the obvious question: How is it possible to speed up near the end of a race when the very reason why the runner's pace has been "limited" in the first part of the race is because the poisoned muscles have been unable to work any harder? If it suddenly becomes possible somehow to overcome this effect when the finish line comes in sight, why was it not possible earlier? And how ever do the muscles or the heart suddenly "know" that the finish line is in sight so that they can begin the final spurt to the line—the heart by suddenly finding a reserve of blood flow it can direct to the muscles; the muscles by suddenly releasing themselves from the restraining grip of lactic acid? Indeed it would be most interesting to know how the heart and the muscles can sense the proximity of the finish, if not through the function of the eyes and the brain.

I first became aware of some of these apparently insoluble paradoxes, so well detailed in this book, in the 1980s, when our group began to evaluate the biological features of athletes in the laboratory. For we wished to understand the biology explaining their success. It soon became clear that there was really no good reason to suppose that they stopped running during maximal exercise because their muscles had become catastrophically "anaerobic" and poisoned by lactic acid. And so began a twenty-five-year study to try to explain exactly what really was going on. In time we came to the conclusion that the brain was in charge and that it regulated the exercise performance specifically to ensure that no organ in the body ever went beyond the limits of its capacity and so lost its homeostasis. For the only time homeostasis fails is when we are no longer alive. And if the goal of the brain is to ensure that homeostasis is retained, it follows that the body always finishes every exercise bout with reserve. Which in turn means that the goal of the athlete's brain is never to reach the race finish in the fastest possible time. Rather it is to reach the end safely, regardless of the time it might take.

And so it was that these writings, which have attracted the attention not so much of our scientific colleagues (whose job it is to be skeptical and so to doubt everything, including new ideas of how the body works during exercise until some "definitive" evidence is available), but of those practical people who saw the relevance of these ideas to their own areas of specialty.

And perhaps the most important such mind to have been activated so far may be that of Matt Fitzgerald. For by combining his experience as a runner and a coach with an intellectual inclination for the unconventional, he has produced a work of rare significance. For in this book he has advanced our understanding of the practical significance of these ideas in ways that many of us could not have imagined. My initial impression is that his book is of seminal importance and will prove to be at least as significant as any book yet published on the training of runners, including those iconic writings from which Matt Fitzgerald has drawn ideas and special inspiration. He proposes nothing other than a fundamental shift in the way we approach the training of runners and, in time, those in other endurance sports.

The basis for my enthusiasm is that Matt may just have solved some of the key training challenges that have evaded all the rest of us.

As is appropriate, his novel ideas and the fundamental change that he advocates can be summarized in just a few lines—lines whose simplicity belies the effort and wisdom in their production. So he posits that "the threshold approach to training is misguided because (according to the model of brain regulation of exercise performance) there are no direct physiological causes of fatigue." So how can we ever "fix" or "adapt" a single physiological limitation to performance when no such limitation exists?

Instead he argues that the "goal of training is not to push back particular physiological causes of fatigue. Rather, the goal of training is simply to gradually increase the speed you can sustain over race distance and the duration you can sustain race speed (or faster) until you are able to sustain your goal pace over the full peak race distance." To do this it is necessary to train the brain and body to push back that "wall of fatigue" used by the brain to ensure that a catastrophic failure does not occur. Thus: "Regardless of the particular factors that may cause you to experience discomfort and slow down in a race, you want to train in a way that enables you to sustain your goal pace all the way to the finish line without slowing and without the overwhelming discomfort that comes with it." This is best done "if you have already done in training more or less what you are attempting to do in the race."

The Fitzgerald approach requires that the runner first decide what is the peak race goal time. The goal of training then becomes to adapt the body and mind "to increase the duration you can sustain your goal pace and to increase the pace you can sustain over the full race distance." The runner begins by identifying a starting level of fitness, the target pace level, on the basis of recent racing performances. Armed with these two pieces of information, the runner can construct an appropriate training program from the wide variety provided in the book. These programs are based on what has been shown to work.

A key component of these programs is that Fitzgerald has arrived at a novel method for determining the intensity of different workouts for athletes at different levels of fitness and with different abilities. Instead of the classic tables, which are based on the catastrophe model and which require the runner to spend different amounts of time training at different "thresholds," thereby supposedly maximizing resistance to the fatiguing effects of lactic acid, for example, Fitzgerald proposes that the key is to adapt the brain (and the body) to work for increasingly longer periods at the exact pace that will be required in the race. The result is that, by the time the race day approaches, those runners who have followed these programs will have spent enough time running at race pace that their brains and bodies will know exactly what will be expected of them in the race. Better still, exposure to frequent runs at race pace will also establish the pace that is indeed sustainable. This information will in turn further encourage the athlete that the target is achievable. And, if not, what altered pace will more likely be successful.

There is much more to this book than just a novel training approach and many different training programs. It represents a real advance since it is based on a solid, albeit novel interpretation of how humans really function during exercise and uses that knowledge to present a training approach that is simple yet beautiful in its design. It appears so logical that we wonder why no one has ever had this idea before.

I expect runners who follow these guidelines to have more successes more frequently than if they were to follow other programs, mine included.

—Timothy David Noakes MBChB, MD, DSc, FACSM
Discovery Health Professor of Exercise and Sports Science, Director UCT/MRC
Research Unit for Exercise Science and Sports Medicine, Department of Human Biology, University of Cape Town and Sports Science Institute of South Africa, Boundary Road, Newlands, Cape Town, South Africa
Author of *Lore of Running* (Human Kinetic Publishers, Champaign, Illinois, 4th edition, 2002)
e-mail noakes@iafrica.com or timothy.noakes@uct.ac.za

PART ◆ I

INTRODUCTION

Forget everything you know—or thought you knew—about running. The conventional wisdom has been turned on its head. Literally. Within the past several years a quiet revolution has occurred in our scientific understanding of how the human body functions during workouts and races and how it responds to regular training. Exercise physiologists have discovered that the role of the brain in running performance is vastly more comprehensive and powerful than was previously known. The brain—which is as much a part of the body as the heart, lungs, and muscles—is now viewed as a "central governor" that has the most votes and the final veto when it comes to determining your running style, how your body adapts to training, how fast and far you can run, when you throw in the towel, and every other aspect of running performance. Or, to paraphrase the title of a recent scientific paper on this revolution, running starts and ends in the brain.

Consider the following points of conventional running wisdom—just a few among many—that have been subverted by the new, brain-centered model of running performance.

Fatigue is caused by energy depletion. Not so. Numerous studies have shown that there is still fuel available to the muscles when fatigue occurs. The actual cause of running fatigue is a reduction in muscle activation by the brain that is influenced in part by declining energy stores. This phenomenon is believed to serve as a protective mechanism that prevents us from running to the point where we seriously harm ourselves.

*   *   *

Good running form can't be learned. Untrue. Running form is controlled by movement "programs" that are stored in the brain. These programs can be modified through a variety of techniques to produce a running stride that is more efficient and powerful.

A runner's race pace is determined by physical capacities, such as VO₂max. Guess again. Physical capacities such as VO_2max (the capacity to consume oxygen during running) do have a strong influence on the pace a runner is able to sustain in a race. Running pace, however, is truly controlled by a type of subconscious brain calculation called teleoanticipation. When you start a race or other maximum-effort run, your brain calculates the maximum pace you can sustain over the planned running distance based on certain measures of your fitness level, past experience, the air temperature, and other factors, and helps guide you toward the appropriate pace by producing feelings of comfort and discomfort.

Running injuries are caused by the high-impact nature of running. Not really. While impact forces are a contributing factor to running injuries, the main culprits are a couple of other factors that cause us to run in ways that contradict the preferred movement patterns stored in our brains and thereby increase our susceptibility to impact-related tissue damage. These two factors are running shoes and the nine-plus hours that most of us spend sitting each day.

As you can see from these examples, the recent discoveries we've made about the role of the brain in running performance have important practical implications for runners. The brain-centered model of running performance encourages us to not be content with the stride we were born with, but instead to actively work to improve our running form. It also spurs us to cast aside our fatalistic attitude toward injuries and undo the negative effects of wearing running shoes (overstriding and heel-first ground striking) and sitting in chairs (muscle imbalances that reduce the stability of key joints).

Here's another example. As I suggested above, most runners think of "hitting the wall" as running out of muscle fuel (specifically glycogen) toward the end of a marathon or other long run. But recent findings suggest that hitting the wall may also be caused by the brain's response to muscle damage. The running muscles incur large amounts of microscopic tearing during especially long workouts and races. As a result of this damage, chemical signals travel to the brain, which triggers exhaustion when it determines that the muscles have had enough.

Preventing (or delaying) this particular cause of fatigue calls for a somewhat different strategy than the methods most runners use to prevent fatigue due to fuel depletion. Runners typically try to prevent hitting the wall by doing long training runs, which enhance glycogen storage and conservation, and by consuming carbohydrates during long runs. It is now clear, however, that runners would benefit even more by supplementing these traditional measures with jumping drills, which are proven to enhance the muscles' resistance to running-induced damage (through a brain-mediated process), and by consuming protein during long runs, which has been shown to drastically reduce muscle damage (also through a brain-centered mechanism).

The average running coach is not well informed about the recent discoveries concerning the role of the brain in running performance and their practical implications for runners. Few, if any, running coaches have taken more interest in these matters than I have. My brother Josh is partly responsible. Also a competitive runner, Josh studied brain science in graduate school and instilled in me a deep fascination with the brain by sharing some of the things he learned (in lay terms I could understand) and suggesting popular science books about the brain.

A runner myself since age eleven, I was in the early stages of my career as an endurance sports coach, expert, and journalist when the new science of the running brain emerged. It immediately captured my interest by appealing to both my abiding interest in the brain and my passion for training innovations. In studying the new science I quickly discovered that it is not only fascinating in itself but also has important implications for how runners train, fuel, race, and equip themselves. In fact, over time I came to the conclusion that the new brain-centered model of running performance does more than suggest a few "à la carte" adjustments to our training methods and other practices. I think it justifies a whole new approach to running. Over the past few years I have worked to develop this approach, which I call brain training.

Perhaps the best way to explain brain training is to distinguish it from mental training, a concept you may be familiar with. Mental training is a set of techniques, including mental rehearsal (also called imaging) and goal setting, that help athletes develop important psychological skills, such as focus and self-confidence. These techniques and skills apply to all sports and have traditionally been treated separately from the physical component of training for each particular sport. Brain training, on the other hand, encompasses both the mental and physical components of training, and in fact tears down the partition between them. It treats running as both a bodily activity and an experience that the brain regulates. A major goal of brain training is to improve your running by using the material of the running experience (body awareness, workout performance, the sensation of fatigue, observation of cause and effect in training) to make the running action more efficient, powerful, fatigue-resistant, and injury-proof. Also, because your brain is the most important organ with respect to your overall health and well-being, an equally important goal of brain training is to use running to enhance your brain health and general well-being (which, in turn, will enhance your running).

The brain training motto is this: Train your brain and the rest will follow. Everything you could possibly do to improve as a runner and enhance your running experience involves your brain in one way or another. As mentioned above, all forms of running fatigue entail signals of impending harm sent from your body to your brain. You can delay running fatigue by training your body to resist these various types of harm and by raising your brain's threshold of response to the body's danger signals. As also mentioned, cooperation between your central nervous system and muscles determines the efficiency and power of your stride; by reprogramming the stride patterns stored in your brain and rewiring the connections between your motor nerves and your muscles, you can make your stride more efficient and powerful.

Your emotions and thoughts can be conditioned to benefit your running too (both directly and indirectly, through enhanced brain health and mental well-being). And don't forget that everything you know about how to train for running, as well as all the objective feedback you use (split times, miles run, and so forth), influences your running by first affecting your brain.

Brain training starts to make a lot of sense when you think of everything that affects the running brain in terms of feedback. There are three basic types of feedback: subjective, objective, and collective. Let's look at each individually.

Subjective feedback comes to your brain from your body. It is more or less how you feel during your workouts and races and while recovering from them (emotions, pains, effort, energy, and other related factors).

Pacing is one example of an important factor in running performance that is grounded in subjective feedback. Exercise scientists use the term "perceived exertion" to describe the specific form of subjective feedback that runners use to pace themselves. Experienced runners develop an exquisite feel for the fastest pace they can maintain evenly over any given distance on any given day. This refined sense of feel was demonstrated in a recent experiment in which well-trained runners performed several workouts featuring repeated high-intensity running intervals. In the first workout the subjects were required to run twenty-four intervals of one minute apiece as fast as they could (with rest periods between intervals). The running intervals grew longer in each subsequent workout while the total workout duration remained the same. The last session featured four intervals of six minutes. Not surprisingly, the runners performed the longer intervals of the later workouts at a slightly slower pace than they did the shorter intervals of the early workouts. But what surprised the researchers was the fact that in each workout, most of the runners ran the final interval of the workout, in which they held nothing back, neither faster nor slower than the preceding intervals in the same workout. This pattern served as evidence of an exquisitely refined mechanism of teleoanticipation, or knowing intuitively just how much to hold back at the beginning of a maximal running effort to complete the effort without anything left in the tank, yet also without any decline in performance.

Subjective feedback allows you to do much more than pace yourself optimally in workouts and races. In the form of pain, subjective feedback can help you nip injuries in the bud. In the form of feelings of comfort and discomfort, subjective feedback can help you choose the right running shoes. It has a role in every conceivable facet of the running experience.

Subjective feedback can come from your brain, which is a part of the body too, of course. An example of brain-to-brain subjective feedback is motivation. Low motivation for running is often your brain's way of telling your mind that something is wrong—perhaps you are overtrained, or you just need a mental break from formal training. Learning to better appreciate and interpret this type of subjective feedback can do wonders for your running as well.

Objective feedback is mainly numbers and includes such things as speed, distance run, heart rate, and the like. This type of feedback benefits your running by enhancing motivation and by making your training more structured and systematic. Having numbers to shoot for in workouts encourages you to put forth a better effort. Research has shown that athletes who consistently gather objective feedback tend to improve faster than athletes who do the same amount of training but without putting numbers on it.

One of the major barriers to improvement in running is your brain's unconscious sense of what your body can and cannot do. You can use objective feedback to retrain this sense in a way that raises the bar. The best illustration of this phenomenon is the progression of world records. For example, no runner was able to run a mile in less than four minutes until Roger Bannister accomplished the feat in 1954. But in the next year and a half, sixteen other runners followed him under the four-minute barrier! The first sub-four-minute mile proved to the others knocking at the door of this threshold that running just a little faster was possible and probably would not kill them, so their brains finally allowed their bodies to do what they had been physically capable of doing all along.

While you are probably not aiming for world records, you can use numbers in a very similar way to improve your running. If you can run ten miles, why not eleven? If you can run a mile in 6:02, why not 5:59?

Collective feedback is the practical knowledge we all get from the collective experience of others and includes training guidelines, injury prevention and treatment methods, and nutrition information. This type of feedback is essentially a distillation of the subjective feedback and the objective feedback gathered by fellow runners, their coaches, and others, including exercise and nutrition scientists. In theory, if you had all the time in the world, you could re-create this great pool of practical knowledge using your own subjective and objective feedback. But since it's already available, you might as well use it.

The key to better running, from the brain training perspective, is to effectively integrate relevant subjective, objective, and collective feedback and apply the aggregated data toward the goal of running better. This process is, to a certain extent, automatic. Every workout is brain training and every thought and feeling that affects your running is brain training. But you will train your brain much more effectively if you do so programmatically instead of merely by default.

I see two big shortcomings in the unconscious brain training of most runners. First, few runners take a systematic approach to using subjective feedback—they don't know how to fully use pain, perceived effort, fatigue, and other signals from the body (including the brain itself). As you'll see in the coming chapters, the potential usefulness of these signals is truly impressive.

Second, on the side of objective feedback, most runners are not aware of how much the rules of running have changed as a result of the new science of the running brain. For example, few runners know that one of the major differences between top runners and average runners is that top runners are actually able to use a much higher percentage of the muscle fibers in their "running muscles." The most effective way to increase the number of usable fibers in your muscles is to run at maximum intensity, and the best time to do this type of running is early in the training process—that is, in the "base phase" of training—so that the added fibers may be used throughout the remainder of the training process. Incorporating maximum-speed running into the base phase of training is definitely not the norm in distance running, but it is standard procedure in brain training.

The purpose of this book is to show you how to harness the full power of your brain for the sake of running better and getting more from your running. In the following chapters I will present a comprehensive brain training program that will help you do everything from increasing the amount of muscle tissue your brain is able to communicate with during running to preventing injuries.

The book is divided into two parts. Part I presents the brain training system. Part II presents a selection of complete brain training plans based on this system.

Within Part I, the first two chapters look at the big picture, covering the many important roles of the running brain and how to integrate subjective and objective feedback in order to become your own coach. The next several chapters deal with concrete matters of physical training—or the running component of brain training, as it were. I'll show you how to do workouts that enhance your resistance to the various causes of fatigue (all of them brain-mediated), how to reprogram your neuromuscular system to run more efficiently and powerfully, how to use cross-training as brain training, how to use objective and subjective feedback to effectively control the intensity of your running, and how to maximize your fitness by "training responsively."

Chapter 7 describes the role of the central nervous system in relation to recovery and presents novel brain training methods of optimizing recovery. Chapter 8 deals with topics that have traditionally been relegated to mental training guides. But in brain training, the difference between physical and mental training collapses—you're always doing both at once. In this chapter I will show you how to master the discomfort associated with hard running, how to harness your emotions to benefit your running performance, and how to use proven psychological tools and techniques to prepare your mind and body for races, overcome prerace nerves, and much more.

Injuries are so common in running that avoiding them is truly half the battle of improving as a runner. In chapter 9 I will show you a foolproof method to "outsmart" injuries by integrating subjective, objective, and collective feedback. And in chapter 10 I will show you a brain training strategy for fueling optimal running performance.

Part II, comprising chapters 11–14, presents a dozen complete brain training plans for four common race distances: 5K, 10K, half marathon, and marathon. I promise that these plans are different from any plans you've done before, and I am confident they will give you better results.

Indeed, many of the techniques and strategies I will teach you in these pages are unusual, and some may even strike you as a little strange, but all of them are based on sound, cutting-edge science, and I practice most of them myself. In fact, if not for some of the brain training techniques in this book, my running career would have ended a few years ago (see chapter 9). Beyond that, thanks to some of the other brain training techniques I've developed, I am running better and enjoying running more than ever. If brain training does half as much for you as it has done for me, your time here will have been well spent.

CHAPTER ◆ 1

BRAIN TRAINING: AN OVERVIEW

Other runners think I'm weird. I don't train like they do. I run hill sprints in January, many weeks before I do my first race of the year. I hit the gym almost as often as I hit the roads. In each run I deliberately modify my natural stride slightly in one specific way or another. I spend a lot of time doing unusual technique drills and very little time doing familiar stretches. Even my sitting and standing posture are consciously controlled for the sake of aiding my running performance.

I routinely abandon runs when I don't like the way one of my muscles feels. While I always plan my training well into the future, all of my key workouts are scheduled "in pencil"—meaning I frequently change the planned workout based on how I feel at the beginning of the session. Many of my easier (recovery) runs are totally unplanned in terms of duration and pace—I just let my body tell me how far and how fast to go. My primary goal in certain tune-up races is to suffer as much as possible. Literally. I never use a heart rate monitor to guide my running pace. Instead, I control my workout intensity by pace, and perform all of my key workouts (except most endurance runs) at my estimated race pace for one of the following race distances: one mile, 3,000 meters, 5 kilometers (5K), 10 kilometers (10K), half marathon, and marathon.

Most other runners don't brain train (yet), but I do, and that's why most of the runners who know me (except those I coach using brain training methods) think I'm weird. That's fine with me, because each of the weird methods that I use in my brain training system is based on one or more specific facts about how the brain works as the "central governor" of running performance. For example, my warm-ups comprise unconventional dynamic stretches and mobility exercises, such as the Tilt Walk (see page 126), instead of popular static stretches, such as touching your toes. They do so because research has shown that, unlike static stretches, dynamic stretches enhance running efficiency by improving brain-muscle communications in ways that minimize wasteful tension in muscles opposing the working muscles at various phases of the stride.

Not everything I do as a brain training runner is unconventional. But whether weird or traditional, all of the methods I use are secondary to the overarching strategy that defines brain training. This strategy puts the brain at the center of every moment of training and racing, as the hub of three feedback loops: the subjective feedback loop, the objective feedback loop, and the collective feedback loop. In the brain training system, achieving maximum success as a runner is as simple a matter as taking control of these feedback loops, integrating them in the best way possible, and applying the aggregated data to the goal of running better. The particular methods used to accomplish this objective are mere details.

In most conventional training systems there is no attempt to organize the various methods under a coherent, overarching strategy. The typical running coach says, "Do X because it works. Do Y because we've always done it this way." In brain training, by contrast, the strategy comes first, and the strategy is, again, to integrate the subjective, objective, and collective feedback loops in your brain and use the amalgamated data to run your best. Adopting this strategy leads to some significant methodological departures from conventional training methods. For example, due to a greater reliance on subjective feedback in steering the course of your training, you will incorporate a lot more flexibility into your workouts and make almost daily adjustments to your planned workouts instead of stubbornly persisting in executing your plan, which is the conventional way to go.

Another key difference between brain training and conventional training systems is that the methods you will use in brain training are based on the new brain-centered model of performance instead of on the old muscle-centered and energy-focused models. Recent advances in our scientific understanding of the role of the brain in running performance have important practical implications for how runners train. These advances certainly don't require a wholesale transformation in training methods, but they do suggest a few innovations. For example, as you'll see in chapter 7, there is no valid rationale for recovery workouts in the old models of running performance, but in the brain-centered model there is more than one. Consequently, recovery workouts take on greater importance in brain training and are performed somewhat differently.

In the following sections of this chapter I will briefly discuss the methods you will employ in using each of the three feedback loops. In the last of these sections, which concerns the subjective feedback loop, I will say a few words about what it means to integrate this loop with the other two.

THE COLLECTIVE FEEDBACK LOOP

The collective feedback loop supplies a runner with information about practices that are known to be beneficial to all runners. The methods of the collective feedback loop include training guidelines, injury prevention and treatment methods, equipment knowledge, and nutrition information. In the present context I will focus only on proven training practices, including effective workout types and training strategies.

Without the collective feedback loop, each of us would have to reinvent the art of training. Lacking guidance from coaches, books, and more experienced runners, we would be forced to suffer through decades of trial and error to figure out how to train as effectively as today's best-informed competitive runners do. Fortunately, this tedious process is not necessary. By learning and applying the training techniques that have been proven most effective in the trial-and-error process undertaken by millions of competitive runners over the past century and more, we can train at the cutting edge without having to learn every lesson the hard way.

Staying current on the most effective training methods is no small task in itself, however, because the art and science of training for distance running continues to evolve. Several worthy innovations have come about within just the past few years. The fraction of competitive runners I consider to be truly up-to-date on running's best practices is fairly small. A further complication is the fact that top runners and coaches don't always agree on training methods. There is plenty of variety in the way top runners train and in the way top coaches prescribe training.

Happily for you, staying current on the most effective training methods is a big part of my job, so I've done the work for you. There are two important filters that I use in selecting methods to incorporate into my system. First, I only try new training methods that have a brain training rationale. Second, among those methods I consider worth trying in my own training and in that of the runners I coach, I only retain those that prove themselves effective. The methods described below are those that have successfully passed through both filters. Most of them, in general terms, are commonly practiced. They are the most battle-tested training practices that have survived more than a century of high-stakes application on the track, roads, and trails. But some of the methods are new and not widely practiced, and even the familiar ones have a special brain training twist.

In later chapters I will have much more to say about how to practice these methods within the brain training system. My objective here is simply to introduce them.

Running a Lot

Research has shown that the training characteristic that has the closest correlation with improvement in running performance is running volume, or the amount of running you do each week. This is only to be expected. Running fitness improves through a process of stress and adaptation. Workouts stress—or challenge—the body, causing it to adapt in ways that render it better able to handle the same stress when it's repeated. The more stress you apply, the more adaptation you get. Of course, there are such things as exceeding one's limits, doing too much too soon, and a law of diminishing returns. But as a general rule, you will run best by doing close to as much running as your body can handle.

Some of the benefits of high-volume running are brain-related. Running is a neuromuscular skill, like swinging a golf club or operating a crane, which improves with lots of practice. As you practice running, your brain and muscles find more efficient ways to communicate, so you can run faster with less energy and run farther before reaching exhaustion.

In the brain training system I encourage runners to do close to as much running as they can handle, but I recognize that various limitations prevent many runners from following a high-volume training regimen. Therefore the brain training system focuses on squeezing the most benefit out of every second spent running. For example, one of the unique features of the brain training system is the use of proprioceptive cues to control and improve the running stride in every workout. This practice effectively adds a second benefit to each run that is absent in conventional training systems.

Training Cycles

For competitive runners, training is usually oriented toward achieving maximum performance in a race of primary importance—which I call a "peak race"—in the near future. The hope is to steadily increase one's running fitness between the present time and race day. With appropriate training, most runners are able to increase their running fitness consistently for four to six months before reaching a temporary limit. After this point, any further attempts to increase fitness by increasing the training workload will fail and may result in overtraining (a state of persistent fatigue with a nervous system component) or injury. Additional improvement may be possible, but only after a period of relative rest and rejuvenation. For this reason, it is necessary to train in four-to-six-month cycles, each culminating in a peak race and followed by a brief period of relative rest.

The brain training plans in Part II range in duration from sixteen weeks (for a 5K peak race) to twenty-four weeks (for a marathon peak race). In addition to simply offering the optimal training duration for each race distance, these plans provide a model for developing your own brain training plans to use in the future.

Key Workouts

Key workouts are runs that are challenging enough to result in a high level of fatigue. They administer a greater training stress and provoke a stronger adaptive response than less challenging runs. Key workouts are therefore a critical feature of any effective training plan. Of course, you can't train to exhaustion every day, because your body will not recover adequately between runs and you'll soon become overtrained or injured. I recommend a training schedule that includes three key workouts per week (usually two high-intensity runs and one long run) for all runners. All of the brain training plans in Part II include three key workouts per week.

There are three general classifications of key workouts used in the brain training system: speed workouts (whose basic purpose is to maximize the number of muscle fibers that can contribute to race-pace running), intensive endurance workouts (whose basic purpose is to maximize efficiency and fatigue resistance at race pace), and extensive endurance workouts (whose basic purpose is to develop a reserve of fatigue resistance—that is, to make it "no problem" to cover the race distance at a pace that's slightly slower than your goal race pace).

A few key workouts—no more than three or four over the course of a training cycle—should be designated as "breakthrough workouts," which are super-challenging runs that take you to the point of complete exhaustion. These workouts serve the special purpose of pushing back the performance limits imposed by self-protective mechanisms in the brain. Tune-up races serve as ideal breakthrough workouts because the competitive atmosphere of races stimulates a higher level of sympathetic nervous system arousal that enables you to work harder than in any regular workout, resulting in a bigger fitness-boosting benefit. In my brain training plans, tune-up races serve as breakthrough workouts.

Progression

In order to improve steadily throughout a training cycle, you must train progressively. This means your workouts have to change from week to week in ways that allow you to build on the fitness gains you've derived from past training. There are two ways you can progressively modify your training from week to week to continuously stimulate fresh training adaptations. The first way is to make your workouts, and especially your key workouts, harder, which usually means longer and/or faster. The second way is to change the types of training you emphasize in a given block of training—that is, to divide the training process into separate phases and emphasize different types of training in each.

The general trend should be toward increasing specificity. In the final weeks of training before your peak race, do key workouts that are similar to your coming peak race in terms of pace and overall duration. Performing well in such workouts will result in adaptations that will pay off on race day when your brain responds to the feedback of sustained race-pace running by saying, in essence, "I've done this before; I can do it again."

The training that precedes the race-specific key workouts you do should simply prepare you to perform well in your race-specific peak workouts. In other words, it should provide an appropriate fitness foundation for your peak-phase key workouts. There are two sides to the challenge of achieving a race goal. First, there's the challenge of running as fast as you want to run over the full race distance. The second challenge is to run as far as you need to run in your peak race at your goal race pace. In short, race-specific fitness has a speed component and a "fatigue-resistance" (or endurance) component.

The race-specific key workouts you do in the final weeks of training need to integrate these two challenges. That's what makes them race-specific. But while building a foundation for these workouts it's best to work on developing the speed and fatigue-resistance components of race fitness individually. Your earliest speed-focused key workouts should be run much faster than your goal race pace, to make it no problem to run at that speed, but these high-speed efforts should be very short so they don't overtax you. The fitness adaptations you derive from these workouts will enable you to move on to speed workouts emphasizing efforts that are a little longer, a little slower, and therefore more race-specific.

Likewise, your earliest endurance-focused workouts should be run much slower than race pace. (Whether they are also much shorter than race distance depends on the distance of your peak race.) In the first phases of the training cycle you will concentrate on making these endurance efforts longer, so that covering the full race distance (at a relatively slow pace) is no problem. Then you will concentrate on increasing the pace of these workouts to make them more race-specific.

My brain training plans are divided into four phases: Base, Build 1, Build 2, and Peak. In the Base phase you will do your fastest speed running to increase the number of muscle fibers you can use in later training and racing. At the same time you will steadily increase your total volume of running (most of it done much slower than race pace) to build a foundation of fatigue resistance. In the Build phases you will steadily increase the specificity of your fitness by moving closer to race distance and race speed in your various key workouts. And finally, in the Peak phase you will do key workouts that are race-specific in both speed and duration.

Base Runs

Base runs are short-to-moderate-duration runs performed at a moderate intensity. They derive their name from their purpose, which is to provide a base or foundation of aerobic fitness, endurance, neuromuscular efficiency, and injury resistance. If you were only allowed to do one type of workout, base runs would be the best choice. While individual base runs do not provide as great a training stress or as strong an adaptive response as faster or longer key workouts, base runs, by virtue of their moderation, lend themselves to high-volume training. And as I mentioned above, total running volume is the most important determinant of running fitness.

Like the other workout types discussed below, base runs are almost universally practiced by competitive runners because they have shown themselves to be beneficial to every runner who's used them properly over the past one hundred–plus years. In contrast to some other training systems, the brain training system largely phases out base runs after the Base phase, replacing them with recovery runs (defined below).

Endurance Runs

Endurance runs are workouts that challenge a runner's resistance to low-intensity fatigue factors, including glycogen depletion and muscle damage. They are usually performed at a steady, moderate pace (termed "base pace" in the brain training system), but there are variable-pace and moderately fast formats as well. Endurance runs are an indispensable means to build a reserve of fatigue resistance in distance runners—especially in those training for longer races.

Endurance runs are used somewhat differently in the brain training system than in some other training systems. Specifically, in the Build and Peak phases, there is a strong emphasis on increasing the pace of these runs to make them more race-specific in this dimension. In the brain training plans in chapters 11–14, all runs (except longer marathon-pace workouts) exceeding ten miles in distance are classified as endurance runs. Base-pace runs of nine miles or fewer are classified as base runs.

Tempo Runs and Cruise Intervals

Tempo runs are workouts featuring one or more sustained segments of moderately fast-paced running (usually equivalent to between 10K and half-marathon race pace). Tempo runs have survived the collective trial-and-error process because they provide highly race-specific fitness benefits, such as heightened aerobic capacity, greater glycogen-burning efficiency, and better maintenance of muscle pH balance at race pace.

Cruise intervals are tempo runs that are divided into two parts, with a short period of "active recovery" between them. For example, in a typical tempo run you might warm up with a mile of easy jogging, run four miles at 10K race pace, and cool down with another mile of easy jogging. In a cruise-intervals version of the same workout the four miles of 10K-pace running might be divided into a pair of two-mile segments at the same pace with a mile of active recovery running separating them.

Traditionally, tempo runs and cruise intervals are performed at "anaerobic threshold" pace, or a pace that is believed to correspond to the pace just above which lactic acid begins to accumulate rapidly in the runner's muscles. From the brain training perspective, this tradition is based on a discredited belief that it's possible to isolate specific, individual causes of fatigue in training. In my system, tempo runs and cruise intervals are performed at estimated half-marathon or 10K race pace. The purpose of using these performance-based pace targets is to encourage runners to work harder in these workouts and thus get more out of them.

Intervals

Intervals are short or relatively short segments of high-intensity running separated by active or passive recovery periods. High-intensity running provides a number of benefits, including improved resistance to muscular acidosis, which is a major contributor to fatigue in all-out efforts lasting thirty seconds to thirty minutes. Interval workouts are more effective than workouts featuring a single, sustained high-intensity effort to exhaustion because the insertion of recovery periods within the overall effort enables the runner to spend more total time running at high intensity before reaching exhaustion.

The best place to run intervals is on a running track, an environment that is conducive to faster running and accurate pace control, given its precise distance. A special type of interval workout that is designed to be performed away from the track is what's called a fartlek workout, in which intervals of a designated duration and pace are arbitrarily scattered throughout an otherwise base-pace run on a road or trail.

Intervals are used in a unique way in the brain training system, becoming more and more race-specific as the training process unfolds. Also, as with tempo runs and cruise intervals, all other interval workouts are performed at one's estimated race pace for a given race distance to motivate greater effort.

Hill Running

Uphill running can be used to increase leg strength and stride power, to enhance hill-running performance in races, and to provide the benefits of high-intensity running with less impact shock than fast running on level ground. There are many ways to incorporate uphill running into your training, from hill sprints (twenty-to-thirty-second full sprints on a steep gradient) to Kenyan mountain runs (long, moderate-pace runs on a very long hill). In my brain training plans, hill sprints are used to increase muscle activation potential (defined in the next chapter) in the Base phase.

Recovery Runs

Recovery runs are relatively short, slow runs performed within twenty-four hours after a key workout. They serve a couple of purposes. First, they increase the total amount of running you do beyond the level you could achieve if you tried to make every run a key workout. In addition, recovery runs enhance neuromuscular efficiency by subjecting your body to the unique challenge of starting a run in a prefatigued state.

Recovery runs in the brain training system are similar to base runs except that they are flexible in terms of duration and pace. They must be short and slow enough to not interfere with recovery from the previous key workout or negatively affect performance in the next key workout, but runners are free to make them as long and fast as they can within these constraints. You will use subjective feedback—how your body feels and responds to training—to determine the best pace and duration for each recovery run.

Technique Training

Running technique is difficult to improve, because every runner's existing running form is deeply ingrained in the brain's motor centers. With consistent, disciplined effort and proper methods, however, all runners can improve their technique. Conventional training programs incorporate very little specific technique work, but technique development is an integral facet of brain training.

Specifically, my system employs various technique drills and proprioceptive cues (images and other sensory cues that enable you to modify your running stride for the better as you think about them while running). All of my brain training plans in Part II include one drill session per week, every week, from start to finish. Also, proprioceptive cues are used in every workout. A different cue is suggested for each week of training.

Cross-Training

Cross-training is any type of exercise besides running that you do for the sake of improving your running. There are three basic types of cross-training that have been proven beneficial to runners: resistance training, flexibility and mobility training, and nonimpact cardiovascular training. Each type of cross-training has a brain training dimension.

Resistance training improves communication between the brain and muscles in ways that enable you to run more efficiently and with less chance of injury. Flexibility and mobility training enhance running efficiency by training your neuromuscular system to eliminate unnecessary muscle tension from your stride. Nonimpact cardiovascular training increases running efficiency and fatigue resistance by training neuromuscular patterns that are similar to but slightly different from those used in running. Your brain can then "transfer" some of these patterns back to running in ways that boost efficiency and fatigue resistance.

Cross-training has a much bigger place in brain training than in most training systems. Nevertheless, in recognition of the fact that most runners would rather run than bicycle, stretch, or lift weights, the brain training plans in Part II incorporate cross-training in a flexible, efficient way.

Tune-up Races

Tune-up races are races that precede your peak race. As mentioned above, they make great breakthrough workouts because the competitive atmosphere of races stimulates a higher level of sympathetic nervous system arousal that enables you to work harder than in any regular workout, resulting in a bigger fitness-boosting benefit. Well-timed tune-up races also build confidence that will enhance peak race performance independently of the fitness benefits they provide. Finally, tune-up races familiarize your brain with prerace nerves, race pain and suffering, and other concrete aspects of the race experience, so you are both consciously and subconsciously less fearful of these things in the context of your peak race. The brain is always less aggressive in self-protectively limiting performance when a particular challenge facing the body or the mind is at least somewhat familiar. That's why my primary goal in some tune-up races is literally to suffer as much as possible!

Each of my brain training plans includes at least one tune-up race/breakthrough workout.

Recovery and Tapering

In order to build maximum fitness during a training cycle, it's not enough to simply do three key workouts per week. You must also perform well in most of these workouts. This requires that you allow your body to recover adequately between key workouts by performing relatively easy runs and/or relatively easy nonimpact cardio cross-training workouts that spare your legs additional impact trauma, and by taking days off when necessary. When you train hard you can't avoid starting some workouts with residual fatigue from previous workouts that hampers your performance. But you mustn't allow yourself to carry so much fatigue that you are unable to perform well in the majority of your key workouts.

Finding the right balance between training hard enough to maximize your fitness and getting enough recovery to avoid injury and overtraining requires a responsive training approach, where you listen to your body and modify planned training accordingly. My brain training plans have built-in flexibility—much more flexibility than conventional training plans—to facilitate responsive training.

Likewise, to perform optimally in important races, your body must be fully recovered from and fully adapted to recent training. This requires that you train very lightly in the final days preceding the race—a process called tapering. The peak race in each of my brain training plans is preceded by a one- or two-week taper.

THE OBJECTIVE FEEDBACK LOOP

Objective feedback consists of data relevant to your individual performance in workouts and races and includes such things as speed, distance covered, and heart rate. This type of feedback benefits your running by enhancing motivation and by making your training more structured and systematic. There are four basic ways objective feedback is used in the brain training system.

Goal Setting

Goal setting is an indispensable tool for maximizing performance. When you set an appropriate performance goal that represents the true current limit of your capabilities, it is much more likely that you will achieve the most you're capable of than if you simply try to do your best without setting an objective, measurable goal.

Your true performance limit is the fastest pace you can sustain over the full race distance without literally killing yourself. The self-protective mechanisms your brain uses to regulate running performance will never allow you to run this hard. There's always a buffer. But the size of this buffer can vary depending on how important a race is. If you're running away from a hungry lion, your brain will allow you to run very nearly to death to escape certain death in the lion's jaws. But if nothing's at stake, your brain won't allow you to run nearly as fast when running "as fast as you can." Goals are simply a way of raising the stakes of a maximum-effort run so that your brain will allow you to run a little harder.

Every competitive runner has had the experience of struggling to beat another runner to the finish line of a race. And every runner who's had such an experience knows that, win or lose, this type of battle results in a better performance than is possible without the spontaneously chosen goal of out-running the other. This is a good example of how a real-world standard makes a higher level of performance possible. A scientific study of this phenomenon found that subjects performed 21 percent better in a maximal exercise test when they competed against other subjects of similar ability than when they did the same test alone.

Time goals function in precisely the same manner. They originate in your cognitive consciousness, but they affect your emotions, your perception of effort, and other brain functions in ways that focus your body toward the pursuit of that standard and thereby enable you to squeeze a little more out of your mind and body. Armed with an appropriate race-time goal, you will reach a bit higher not only on race day but also throughout the training cycle. Similarly, pace-based key workout goals will enable you to give a greater effort and achieve a higher level of performance in each key workout.

Goal setting is only effective, however, if goals are well chosen. A well-chosen goal is one you believe you can achieve but are not quite certain you can achieve, based on your past performances as a runner. Almost every competitive runner naturally becomes a pretty good goal setter by accumulating racing experience. In chapter 4 I will provide some tools to help you establish peak race-time goals and workout "target pace" goals.

Customization of Training

Each runner is unique. No two runners respond in precisely the same way to the same training, even when they are more or less equal in ability. Because each runner is unique, training must be customized to the individual to yield optimal race performance. Some runners can handle more mileage than others. Some recover faster from high-intensity running than others. Some are more susceptible to injuries than others. Such factors and numerous others must be accounted for in the process of creating an individualized training plan.

This doesn't mean you have to create your training plans from a blank slate. We're all human and we all respond to training in the same general manner. So you can get a good start on creating a customized training plan by starting with the proven training methods described in the previous section—or by starting with one of the twelve training plans provided in Part II of this book. But the details—including how much you run, how hard your key workouts are, which types of key workouts you emphasize most, and so forth—must be determined by your knowledge of yourself as a runner. If you're relatively new to the sport, you might not know enough to do much customization, but as you execute your plan you will learn about your strengths, weaknesses, and needs and become better able to account for them in planning your future training.

This process is never-ending. No matter how experienced you are, you will never stop learning about yourself as a runner—nor will you ever stop changing as a runner—so there will always be a need for further customization.

Monitoring and Controlling Running Pace and Intensity

The most important type of objective feedback you can use while running is pace information (minutes and seconds per mile). Knowing how fast you're running during workouts enables you to ensure you're doing workouts appropriately, to assess your performance, and to measure your progress. You should have a target pace and/or goal time for each key workout. These targets will be based on your current fitness level and will gradually become faster (relative to distance) as your fitness improves. In addition to helping you keep your training on track, pace and time targets also function as performance goals that will motivate you to perform better than you would if you ran by feel alone. A further benefit of training by pace is that it helps you develop a sophisticated sense of pacing that will help you set appropriate race goals and execute your race plans effectively.

Pace-based workouts are one of the most important and unique features of the brain training method. The whole system is oriented toward the goal of convincing your brain that you can sustain your goal pace all the way to the finish line of your next big race, so it just makes sense that each workout has a target pace with a definite relationship to that goal pace.

Keeping a Training Log

Keeping a training log is essential to getting the most out of your training. The human memory is faulty. You can't rely on your memory to keep an accurate and complete record of your training. But you can always rely on a training log. Having such a record available whenever you need it offers several benefits. First of all, it helps ensure that you are actually training according to plan. A training log also helps you identify patterns that you can use to make changes when necessary. For example, if you develop an injury you can look at your training log to see if your training changed—and if so, how—in the days preceding its onset. A training log also provides the purely psychological benefits of enhancing self-efficacy, as discussed in the next chapter. It provides evidence that you can achieve your peak race goal. I always get a big confidence boost from looking back at all the training I have accomplished as a peak race approaches.

THE SUBJECTIVE FEEDBACK LOOP

Subjective feedback is experience, or what neuroscientists and philosophers call qualia: feelings, emotions, thoughts—anything that lets you know you're alive. Subjective feedback comes to your brain from your body, which includes your brain itself. It is more or less how you feel during your workouts and races and while recovering from them. The emergence of knee pain during a run, the exhilaration of running fast and feeling strong, and that burning sensation that develops in your legs as they become acidic during high-intensity running are all examples of subjective feedback. These types of information can be extremely valuable if you know how to use them. You will use subjective feedback in five specific ways in the brain training system.

Responsive Training

It is impossible to predict ahead of time exactly how your body will respond to the training you do. Sometimes it takes you longer to recover from a hard workout or a hard training week than you expect it will, so that you're just not ready for the next hard workout your plan calls for when your plan calls for it. Other times you feel unexpectedly strong—ready for more than the short recovery run on your schedule. In either of these cases, persisting with the plan instead of changing it to answer your body's present needs is a mistake.

Training is most effective when you do just the right workout—the precise workout your body needs and is ready for—every day. With careful planning, the workout on your training schedule will be the workout you need more often than not. But when you find that it's not, you must be willing and prepared to make a change. This approach is called training responsively: assessing the state of your body immediately before or after beginning a planned workout and, if necessary, changing it to administer the training stimulus you truly need.

Too many runners stubbornly persist in training according to the plan they set out for themselves despite subjective feedback from their bodies telling them they ought to do otherwise. You'll make much more progress in the long run if you replace a planned run with an easier run (or even a day off) on days when you feel unexpectedly bad, and run a little harder than planned on days when you feel unexpectedly good. I'll provide specific responsive training tips in chapter 7.

Heeding Pain

In addition to residual fatigue from recent training, another form of subjective feedback that runners too often try to ignore is running-related pain. Such pain is almost always a sign of an incipient overuse injury, and trying to push through it almost always results in a worsening of the injury and a training interruption that might have been avoided. It is important to stop running before pain becomes so severe that you have no choice. By doing so you will limit the damage and miss less running overall.

It is also important to integrate subjective feedback concerning the specific nature of your injury symptoms with objective information concerning its onset (Did it follow a sudden increase in mileage? A switch to different shoes?) and with collective information concerning the known causes and effective treatments for running injuries. In chapter 9 you'll learn a foolproof brain training method of preventing injuries by integrating subjective, objective, and collective feedback.

Running by Feel

Many runners greatly underestimate the importance of perception of effort—how hard running feels—in training and racing. Look at it this way: The goal in racing is to reach the finish line as fast as you can. How do you know how fast you can go—not only in terms of average pace, but at various points throughout a race, such as when you climb a hill or try to surge ahead of a competitor? Past race times and recent workout times will certainly give you some indication, but what you rely on most of all is perception of effort—an indescribable sense of how hard running ought to feel at any given moment in a workout or race.

If you've ever had the experience of a breakthrough race—running much faster than you expected to—then you have some idea how important it is to let perception of effort guide you and not to let numbers hold you back. Of course, it works the other way, too: Sometimes your body tells you that you aren't going to be able to run as fast as past numbers suggested you could. While that's disappointing, you'll still get to the finish line faster in such cases by listening to your body and playing it safe instead of sticking to the numbers and consequently falling apart well before you reach the finish line.

Developing the ability to "run by feel" is an automatic outcome of running experience, to some degree, but you will develop it faster by consciously nurturing the ability. By being as mindful as possible of your perception of effort during running you will not only do your best in every race and key workout, but you will also practice responsive training more effectively, because you will have a keener sense of what sort of workout your body is ready for on any given day.

Monitoring and Controlling Your Running Form

"Proprioception" is a scientific term that refers to the sense of where your body parts are in space and how they are moving. The proprioceptive system includes proprioceptive nerves located in skeletal muscle and joint tissue throughout your body, the visual system, and the equilibrium system of the inner ear—all of which provide electrical and chemical feedback to your brain, which processes it and produces feelings that your mind experiences. Your mind is free to pay varying degrees of attention to this feedback. By paying close attention to the feel of your body's movement when you're running, you can consciously work to maintain proper form or even improve your form.

Making effective use of this strategy requires that you integrate proprioceptive feedback with objective feedback about the faults in your stride and collective information about correct running form.

Staying Positive

Many of the things that the brain does when we run have only recently been discovered, but two things we've always known that the brain does during running are thinking and experiencing emotions. We humans are capable of having all manner of thoughts as we run, from considering whether to surge ahead of a competitor who's currently running on our shoulder to wondering what to make for dinner tonight. Likewise, our emotions can run the gamut from euphoria to despair.

Some thoughts and emotions are helpful to performance, while others have the opposite effect. Among the types of thoughts that tend to enhance performance are believing in the achievability of a goal and focusing on the mechanics of performance (paying attention to split times, for example). Doubting and worrying thoughts, on the other hand, tend to hamper performance. Among the helpful emotions are confidence and motivation, while fear, apathy, and other such negative emotions are known to sabotage performance.

You will perform better if you actively control your thoughts and emotions to cultivate those that help and quash those that hurt. This effort will be aided if you integrate the subjective feedback of your thoughts and emotions with objective feedback about your thought patterns (for example, are you an optimist or a pessimist?) and collective feedback about thoughts and emotions that are known to boost and hinder performance.

CHAPTER ◆ 2

THE RUNNING BRAIN

Most runners understandably have little knowledge of how the brain controls running performance and fitness adaptations. In fact, many professionals in the field of exercise physiology are rather fuzzy on the details of the new, brain-centered conception of exercise performance that has recently invalidated much of what they were taught in graduate school. In this chapter I will provide a basic explanation of the brain's running-related functions without getting too deep into neuroscientific jargon, which I'm not entirely comfortable with myself.

My main objective in bringing you up-to-date on current scientific knowledge regarding the role of the brain in running performance and fitness development is to get you excited about brain training: the first and only training system for runners that is based on the new brain-centered theory of exercise performance. If you're already excited about brain training and if biology was your least favorite subject in school, feel free to skim or skip over this chapter and go straight to learning how to practice brain training in chapter 3.

A Quick Tour of the Human Brain

The average human brain weighs approximately three pounds. It is made up of two main types of cells: neurons and glia. Neurons are the active cells in the brain that regulate the nervous system and produce the five senses, feelings, emotions, and thoughts by sharing electrical and chemical signals. Glia are essentially support cells that help connect neurons, insulate and protect them, and enable them to function more efficiently. There are believed to be roughly 10 billion neurons in the human brain and perhaps ten glia for each neuron.

The human brain comprises numerous individual structures with disparate functional roles. The brain stem is the most primitive part of the brain and connects the rest of the brain to the spinal cord. It is responsible for regulating many automatic body functions, including breathing, heartbeat, and blood vessel dilation. The cerebellum, another primitive structure in the lower part of the brain, is mainly responsible for integrating sensory perception and motor output (muscle activation). The hippocampus is involved in spatial navigation and the formation of long-term memories. The motor cortex handles most aspects of planning, coordinating, initiating, and adjusting movements. The most recently evolved and human-specific part of the brain is the frontal lobe, at the very front of the brain, which specializes in planning, impulse control, problem solving, language, and complex social behavior. There are many other parts of the brain that I have skipped over (hey, this isn't medical school!), but this sampling of functionally focused structures should give you a sense of how the brain is organized.

All of the brain activity that makes you a living, moving, feeling, thinking being consists of communication among large numbers of neurons. The points where individual neurons connect to one another are called synapses.

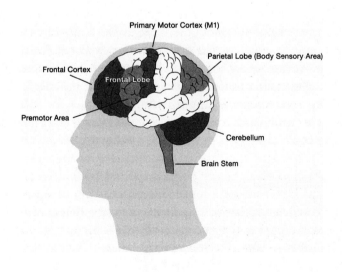

Each neuron has wirelike input channels called dendrites and wirelike output channels called axons. A synapse forms where the axon of one neuron meets the dendrite of another.

Neurons communicate with each other through electrical-chemical signals, called action potentials, which travel through synapses. When a neuron is stimulated in the right way by input from other neurons, its internal electrical charge suddenly changes, creating a sort of current that travels in wavelike fashion down the length of its axons until it reaches their terminal points. The arrival of the electrical signal at the axon terminal causes the release of chemicals called neurotransmitters, which cross over to the dendrite of the adjoining neuron, initiating electrical events there. This whole process unfolds within thousandths of a second.

One of the most celebrated characteristics of the brain is something called neural plasticity. What this means, essentially, is that individual neurons are very flexible in terms of the jobs they perform. Every time you form a new memory, learn a new word, learn a new skill, taste a new food, or experience novelty in any form, neurons in your brain change their function to accommodate the experience.

The brain is most plastic at birth, when most of the brain cells have not yet found any kind of functional specialty. The brain is so adaptable at this stage that infants with brain damage have been known to develop normally after having half of their entire brain removed. While neurons become more and more stuck in their ways as we mature, they still maintain a high degree of plasticity. For example, neurons involved in vision may become involved in hearing in an adult who loses his or her sight.

Each and every conscious experience that a human being has is associated with what's called an activation pattern in the brain—a complex pattern of communication among millions of neurons that essentially *is* that experience. Sights, sounds, scents, feelings, body states, and thoughts are all wrapped up into these activation patterns, which exist only for milliseconds before fluidly evolving to represent the next experience.

Conscious experience is only the tip of the iceberg of total brain activity. Even many of the things you experience as being consciously controlled are not. For example, high-speed reflex actions, such as swinging a bat at a baseball pitch, occur without the aid of conscious vision, which is far too slow to be helpful in such situations. Instead, visual cues from the pitcher's movements *prior to releasing the ball* are processed in the brain's preconscious visual centers and used to trigger a "decision" to swing or not to swing before these cues are even consciously registered.

When a given moment of conscious experience gives way to the next experience, the activity pattern that was associated with it does not simply disappear without a trace. Each experience strengthens the neural communication channels that are involved in the activation patterns that correlate with the experience. As a result, chunks of neural activity that represent different aspects of a particular experience become linked, increasing the likelihood that when one of these chunks of activity recurs in the future, the others will also. For example, if your mother wore red frequently when you were a child, and if, as most children do, you often experienced feelings of comfort and safety in your mother's presence, you may experience feelings of comfort and safety sometimes when you see the color red as an adult. Neuroscientists have an expression that describes this phenomenon: "Neurons that fire together wire together."

The brain is deeply interconnected with every part of the body. For example, it interconnects with the muscular system through motor nerves that transmit movement impulses from the brain to the muscles and sensory nerves that send information from the muscles and connective tissues back to the brain. The brain is also deeply interconnected with the endocrine, or hormonal, system. The two most important glands of the hormonal system, the hypothalamus and the pituitary gland, are located inside the brain. These glands release a variety of hormones that travel through the bloodstream to every other organ of the body, where they act as chemical messengers.

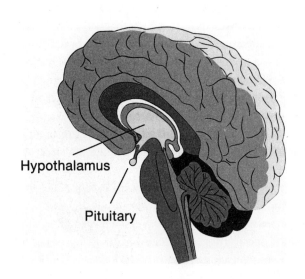

Hypothalamus

Pituitary

Likewise, the brain interconnects with the immune system, the circulatory system, the digestive system, and every other functional system of the body. In fact, it's really not accurate to define any functional system of the body as distinct from the nervous system. It's more accurate to speak of the neuro-muscular system, the neuroendocrine system, and even the neurodigestive system.

The human brain is often compared to computers. Like a computer, the brain stores and processes information and runs "programs," such as executing learned motor skills that are stored in the brain's motor centers. But the brain actually works very differently from a computer. For example, in a computer there are obvious distinctions among the physical hardware of the machine, the information it stores, and the processes it enacts. In the brain, however, there are no such distinctions. The stuff the brain is made out of is indistinguishable from the information it stores and the processes it enacts.

One major consequence of this difference is that everything the brain does actually changes its physical structure and makeup. Computers are static. You can put information and programs in them, move them around, and take them out, but the machine remains essentially the same. The brain, on the other hand, is dynamic and ever evolving. It's as if every time your brain runs a program, the program changes the "machine" that ran it, which in turn changes the program.

The brain is much like other organs in that it consumes and requires energy. Its favorite fuel is glucose, but it can also process other fuels. Like other

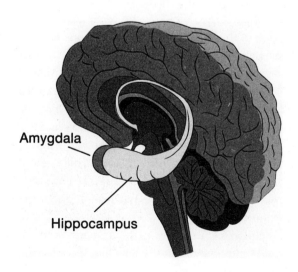

organs it requires oxygen to fully metabolize its fuels. And like other organs, the brain receives glucose, other fuels, and oxygen through the bloodstream.

As you might expect from such a powerful and busy organ, the brain consumes and requires a tremendous amount of fuel compared to other organs. Although it accounts for only 2 percent of our body weight, it burns up 20 percent of our food energy and oxygen—at rest and during exercise.

Your Brain on the Run

There are six major jobs that your brain must perform while you run: motor output, stride adjustment, metabolic regulation, perception of effort, cognition, and attentional focus. Let's take a close look at each of them.

Motor Output

Running requires a breathtakingly complex coordination of muscle activation patterns. All muscle activation originates in the brain, but only a tiny fraction of it is consciously controlled. None of us would ever learn to run if we had to consciously control the coordinated activation and relaxation of each individual motor unit (a bundle of muscle fibers fed by a single motor nerve).

Unlike all other animals that are capable of running, humans usually run by plan. We have a conscious intent to run at a certain time, then we take steps to make this chosen running opportunity come about, and then we start running. (Sometimes, though, we do run spontaneously, without prior planning, as when a dog comes charging at us from out of nowhere and we take sudden flight.) The plan and intent to run begin in a part of the human brain called the frontal cortex, which is the outer layer of the frontal lobe of the brain. This area of the brain handles all conscious planning and decision making and seems to be mostly or entirely lacking in all other animals. The conscious command to run travels as an electrical impulse to the brain's motor centers, which transform the general intent to run into a detailed muscle action plan. The supplementary motor area contains information about the running you've done in the past and adds this to the plan. It also links to the brain's body sensory areas, housed mainly in the parietal lobe, enabling it to generate planning imagery. The premotor area handles the coordination of muscle stimulation patterns that will be required to execute the plan. It also connects to sensory areas that provide information about the body's immediate physical environment.

From here, the plan to run travels to the primary motor cortex, which assembles the relevant information. In the final milliseconds before the running command leaves the brain through the brain stem, the cerebellum adds a final bit of "smoothing" in the form of motor habits developed through past experience. The last stop is a part of the primary motor cortex called M1, which contains a neuronal map of the entire body. When the part of this map that represents your right pinky finger is activated, your right pinky finger moves. The brain is the puppet master; the muscles are merely the puppets. If you're skeptical on this point, consider the fact that it is now possible for paralyzed humans and restrained monkeys to control devices such as computer cursors and robotic arms by *thought* with the help of electrodes implanted in their motor centers or special caps that sense neural activity.

A muscle contracts, or shortens, when electrical impulses are sent from the motor centers of the brain and travel through nerves that snake through the spinal cord and into the targeted muscle, where they eventually reach the neuromuscular junctions of individual motor units (each of which contains between several dozen and many hundreds of individual muscle fibers).

I will pass over the complexities of how muscle fibers contract once the motor impulse enters them. It's an incredibly intricate process. But even more complex is how the contraction and relaxation of thousands of muscle fibers is coordinated to produce an action such as running. To spend time studying the biomechanics of running, as I have done, is to develop a profound appreciation for the intelligence of the entire human body.

One brief example will give you a sense of what I'm talking about. The most powerful thrust-generating muscle during running is the gluteus maximus: the large muscle in each of your buttocks. This muscle is most active during the stance phase of running, when your foot is in contact with the ground. The gluteus maximus is a hip extensor, which means it pulls your thigh backward. But during running it works a little differently. Since your body has forward momentum when your foot makes contact with the ground, your stance leg becomes a fulcrum. So when your gluteus maximus contracts, the effect of pulling your thigh backward is actually to pull your body forward in relation to your foot. But there's a problem. Under these circumstances, contracting the gluteus maximus tends to extend the knee, which is slightly bent on ground contact during running. If this leg-straightening effect were allowed to happen, a lot of the energy that the gluteus maximus was trying to convert into forward thrust would be wasted, as if your legs had been replaced with cooked noodles. But the hamstrings—the muscles that run along the back of the thigh, and act to bend the knee—prevent such waste by tensing up just enough at just the right time to prevent knee extension. It's not something you have to think about; it just happens. This example of precision cooperation between the gluteus maximus and hamstring muscles is just one example of dozens of ways your muscles, tendons, and other tissues cooperate to enable you to run efficiently.

As a complex motor skill, running is not genetically "hardwired" or preprogrammed in the brain. Human beings who are not shown or taught how to run (or even walk, for that matter) will never learn how on their own. The average child develops the ability to run at twenty to twenty-four months of age, or about six months after first learning to walk. At first the child is able to run only very short distances and falls often, but by their third birthday most children can run fairly well.

As children become increasingly proficient in running, their improved efficiency is easily observed. Changes in the brain that correspond to such improvement are equally significant. Research has shown that when animals, including humans, learn new motor skills, the areas of the motor cortex that map to the muscles involved increase in size. At the same time, a fatty sheath called myelin that insulates axon-dendrite connections the way rubber insulation surrounds electrical wires becomes thicker around those connections that are most often used in the performance of a motor skill. As a result, nerve impulses travel faster along the nerves and can be more precisely timed, resulting in more efficient movement. Even more interesting, as a person gains proficiency in a motor skill such as running, the amount of brain activity that is required for the performance of this skill decreases. This decrease in brain activity represents two things. First, as skills become increasingly automatic, less brain activity is required to repeat them. Also, the more you practice a motor skill, the more ways your neuromuscular system finds to eliminate unnecessary muscle activation from the performance of the skill, and as muscle activation decreases, so too does the brain activity that causes muscle activation.

Children normally become increasingly efficient runners throughout their preteen years, reducing a tendency to overstride, trimming waste from their upper body movements, and so forth. Efficiency may continue to improve in ever-subtler ways well into adulthood in those who become habitual runners. Many of these efficiency gains come from improvements in a runner's ability to capture and reuse energy provided in the form of ground impact forces. As the foot makes contact with the ground, tendons and elastic components of certain muscles stretch beyond their natural length, thereby capturing and storing energy from the impact. As these tissues return to their natural length, their stored elastic energy is released. Exquisitely timed and coordinated muscle actions direct the energy back into the ground, sending the runner's body upward and forward. The more you run, the more ways your neuromuscular system finds to turn borrowed energy into forward thrust.

An interesting question is whether there are properties intrinsic to the brains of individual runners that affect their ability to learn new stride efficiencies, or whether the brain is totally dependent on the structure of the muscles, skeletal frame, and connective tissues in this regard. It is a well-established fact that certain structural characteristics, such as greater muscle and tendon elasticity, translate into better running efficiency. But there is also evidence that two runners with more or less identical bodies may gain running efficiency at different rates due to differences in the motor systems of their individual brains. Recent research in the field of motor learning shows that individuals who gain proficiency in particular motor skills (such as throwing a Frisbee at a target) more quickly exhibit a natural, unconscious tendency to vary their technique more in the early stages of learning. The innate "neuromuscular restlessness" in these fast learners enables them to stumble upon more effective coordination patterns faster than slower learners.

Because running is as complex a motor skill as throwing a Frisbee, there is every reason to believe that the same phenomenon is manifest in runners. The brains of individual runners probably have widely varying propensities to try out subtly different ways of coordinating the muscles during running. Those with the most "play" in their muscle recruitment patterns probably learn new efficiencies the fastest.

Stride Adjustment

Motor output is really only half of the stride production formula. The other half is a continuous process of adjustments to the stride that results from sensory feedback sent to the brain from nerves in the muscles, joints, and elsewhere throughout the body. The most important type of sensory feedback for stride adjustment is proprioception, or the feeling of the body's position and movement in space. Proprioceptive nerves in the muscles and joints tell your brain where your body is in the running action (muscle lengths, joint angles, amount of tension in tendons) and how the external environment is affecting the execution of your running (whether you're on a soft or hard surface, a smooth or rough surface, running uphill or downhill or on level ground, and other such information).

The best way to run in any given moment depends on how your body's execution of the running plan is going and on how the environment is affecting it. So the raw motor output patterns that control running are actually incomplete, allowing plenty of room for fine-tuning and continual adjustments. It is left to the proprioceptive feedback system to fill in the details and provide information needed to make proper adjustments.

For example, like many runners, you may often have the experience of feeling somewhat clumsy and awkward as you begin a run. Your brain can use this proprioceptive feedback to make small adjustments that help you find a comfortable groove. Similarly, during a run you might turn onto a new street and encounter a fierce headwind. Proprioceptive nerves near your skin will sense the air pressure and transmit information about it to your brain, which will use the feedback to alter your stride in a manner that minimizes the effect of wind resistance on you. (You'll probably crouch and lean forward a bit.)

The equilibrium system of the inner ear and the visual system provide proprioceptive feedback as well. Almost all proprioceptive feedback processing occurs on a subconscious level, allowing for more rapid and numerous stride adjustments than could ever be possible if proprioception required conscious control. Because rapid and numerous adjustments are possible, and because running is a cyclical motion, repeated over and over, proprioceptive feedback from every single stride is used to make adjustments to the next stride.

Metabolic Regulation

One of the most salient changes that occur during running is a dramatic increase in the metabolic rate. The body consumes ten to twenty times more fuel and oxygen during sustained running than it does at rest. The working skeletal muscles, especially those in the legs, the heart muscle, and the respiratory muscles, all consume fuel and oxygen at a high rate. So does the brain. The motor centers of the brain become intensely active during running, and like the muscle cells, the neurons can only remain intensely active with a steady, abundant supply of fuel and oxygen.

To meet the demand for oxygen, the brain stem sends commands to the heart to increase its pumping rate and to the respiratory muscles to increase ventilation. Recent research has demonstrated that a part of the mid-brain called the periaqueductal gray area initiates these increases before the onset of exercise, and becomes more active during exercise. The rate at which the human body can supply oxygen to its tissues is limited. An exceptional ability to supply oxygen at high rates (or aerobic capacity) is one of the hallmark characteristics of elite endurance athletes, but even these men and women have limits. Failure to supply adequate oxygen to muscle tissues would quickly result in their death, and failure to supply adequate oxygen to the brain or heart would quickly result in the death of the runner. Therefore, in addition to keeping the heart rate high enough to supply needed oxygen during running, the brain also limits the number of muscle motor units it recruits based on afferent feedback from the blood, muscles, and other organs to ensure that demand never outpaces supply for long. (The word "afferent" refers to any mechanism that provides chemical or electrical information to the brain from other parts of the body.)

The brain also plays a critical role in increasing the availability of fuel during running. The hypothalamus and pituitary glands in the brain stimulate the adrenal glands (located in the pancreas) to release catabolic hormones, mainly cortisol and adrenocorticotropin, which facilitate the breakdown of muscle glycogen (a crucial carbohydrate-based energy source during intense running) and other fuels. The hypothalamus-pituitary-adrenal (or HPA) axis also releases a hormone that causes blood vessels to dilate, increasing blood flow and with it the rate of oxygen and fuel supply to the muscles and brain.

Conventional wisdom in exercise physiology holds that fatigue usually occurs when the working muscles run out of a critical fuel (such as adenosine triphosphate during maximum-intensity exercise, or muscle glycogen during submaximal exercise). Recent research, however, suggests that fatigue always occurs when there is fuel still available in the muscles. Rather, it is more often the brain that encounters a shortage of energy, causing it to reduce muscle activation, which precipitates the involuntary slowing that comes with running fatigue.

Perception of Effort

One of the most prominent aspects of the experience of running is perception of effort, or how difficult running feels. Perception of effort encompasses two distinct but related sensory experiences: perception of exercise intensity and perception of fatigue. The faster (or more intensely) you run, the more difficult it feels, even before fatigue sets in. But it is possible to feel "good" even at very high running intensities prior to the onset of fatigue. When fatigue does manifest, running feels hard at any intensity level. Even walking is perceived as a maximal effort if sustained long enough.

In the traditional scientific understanding of exercise performance, perception of fatigue was considered only a *sign* of fatigue that happens to coincide with the performance decline associated with fatigue but serves no function. Recent discoveries have made it clear that perception of fatigue is also a major *cause* of performance decline. The emerging belief is that, based on chemical events in the brain and afferent feedback from other organs, the brain produces feelings of discomfort, pain, and loss of motivation in order to make the runner voluntarily slow down or stop, thus reinforcing the involuntary slowing aspect of fatigue.

Evidence in support of the notion that perceived effort contributes causally to fatigue comes from the discovery that when the drug naloxone is administered to athletes, they experience a higher level of perceived effort during exercise and fatigue more quickly without any measurable changes occurring in the muscles, blood, or heart rate. Also, studies have shown that athletes perceive maximum-intensity exercise as being "easier" and perform better when receiving encouragement from others—a stimulus that clearly acts on the brain's sensory areas, not on the muscles. And finally, researchers have found variations in the activation of the brain's insular cortex at different exercise intensities that are associated with changes in cardiovascular function *and* perception of effort.

Cognition

The stream of consciousness that flows continuously at rest continues to flow during running, but it does tend to change form. The brain centers that are mainly responsible for producing conscious thought, or cognition, are the frontal lobes. But other brain regions have a tremendous influence on the form and content of our thoughts. Afferent feedback from our bodies, as well as brain activity in the regions of the brain that govern body actions, are among the factors that influence cognition. Running is, of course, a specific type of body action involving characteristic sorts of afferent feedback and characteristic patterns of activity in the motor and sensory centers of the brain, and for this reason there are some characteristic types of thought that are associated with running.

At comfortable running intensities, runners usually experience a state of wandering thoughts that seem to go wherever the wind blows them. Research studies using electroencephalogram (EEG) technology have shown that this state is associated with alpha-wave activity in the frontal lobes. Neural activity has a rhythmical nature to it that results from large numbers of neurons firing synchronously. Various rhythm patterns have been identified and classified as wave states. The alpha-wave state is associated with a relaxed, meditative consciousness.

During more intense running, especially in fitter runners who are performing well, thoughts tend to become focused on the sensory experience of running, sometimes to the point where runners feel they have "become" the act of running. Athletes in all sports, as well as musicians, video game players, surgeons, and others describe a similar experience when they are doing what they do best or most enjoy doing. The state of becoming what you're doing is popularly referred to as being "in the zone." EEG data have revealed that the zone is associated with a state of widespread *inactivity* in the frontal lobes and virtually every other brain area not directly involved in the task at hand. In other words, these data confirm objectively what runners in the zone experience subjectively: that they are *not* thinking; they're just doing.

At extremely high running intensities, and whenever a runner is near exhaustion, cognition becomes fractured and scrambled. If you're a veteran runner you've almost certainly had the experience of your consciousness seemingly narrowing to a point as you begin to bonk in a long workout or race. Your mind is cloudy, and each new thought scarcely has a chance to get off the ground before it's shot down by the distraction of your physical suffering. Some researchers have recently suggested that this phenomenon may occur because, as exhaustion approaches, the brain literally doesn't have the energy left to think straight.

Attentional Focus

The human mind is capable of sustaining only one top priority of attention at a time. You can be aware of how your big toe feels anytime you choose, but unless you so choose, or unless the feeling of your big toe draws attention to itself for some reason (perhaps it just got stung by a bee), then you will not be aware of it, or of dozens of other parts of experience that you could be aware of, due to the extreme limits of attentional focus.

Owing in large part to all of the recent public concern about attention deficit disorder, the phenomenon of attention has been hotly researched in the past several years by neuroscientists and psychologists, who have learned much about it. What they've discovered above all is that attention is very complicated, involving numerous brain regions and encompassing a whole range of disparate skills and functions. Attention involves the sensory perceptions; something called working memory, which is housed in the frontal lobes and allows you (for example) to remember what someone has said to you long enough to reply appropriately; and supervisory attention, also seated in the frontal lobes, which is the faculty that enables you to (often but not always) choose what you pay attention to.

What's also clear about the nature of attention is that different people have different attentional profiles. Some people are much better at focusing on faces than on voices, while others are the opposite. Some people have a greater ability to switch from one attentional focus to another than to sustain their attention on a single object, while for others the reverse is true. Differences in attentional profiles may partly explain why some people find running boring while you and I find it quite entertaining.

Attentional profiles, skills, and habits have a strong bearing on running performance. For example, sports psychology research has found that faster runners tend to focus their attention on the concrete experience of running during competition, whereas slower runners tend to dissociate their attention from the feel of running and their immediate environment, preferring to make shopping lists and play songs in their heads.

Your Brain and Fitness

In addition to governing virtually every aspect of the act of running, the brain is also centrally involved in many of the fitness adaptations that occur in response to training. There are five brain-related adaptations to running that are especially noteworthy: greater muscle activation capacity, improved neuromuscular efficiency, elevated fatigue signaling thresholds, increased self-efficacy, and better all-around brain health.

Greater Muscle Activation Capacity

The physiological essence of running is communication between the brain and the muscles. The brain sends motor signals to the muscles, which in turn send proprioceptive and other afferent feedback signals to the brain, which uses this information to modify the stride, change pace, produce feelings of energy or fatigue, and so forth. To train for running is to practice communications between your brain and your muscles. By engaging in such practice you will improve these communications in ways that make you a stronger runner.

For example, training increases the number of motor units that your brain is able to access and use to contribute to running. Some very interesting studies have shown how improvements in muscle performance derive from a simple boost in the amount of tissue the brain is able to recruit during exercise—an adaptation that is completely independent of structural changes within the muscles themselves. In one study subjects engaged in a strength training program for the calf muscles of only one leg, while leaving the other leg alone. After six weeks, maximum voluntary contraction force was improved in *both* legs. The improvement in the untrained leg was clearly correlated with increased neuromotor input received from the brain.

Increasing the number of motor units capable of involvement in the running stride—or muscle activation capacity—carries a couple of benefits.

First, it enables you to generate more force at key moments of the stride. There are actually moments of the stride when particular muscles are required to contract even harder than you can voluntarily contract them using all of your strength while standing still. Runners who can contract these muscles more forcefully at such moments will run better because of it. A team of Finnish researchers has shown that higher-caliber runners generate stronger muscle contractions in the moment preceding footstrike, stiffening their legs in a way that enables them to capture and reuse more elastic energy, spend less time with their foot on the ground, and therefore run faster.

Greater muscle activation capacity also enhances endurance, due to a phenomenon known as motor unit cycling. During sustained running, your brain seldom activates more than 30 percent of the motor units in the working muscles simultaneously. It constantly changes the specific motor units it activates, however, allowing some to rest while others take their turn. By increasing the pool of muscle fibers capable of contributing to the stride, you increase the amount of rest opportunity for each, so you can sustain any given speed longer before motor units begin to fatigue.

Improved Neuromuscular Efficiency

An improvement in neuromuscular efficiency can come from a reduction in the amount of motor output or muscle activity required to run a certain speed, or from an increase in the running speed that is achieved from a given amount of motor output or muscle activity. Like the gains in muscle activation capacity described above, improvements in neuromuscular efficiency result from better communications between the brain and the muscles.

The running stride becomes more efficient essentially by becoming more ballistic. Your brain learns how to contract fewer motor units more forcefully and for shorter periods of time without losing forward thrust. As a result, more of your muscles spend more time relaxing. Studies have shown that one of the main reasons children are less efficient runners than adults is that kids have a tendency to contract the muscles opposing their main working muscles, creating a sort of internal resistance in their stride that wastes a lot of energy. Even the most experienced adult runners may continue to improve their efficiency by reducing the amount of so-called co-contraction in their stride.

Elevated Fatigue Signaling Thresholds

Maximum performance is not a hard limit but a fuzzy border. The ultimate limit of any runner's performance capacity is irreversible tissue damage, organ failure, or death. Fortunately, your brain will never allow you to run that hard. Exactly how close to this limit your brain allows you to go is modifiable by training, however. For example, in prolonged running, fatigue is often associated with sharply reduced levels of glycogen in the working muscles. No runner is ever able to run to the point of completely depleting this fuel, which would cause catastrophic damage, but highly fit runners are able to come closer to depleting it than are less fit runners. In runners who are less fit or experienced, the brain is somewhat overprotective, causing fatigue to occur when the muscle glycogen level is low but far from depleted. Through training experience, the brain becomes less cautious, allowing the runner to continue running until muscle glycogen is a little closer to a dangerous level of depletion before causing fatigue.

Training also produces changes in the muscles and other organs and systems that enhance performance by attenuating the fatigue-causing signals that these organs and systems send to the brain during running. For example, training greatly increases the amount of glycogen the muscles and liver store. Because they have a larger supply of glycogen, highly fit runners can run longer before the brain receives signals of impending glycogen depletion that trigger fatigue.

Increased Self-Efficacy

"If you believe it, you can achieve it." Athletes and coaches with an appreciation for the psychological dimension of sports performance have spoken this platitude and similar ones for generations. Most of them don't know how right they are. Recent science has shown that the brain allows the body to exercise as long and hard as it "believes" the body can go without harming itself. The brain's sense of what the body can safely do is defined primarily by afferent feedback signals received from the body and by the establishment and adjustment of "set points" through exercise experience. But purely psychological phenomena, such as beliefs, can have an effect, too. If you truly, consciously believe that you can achieve a certain running performance, this belief may relax your brain's self-protective limiters and allow your body to run closer to the point of self-harm than it otherwise would.

We get a glimpse of the power of belief from studies demonstrating a performance-enhancing placebo effect in runners. In one such study, time trial performance was enhanced in runners who watched a bogus video that presented the amazing performance benefits of super-oxygenated water (which does exist but offers no physical benefits beyond those of regular tap water). These runners were given plain tap water before running the time trial, but were told it was super-oxygenated water. They ran faster because they believed it would make them run faster.

One of the important benefits of training is that it enhances self-efficacy, or your beliefs about the running goals you can achieve. Although these changes in beliefs are caused primarily by the changes in your physical fitness that make your body capable of better performances, there is a psychological component as well. Elite runners often speak of drawing confidence during races from thinking about all of the hard training they've done leading up to the race, and the fine workout performances they've achieved.

Better All-Around Brain Health

Cardiovascular exercise is scientifically proven to enhance brain health in a number of ways. Exercise stimulates the growth of neurons and strengthens their interconnections. It has been shown to enhance cognitive function, including memory, attention and concentration, and executive function (that is, planning and decision making). Exercise slows brain aging, reduces symptoms of depression, lowers the risk of Alzheimer's disease and dementia (and also delays their onset and slows their progression), and enhances subjective well-being (which is essentially the scientific term for happiness).

The mechanisms by which aerobic exercise produces these effects are various and complex, and most remain only dimly understood. Clearly, some of the benefits are related to the increase in blood flow and oxygen supply to the brain that result from exercise. Other mechanisms are more unique to the brain. To give one example, recent research has shown that exercise interacts with estrogen to regulate brain-derived neurotrophic factor (BDNF) in the hippocampus. BDNF enhances neural plasticity and neuron function.

The brain is not just the most important organ for running performance; it's also the most important organ for life. Enhancing your brain health is one of the best things you can do to boost your overall health. What's more, I firmly believe that any factor that positively affects the overall health of runners will ultimately benefit their running. So looking after the general well-being of your brain is good for your training and racing.

CHAPTER ◆ 3

BREAKING THROUGH THE WALL

Every runner's greatest opponent is the wall—the wall of fatigue, that is. The goal of training is to push back the wall of fatigue by increasing the maximum pace one can sustain from the start line to the finish line of a race. The goal of race execution is to actually run as fast as possible without hitting the wall before reaching the finish line. It's that simple.

In team sports such as football, the virtue of knowing your opponent is often preached. The more aware you are of your opponent's strengths and weaknesses, the better you can exploit that team's weaknesses and the better you can protect yourself against that team's strengths. We runners can also benefit from knowing our opponent. Most runners take it for granted that they know what fatigue is and how it works. But the conventional scientific conception of exercise fatigue that most runners' beliefs and assumptions about fatigue are based on has been falsified by recent discoveries concerning the role of the brain in exercise performance. The new, brain-centered conception of fatigue gives us a very different view of our common opponent and suggests a different way of training to break through the wall.

Throughout the twentieth century, the prevailing conception of exercise fatigue was the so-called catastrophe theory. According to this conception, fatigue is an involuntary drop in performance caused by the loss of homeostasis (or balance) somewhere in the body. For example, lactic acid buildup causes the muscles to lose their normal pH balance, and they become too acidic to function properly. Or the muscles become glycogen depleted, so there's no longer sufficient energy available to sustain performance. This conception of fatigue has been referred to as the catastrophe theory because it associates fatigue with a short-term "catastrophic" functional breakdown in the muscles.

In the 1980s, a new generation of exercise scientists led by Tim Noakes, M.D., of the University of Cape Town, South Africa, began to poke holes in the catastrophe theory and eventually proposed an alternative, brain-centered conception of exercise fatigue. According to this new conception, fatigue is a self-protective mechanism that the brain uses to *prevent* a catastrophic loss of homeostasis from occurring during exercise. Fatigue happens when feed-back signals from the body to the brain indicate the imminent likelihood of a catastrophic loss of homeostasis if exercise continues at the current intensity level. In response to these signals, the brain decreases muscle activation and produces feelings of discomfort and loss of motivation, resulting in reduced exercise performance.

Let's take a closer look at the differences between the catastrophe theory of exercise fatigue and the brain-centered conception, and at some of the ev-idence against the former and in favor of the latter. Then we'll discuss the brain training approach to breaking through the wall of fatigue as defined by the newer, better scientific understanding of every runner's greatest oppo-nent.

CATASTROPHE AVERTED

There are two major arguments against the catastrophe theory of fatigue. First, the various specific functional breakdowns that have been put forward as direct causes of fatigue never actually occur. Second, the catastrophe the-ory cannot explain some commonly observed realities of maximum exercise performance, including performance in running races of all distances.

It is widely assumed by proponents of the catastrophe theory of exercise fatigue (and there are still many) that fatigue in short, maximum-intensity ex-ercise efforts is caused by the muscles' inability to produce its fundamental energy currency, adenosine triphosphate (ATP), as fast as it's being used. Exercise-related ATP depletion has never been shown to exceed even 50 per-cent in healthy subjects, however. Similarly, fatigue in prolonged exercise is "supposed" to be caused by glycogen depletion, but in reality there's always glycogen left over in the working muscles of "exhausted" athletes. If total glycogen depletion ever did occur, ATP depletion would soon follow, because glycogen is not a direct muscle fuel, but is rather a source of ATP replenishment. And if ATP depletion ever did occur, the result would be muscle rigor—that is, the working muscles would become locked in a state of full contraction and the athlete would be essentially paralyzed. I doubt you've ever seen this happen.

Another proposed cause of catastrophic fatigue is muscular acidosis. The muscles produce lactic acid faster than they can metabolize it, and as a result the muscles become too acidic to function properly. If muscular acidosis were a direct cause of fatigue, then fatigue in any given runner would always occur at the same level of lactic acid concentration in the blood. But it does not. For example, studies have shown that, with increasing altitude, fatigue occurs at lower and lower blood lactate concentrations.

So much for the catastrophes that never happen. Now let's talk about some of the realities of maximum exercise performance that the catastrophe theory fails to explain.

Believe it or not, the catastrophe theory of exercise fatigue cannot explain why runners run faster in shorter races than they do in longer races. In other words, it cannot account for the phenomenon of pacing. As every runner knows, whenever the race distance exceeds a short sprint, a runner achieves maximum performance by "holding something back"—that is, by running not at absolute maximum speed but at the maximum speed that can be sustained to the finish line and no farther. This pacing phenomenon cannot be accounted for without reference to the brain. Only the brain can hold the muscles back. If maximum efforts were controlled entirely by the muscles and cardiovascular system, then runners would run (or at least start) every race, regardless of distance, at the same speed. The catastrophe theory of exercise fatigue simply cannot formulate a concept of maximum performance that is relative to exercise duration. Maximum effort is maximum effort.

Furthermore, if maximum efforts were controlled entirely by the muscles and cardiovascular system, then fatigue would always occur when the muscles were working *absolutely* as hard as possible. In scientific terms, a muscle is working absolutely as hard as it can if 100 percent of the motor units within the muscle are active. So the catastrophe conception of fatigue predicts that 100 percent of the motor units in the working muscles will be active whenever fatigue occurs, regardless of the duration or intensity of exercise. In reality, however, activation of available motor units never exceeds 50 percent at fatigue in prolonged exercise.

When confronted by the catastrophe theory's inability to account for pacing, some of its proponents spontaneously offer the commonsense explanation that runners consciously control their pace in competition based on target split times derived from training and past racing experience. But a realistic consideration of how split times are used in racing yields the inevitable conclusion that runners rely on a subconscious feel for pace to a far greater extent than they rely on the clock. A 5K road race is 30 percent over with by the time you get your first mile split. In the last ten miles of a marathon, most runners are just hanging on rather than trying to nail particular mile split times. And in cross-country races, split times are scarcely used at all. Studies in which inaccurate time and distance information has failed to affect the performance of runners provide further evidence that subconscious feel, not conscious calculation, governs pacing.

The catastrophe theory of exercise fatigue also cannot account for the well-known phenomenon of the finishing kick, or "end spurt." That's because the catastrophe theory predicts that fatigue is always absolute. Once your body loses homeostasis in some area that's critical to performance, that's it—you must stop running or at least slow down until your body can recover homeostasis. But the end spurt phenomenon belies this prediction. Runners routinely begin to experience fatigue and perhaps even start to slow down in the latter stages of a race, only to find the wherewithal to sprint the final straightaway. According to the catastrophe theory of fatigue, this phenomenon is impossible.

The end spurt phenomenon has been scientifically demonstrated in a few noteworthy experiments. In one of these studies, Australian researchers put a group of subjects through a sixty-minute simulated time trial on stationary bikes. They interspersed six all-out sprints throughout the hour-long effort. The purpose of these sprints was to establish when fatigue began to occur, which is otherwise difficult to do in a sustained, submaximal effort (due to the very pacing phenomenon discussed above).

The results showed that while overall power output remained steady throughout the time trial (thanks to good pacing), maximum power output began to decline in the second sprint, indicating a very early onset of initial fatigue. Maximum power continued to decrease through the fifth sprint, and then suddenly shot upward in the sixth and final sprint. If the fatigue that began to set in as early as the second sprint had been caused by a catastrophic loss of homeostasis in the muscles, this final surge could not have happened.

IT'S ALL IN YOUR HEAD

As I stated above, the new, brain-centered model of exercise performance argues that fatigue is not an involuntary drop in performance caused by the loss of homoeostasis somewhere in the body. Instead, it is an effort by the brain to *prevent* a dangerous loss of homeostasis by reducing muscle activity and by producing feelings of discomfort and loss of motivation. Throughout exercise, the brain continually reads feedback signals from the muscles, blood, and elsewhere in order to answer the question, How much longer can my body go at the present work level before something terrible happens? When the answer received through the various feedback channels is, in essence, Not much longer, the brain reduces motor output to the muscles and generates those familiar feelings of pain and suffering to reinforce the reduction in output.

When it comes to maximum-intensity running, fatigue thus defined functions as a certain type of pacing strategy known as teleoanticipation. Here's how it works: Running is almost always initiated with an anticipated endpoint in mind—either a total distance or a total duration or both. (This is a fundamental fact of training and racing that the catastrophe theory completely overlooks.) The brain uses this anticipated endpoint to calculate the maximum amount of muscle activation the runner can sustain from start to finish without a loss of homeostasis in the muscles or other organs. This calculation is based on fatigue set points (such as the maximum core body temperature that is allowable without organ damage), afferent feedback (such as chemical signals indicating the amount of glycogen available in the muscles), past experiences (such as explicit knowledge of past performance limits), and environmental factors (such as air temperature). Throughout exercise, the amount of muscle activation continually changes based on ongoing communication among the brain, the body, and the environment.

In most cases, a runner begins running at a very low level of fatigue. In the case of a race or other maximal effort covering any fixed distance, the fatigue level (measured as a rating of perceived exertion, or RPE) subsequently increases in a linear way throughout the run. If the effort is well paced, the runner reaches maximum perceived exertion (the RPE level corresponding to exhaustion) at the finish line. If the runner miscalculates and reaches maximum RPE before the finish line, the runner will begin to slow down, seemingly involuntarily. Exhaustion occurs at many different levels of muscle activation, blood lactate concentration, heart rate, dehydration, core body temperature, muscle pH, ATP depletion, and glycogen depletion, and these levels never exceed homeostatic limits, but exhaustion always occurs when the runner *feels* completely exhausted—because that feeling of exhaustion is what fatigue really is!

Indeed, in stark contrast to the catastrophe theory of exercise fatigue, which ignores both the brain and the mind, the brain-centered conception of exercise fatigue suggests that pacing during prolonged maximum-intensity running is really governed by feel. This feel for pacing is both an innate capacity and a learned skill, and is an excellent example of the neuroscientific maxim "Neurons that fire together wire together." During hard workouts and races that leave a runner exhausted, the feeling of running at a certain pace becomes associated with a subconscious memory of how long that pace was maintained before fatigue set in, and also with the particular afferent feedback signals from the body that preceded fatigue in that situation. The forging of these neural connections serves to calibrate the brain's pacing mechanism. The more times you experience running fatigue, the more your brain learns about how long your body can sustain any given running pace. As a result, when you start a race of a given distance, you are able to feel your way into the appropriate pace—which is your current maximum speed relative to the distance. Your brain knows just how much to hold back so that the finish line is within sight when your RPE level maxes out.

Science has only just begun the process of validating the new, brain-centered conception of exercise fatigue. There's still a lot more evidence disproving the old theory than there is proving the new one. And we still know very little about how it all works. But all of the recent studies designed to test the brain-centered fatigue conception have indeed supported it. For example, studies involving simulated races (usually on stationary bikes) have shown that a decline in performance due to fatigue almost always coincides with a drop in electrical activity in the muscles. This observation is significant

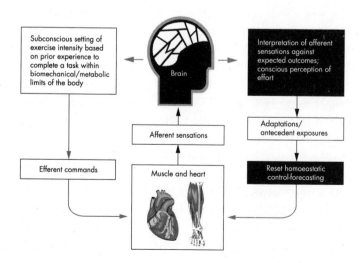

because it indicates that the cause of slowing is reduced electrical input to the muscles from the brain. If the cause of fatigue were some factor inside the muscles (such as lactic acid buildup), the athlete would slow down despite a steady level of electrical activity in the muscles.

RETHINKING THE WALL

The new, brain-centered fatigue conception does not wipe away everything we thought we knew about exercise fatigue. Several of the physiological factors that were previously believed to be direct causes of fatigue remain relevant to the brain-centered conception as indirect causes of fatigue. Whereas in the past these factors were believed to cause muscle dysfunction through loss of homeostasis, they are now understood to contribute to fatigue by sending signals to the brain that warn of impending loss of homeostasis. These factors include muscular acidosis, muscle depolarization, glycogen depletion, muscle damage, and heat accumulation. There are also others that I will not discuss here, because they are less important from a practical perspective.

I will forewarn you that there is some fairly heavy physiology in this section. If you are not quite as fascinated by the workings of the human body (especially during running) as I am, go ahead and skip to the next section, where you will learn what all of this physiology means for your training.

Muscular Acidosis

When I was a beginning student of the sport of running, every book I read taught me that lactic acid (or lactate) buildup was the primary cause of fatigue during efforts lasting more than thirty seconds and less than thirty minutes. Exercise physiologists have since demonstrated that, far from being a cause of fatigue, lactate is an important fuel during exercise. Nor is lactic acid the direct cause of increasing muscle acidity during high-intensity running. It's the hydrogen ions produced along with lactic acid that do so.

What's more, the muscles never reach a level of acidity that would directly cause dysfunction (or fatigue) of the muscle fibers. The body's normal pH at rest is approximately 7.4. During intense exercise, as the muscles become more acidic, pH may drop as low as 7.0 at the point of exhaustion. When muscle cells are electrically stimulated outside the body, however, mechanical failure only occurs when the pH drops all the way down to 6.8. This observation suggests that fatigue always occurs before a catastrophic loss of acid-base homeostasis in the muscles takes place.

It certainly stands to reason that the brain would inhibit the muscles from working to the point of catastrophic acidity. Acid-base (or pH) balance is one of the most important types of homeostasis in the body. If organ tissues become either too acidic (too positively charged) or too alkaline (too negatively charged), irreparable damage ensues.

How does the brain know that the muscles are approaching a dangerous level of acidity? Lactate might act as a brain signal of muscular acidosis, thereby contributing to fatigue indirectly. Lactic acid acts on acid-sensing nerves in muscle tissue that connect to pain centers in the brain. It is believed that this effect accounts for the burning sensation in the working muscles that is commonly felt by athletes engaging in high-intensity exercise. The feeling of pain may trigger a reduction in motor output from the brain to the muscles.

There's also a second indirect mechanism by which lactic acid production might cause brain-mediated fatigue during intense running. The body contains various buffering systems that neutralize excess hydrogen ions and help the body maintain pH balance. One of them is sodium bicarbonate—that's right: baking soda. When sodium bicarbonate buffers lactic acid, carbonic acid is formed. When carbonic acid reaches the lungs, it breaks down into carbon dioxide and water. Carbon dioxide is a potent breathing stimulator. Thus, rapid lactic acid production causes a dramatic increase in breathing stress that may hasten fatigue, also through discomfort.

Muscle Depolarization

Another potential contributor to fatigue during very high-intensity running is muscle depolarization. Muscle cells work somewhat like batteries. Their potential to release energy and perform mechanical work depends on a difference in atomic charges between the inside of the muscle cell and the outside. When the positive charge inside the muscle cell is much greater than the positive charge outside it—as is normally the case at rest—the muscle cell membrane is said to be highly excitable, meaning it is very easy for electrical impulses to enter the muscle cell.

The difference in electrical charges between the inside of the cell and the outside of the cell is referred to as an ion concentration gradient. When the concentration gradient is high, the cell membrane is very excitable and nerve impulses pass through very efficiently. When the concentration gradient is low, the cell membrane is less excitable and nerve impulses lose effectiveness. During very high-intensity exercise, there is a steady decline in the concentration gradient in muscles and in muscle cell membrane excitability that is strongly correlated to fatigue.

Unlike the other fatigue-contributing factors discussed in this section, muscle depolarization relates to the peripheral nervous system—where nerve cells meet muscle cells—rather than to the central nervous system (within the brain itself).

Glycogen Depletion

Glycogen consists of long chains of glucose molecules stored in the muscles and liver. Muscle glycogen supplies glucose directly to the muscles, while liver glycogen is used to maintain stable blood glucose levels, supply the brain with glucose, and send glucose wherever else it may be needed in the body. The glycogen storage capacity of the human body is small. The average adult stores about five hundred grams of glycogen (four hundred grams in the muscles and another one hundred grams in the liver), as compared to twelve to eighteen kilograms of fat. The glycogen supply becomes a performance limiter when runners try to maintain a fairly aggressive pace for an extended period of time—for example, when chasing a personal best time in a marathon. This is because glycogen supplies energy faster than fat, so the higher the intensity of exercise, the more the muscles have to rely on glycogen.

For many years, exercise scientists believed that glycogen depletion was *the* performance limiter in prolonged exercise. Now it's clear that glycogen depletion never actually occurs—the body always holds some in reserve even at the point of complete exhaustion—and that there are other causes of fatigue in prolonged exercise. Nevertheless, there is evidence that the brain is able to monitor glycogen stores and the rate of glycogen usage in various ways and use this information in the calculations made to produce an appropriate pacing strategy and, as necessary, symptoms of fatigue. Exercise scientists refer to these mechanisms as "glycostats."

For example, the rate of glucose usage by the brain is linked to the rate of glycogen usage by the muscles during running, and could function as a glycostat. Another possible glycostat is interleukin-6, an intercellular signaling compound that is released from muscle cells in proportion to glycogen depletion. It travels through the bloodstream and enters the brain. High brain concentrations of interleukin-6 have been shown to cause fatigue in runners.

Muscle Damage

Muscle cells routinely suffer microscopic damage during running. The accumulation of such damage is likely to be a major cause of fatigue during prolonged running. Whenever you complete a run feeling sore, you know you experienced significant muscle damage. And whenever you finish a run feeling sore *and* exhausted, you can be reasonably certain that muscle damage has been a major cause of your exhaustion.

Interestingly, interleukin-6, which I mentioned above in connection with its potential role as a signal of muscle glycogen depletion, may also send the brain a red flag related to muscle damage, since muscle cell membrane rupture causes interleukin-6 to leak from muscle cells. There are also many other candidates for muscle damage–related contributors to fatigue. The pain associated with muscle damage appears to be an independent cause of fatigue. In one study, muscle pain induced by the injection of saline solution in cyclists caused a significant reduction in muscle activation without causing any biochemical changes that could explain it.

Heat Accumulation

Only 25 percent of the energy that the muscles release during running is used for muscle contractions. The other 75 percent is lost as heat waste. In cold and temperate conditions, the body has little trouble dissipating most of this heat, but when the air temperature exceeds approximately seventy-eight degrees Fahrenheit, heat accumulates in the muscles and contributes to fatigue.

There is plenty of evidence that the brain limits muscle activation to keep muscle temperature within safe limits. An interesting study from the University of Cape Town, South Africa, shed some light on the role of the brain in relation to exercise performance in the heat. Ten male cyclists completed a pair of thirty-five-kilometer time trials—one in a cool environment (59°F) and one in a hot environment (95°F). The researchers recorded the time it took to complete each time trial and measured body temperature at a couple of points within it. They also attached EMG sensors to various muscles of the legs. These sensors recorded the amount of electricity present in the muscles. The brain activates muscles by sending electrical signals to them, so EMG sensors are an excellent means of measuring "motor" output from the brain to the muscles.

As expected, the hot environment had a negative effect on time trial performance. The cyclists took longer to complete it and were not able to produce as much power throughout it. The amount of muscle activity as measured by EMG was also lower in the hot time trial, indicating that fatigue was caused not by factors within the muscles but by reduced activation of the muscles by the brain. Equally interesting was the observation that body temperature rose to almost exactly the same level in both time trials. Taken together, these results suggest that exercise performance in the heat is hampered not because athletes become hotter, causing a temperature-related decline in muscle performance, but because the brain reduces motor output to the muscles to *prevent* the body from becoming too hot.

Curiously, hot-weather racing is the only circumstance in which the brain's self-protective fatigue mechanisms sometimes fail to prevent runners from seriously harming themselves. While not common, heat illness, which is potentially fatal, does affect some runners when exerting maximum efforts in hot environments. Research suggests that elevated core body temperature accelerates nerve impulse transmission, potentially causing the protective inhibition of muscle activation to lag behind motor signals ordering continued work at the same intensity.

PUSHING BACK THE THRESHOLD

When I explain to my fellow runners that exercise fatigue is caused by the brain, they often misunderstand my point and draw the conclusion that fatigue is some type of illusion. Then they vow to ignore this illusion the next time they race, and thus push on to faster times. But the fact that exercise fatigue is brain-centered rather than muscle-based does not make it any less real or any more surmountable by willpower. The reality of brain-centered fatigue is as inexorable as the myth of muscle fatigue. For the sake of your safety, I would caution you against acting otherwise and trying to will your way beyond brain-centered fatigue, but that's just my point: You can't, because brain-centered exercise fatigue is itself a virtually infallible safety mechanism.

Actually, there are some mental strategies you can use, not to ignore fatigue but to push back the wall of fatigue, which I will discuss in chapter 8. But in the remainder of this chapter I wish to outline the more important practical training ramifications of switching from the catastrophic theory to the brain-centered conception of exercise fatigue.

If the new conception is accurate—and I'm certain it is—then the training methods we use to prevent hitting the wall should be adjusted. Traditional training methods in running have focused on doing workouts designed to address individual physiological causes of fatigue, such as glycogen depletion. The result has been a heavy emphasis on training at precise intensity thresholds that maximize a runner's exposure to specific causes of fatigue and thus, in theory, maximize adaptations that enable the runner to resist these specific causes of fatigue in the future. The use of heart rate zones in workouts is almost entirely based on this training approach.

The brain-centered conception of fatigue suggests that the "thresholds" approach is misguided, because there really are no direct physiological causes of fatigue. True, the brain triggers fatigue in response to physiological signals of impending danger sent from the muscles, blood, and so forth, but the whole system is so incredibly complex that you can't possibly train to push back individual fatigue factors. What the new science proposes is that we forget about the physiological mechanisms (really the neurophysiological mechanisms) of fatigue and focus instead on preventing fatigue itself (the pain and suffering, the slowing down) in races. Regardless of the particular factors that may cause you to experience discomfort and slow down in a race, you want to train in a way that enables you to sustain your goal pace all the way to the finish line without slowing and without the overwhelming discomfort that comes with it. You can train optimally to achieve this objective without having any idea what's going on inside your body.

According to the brain-centered model of exercise performance, a runner achieves his race goal when his brain calculates that achieving the race goal is possible without catastrophic self-harm. It's as simple as that. A runner's brain achieves this desirable state of confidence when the various forms of feedback that the brain uses in its teleoanticipatory calculations— fatigue set points established in training, knowledge of recent training results, and afferent feedback sent from various parts of the body throughout the race—raise no red flags from start to finish. This result is most likely to occur if you have already done in training more or less what you are attempting to do in the race. It follows, then, that the single most important practical response to the new, brain-centered conception of exercise fatigue that you can apply to your training is to formulate and execute training plans that culminate in challenging, race-specific key workouts that closely simulate the demands of your peak race. Performing race-specific key workouts in the final weeks of training for a peak race will establish the fatigue set points, provide the training experiences, and produce the physiological adaptations needed to supply the right feedback to your brain during the peak race.

A key workout is race-specific when it combines both the pace and the duration demands of your coming peak race. So the most important first step in the brain training process is to establish a goal pace for that race (since the distance is already established). A goal pace is an average running pace (per mile) associated with a time goal for a race. If your goal is to run a 3:45 marathon, your goal pace is 8:35 per mile. If your goal is to run a 39:59 10K race, your goal pace is 6:26 per mile. And so forth. Your primary training objective is to cause your brain and body to adapt from their current state to a state that makes this goal achievable. In simple terms, the training process must (1) increase the duration you can sustain your goal pace (up to the full race duration), and (2) increase the pace you can sustain over the full race distance (up to the goal pace).

In my experience, most runners—thanks to the highly evolved teleoanticipation mechanisms in their brains—are pretty good at selecting appropriate goal times. There's no need to complicate the process with a lot of pseudoscience. If you've raced previously at the distance of your goal event, these performances will obviously provide a solid foundation for goal setting. If you're racing at a new distance, various performance equivalence tables and race-time calculators can help you set an appropriate time goal. These tables and calculators are based on known mathematical relationships between individual runners' average pace levels at various distances. Table 4.1 on page 71 can be used to select an appropriate time goal for any of four distances using a recent finishing time from one of the other three. Once you've done so, all you have to do is convert the finishing time to a goal pace per mile.

Regardless of how you come up with your goal pace, you can always adjust your time goal for a peak race—based on your performances in training and tune-up races—as you get closer to it. The purpose of selecting a time goal before you even start training for a peak race is not to lock yourself into that goal time but rather to establish appropriate pace goals for various workouts. It also helps you design a progressive training program that increases your fitness level step by step toward the level needed to enable you to achieve your peak race goal.

Once you have established a goal pace, the next step is to create a training plan that will increase the duration you can sustain your goal pace, up to the full race duration, and increase the pace you can sustain over the full race distance, up to the goal pace. The most sensible way to ensure that you achieve your race goal is to perform key workouts in the final weeks of training that are highly race-specific in terms of their *combined pace and distance demands*. If you're fit enough to perform at the desired level in very race-specific workouts in the final weeks before your peak race, you'll probably be fit enough to perform at the desired level in the peak race itself.

Race-specific key workouts for the 5K race distance include 5K tune-up races and interval workouts featuring moderately long intervals at your 5K goal pace and fairly short jogging recovery periods (for example, 5×1K @ 5K goal pace with 90-second jogging recoveries). Race-specific key workouts for the 10K race distance include 5K and 10K tune-up races and interval workouts featuring long intervals at goal pace and fairly short jogging recovery periods (for example, 3×3K @ 10K goal pace with 2-minute jogging recoveries). Effective peak workouts for the half-marathon race distance include long tempo runs and cruise interval workouts at half-marathon goal pace (for example, 13 miles with 2×20-minute segments @ half-marathon goal pace). And for the marathon distance, I recommend peak long runs that match your marathon goal time but are run at a pace that's 10–15 percent slower, and moderately long marathon-pace runs, such as sixteen miles with the middle fourteen run at marathon pace.

The objective of all of the training that precedes these race-specific key workouts performed in the Peak phase of training is simply to prepare you for these workouts step by step. Your Base phase and Build phase training create a general foundation for the specific training that in turn gives you the ability to run the full race distance at your goal pace.

The main drivers of your fitness development in all three phases are your key workouts. There are three basic categories of key workouts: speed workouts (hill repetitions, fartlek runs, interval workouts), which feature short efforts that are equal to or faster than goal race pace; intensive endurance workouts (interval workouts, tempo runs, cruise intervals), which feature efforts that are equal to or slightly slower than goal race pace; and extensive endurance workouts (long runs, progression runs, marathon-pace runs, tempo runs, cruise intervals), which feature long efforts that are usually substantially slower than goal race pace, but may include some race-pace running in the latter phases of training. I recommend that all runners perform one workout of each category throughout the training cycle. The structure of each will necessarily vary widely depending on the distance of your goal event, your fitness level, and the phase of training.

When training for goal events of 10K distance and shorter, your training should emphasize increasing your maximum sustainable pace, because in such events the pace is more challenging than the distance. When training for a half marathon or marathon, either speed or distance may be the greater challenge, depending on your goal, your background, and your individual strengths and weaknesses. In any case, you will want to balance the speed and endurance components of race fitness more evenly than you would when training for shorter goal events.

Nevertheless, the general strategy for key workouts is the same for all runners. The first speed workouts should feature very short, very high-intensity efforts; the number or duration of these efforts should increase gradually with each repetition of the workout. These workouts will build a foundation to perform slightly longer, slightly slower speed workouts in the next phase of training. The number and/or duration of speed efforts again increases within the phase, building a foundation for speed workouts featuring intervals that are, once more, slightly slower but substantially longer. The overall objective is to extend your speed over distance.

The objective of intensive endurance workouts is the same, but in these workouts extension is prioritized over speed. For 5K and 10K runners, efforts never exceed goal pace in these workouts, but become longer and longer as the training cycle unfolds. For half-marathon and marathon runners, efforts never exceed 10K race pace, move downward toward race pace as the training cycle unfolds, and become steadily longer.

The first priority of extensive endurance workouts is to ensure the runner is able to complete the full goal event distance. For experienced runners training for shorter races, this priority is taken care of very quickly, if not before the training cycle even begins. But for beginning runners and those training for longer races, building sufficient endurance to "go the distance" may be the most important training challenge. Once a solid foundation of endurance has been built, the emphasis of extensive endurance workouts turns toward running long distances at faster speeds.

The following table provides examples of how to structure the training cycle for each of four goal event distances according to the guidelines I've just given you. The training cycle is divided into four phases (or three phases, with the middle phase itself divided into two subphases): Base, Build 1, Build 2, and Peak. Three key workouts—a speed run, an intensive endurance run, and an extensive endurance run—are performed each week in every phase.

At all four distances, speed training begins with short hill repeats that become longer over the course of the phase. The only difference is that their maximum length is greater for longer-distance goal events. In Build 1, speed workouts are more or less the same for all distances, featuring faster-than-goal-pace efforts that increase muscle activation capacity. In Build 2, speed workouts feature slightly longer, slightly slower efforts at longer distances. In the Peak phase, everyone does mixed intervals, but the pace levels that are emphasized differ by goal race distance. Naturally, those training for shorter races focus on faster paces. I like to prescribe mixed interval workouts in the Peak phase because they help runners maintain the adaptations they gained by doing fast intervals earlier in the training process while emphasizing efforts at or near goal race pace.

Intensive endurance training starts with fartlek workouts at all distances. The Base phase begins with fartlek workouts featuring short, fast efforts. But those training for longer race distances increase the duration and reduce the pace of these efforts more as the Base phase unfolds. Those training for a 5K peak race focus on goal pace training in their Build and Peak phase intensive endurance workouts. The length of the intervals increases. Those training for a 10K peak race do intervals of increasing distance at 10K goal pace. And those training for both the half-marathon and marathon distances do intensive endurance workouts at 10K pace in the Build phase and at half-marathon pace in the Peak phase.

As for extensive endurance workouts, all runners do easy endurance runs of increasing distance throughout the Base phase. Those training for longer goal events increase the distance of these runs more. In Build 1, 5K runners stop increasing the distance of their long runs and instead increase the pace to marathon pace; 10K runners perform longer endurance runs at variable paces (between base and marathon pace). Half-marathon and marathon runners continue to increase the distance of these runs in Build 1.

In Build 2, 5K runners increase the pace of their extensive endurance workouts even further, transforming them into half-marathon-pace tempo runs, and in the Peak phase they crank up the intensity still more with 10K-pace tempo runs; 10K runners follow a similar progression with marathon-pace endurance runs in Build 1 and half-marathon-pace tempo runs in the Peak phase. Half-marathon runners do variable-pace endurance runs in Build 2 and marathon-pace long runs in the Peak phase. Marathon runners do a mix of variable-pace and easy long runs in Build 2 and a mix of moderately long marathon-pace and very long moderate-pace endurance runs in the Peak phase.

A NOTE ON PACING

In reading through the previous section, and in perusing Table 3.1, you were probably struck by the fact that nearly all of the key workouts described use pace levels associated with various race distances as pacing guidelines instead of more commonly used guidelines, such as anaerobic threshold pace, VO_2max pace, and so forth. Because there is a definite mathematical relationship between race pace levels at various distances (for example, every runner's 3,000m pace is slightly faster than his or her 5K pace),

TABLE 3.1 ◆ A Sample Brain Training Key Workout Progression
at Four Race Distances

The primary purpose of this table is to demonstrate the brain training approach to structuring a training cycle to achieve the goal pace objective. It is not meant to provide a comprehensive training plan. For example, it does not incorporate such important factors as variations in total running volume and nonkey workouts (base runs, recovery runs) that also contribute to fitness development in crucial ways.

GOAL EVENT DISTANCE	TRAINING PHASE	SPEED WORKOUTS	INTENSIVE ENDURANCE WORKOUTS	EXTENSIVE ENDURANCE WORKOUTS
5K	Base	Hill repeats (100–200m)	Fartlek (100–400m efforts)	Endurance run
	Build 1	400m intervals @ 1-mile pace	30/30 intervals @ 5K goal pace	Marathon-pace run
	Build 2	600m intervals @ 3,000m pace	60/60 intervals @ 5K goal pace	Tempo run @ half-marathon pace
	Peak	Mixed intervals @ 10K pace to 1-mile pace	1K intervals @ 5K goal pace	Tempo run @ 10K pace
10K	Base	Hill repeats (100–300m)	Fartlek (100–600m efforts)	Endurance run
	Build 1	400m intervals @ 1-mile pace	1K intervals @ 10K goal pace	Variable-pace endurance run
	Build 2	1K intervals @ 5K pace	2K intervals @ 10K goal pace	Marathon-pace run
	Peak	Mixed intervals @ 10K pace to 3,000m pace	3K intervals @ 10K goal pace	Tempo run @ half-marathon pace
Half Marathon	Base	Hill repeats (100–400m)	Fartlek (200–800m efforts)	Endurance run
	Build 1	600m intervals @ 3,000m pace	1-mile intervals @ 10K pace	Endurance run
	Build 2	1K intervals @ 5K pace	Tempo run @ 10K pace	Variable-pace endurance run

GOAL EVENT DISTANCE	TRAINING PHASE	SPEED WORKOUTS	INTENSIVE ENDURANCE WORKOUTS	EXTENSIVE ENDURANCE WORKOUTS
Half Marathon	Peak	Mixed intervals @ half-marathon pace to 3,000m pace	Tempo run @ half-marathon pace	Marathon-pace run
Marathon	Base	Hill repeats (100–600m)	Fartlek (200 m–1K efforts)	Endurance run
	Build 1	600m intervals @ 3,000m pace	1-mile intervals @ 10K pace	Endurance run
	Build 2	1K intervals @ 5K pace	Tempo run @ 10K pace	Variable-pace endurance run and/or long + easy run
	Peak	Mixed intervals @ half-marathon race pace to 3,000m pace	Tempo run @ half-marathon pace	Marathon-pace run and/or long + easy run

I find that using race-pace levels as workout pacing guidelines is the most reliable way to ensure that the pace of your key workouts moves incrementally closer to your goal race pace over the course of the training cycle. Also, I find that performance-based pace targets motivate a greater effort in key workouts by making them more racelike. And remember, in the brain training approach there is no longer any point in using physiologically based pace targets, including anaerobic threshold pace.

The next chapter provides a detailed description of the brain training method of monitoring and controlling pace in workouts, which I call the target pace method.

CHAPTER ◆ 4

TARGET PACE TRAINING

In the autumn of 2004 I received a phone call from Donavon Guyot, the young CEO of Training Peaks, a small company that provides online tools for endurance athletes and coaches. Donavon told me Training Peaks had recently signed a deal with Garmin, the manufacturer of global positioning system (GPS) equipment, in connection with a new GPS device for runners that allowed them to monitor their pace and distance in real time anywhere on earth. The deal called for Training Peaks to create pace-based training plans that runners could download from TrainingPeaks.com right onto these devices, which would then guide the user through each pace-based workout for the entire duration of the training plan. Donavon asked me whether I might be interested in developing these plans, and without hesitation I told him I would.

I was excited about this opportunity for two reasons. First of all, I was already a great admirer of Training Peaks as a company. Their online training and coaching platforms were by far the best I had experienced. Unlike many technology companies, Training Peaks takes its time to do things right instead of rushing new products and services to market and then trying to fix all the bugs afterward.

An additional reason for my excitement was the fact that, at this time, I had recently begun to develop my brain training system, and I had decided that systematic monitoring and controlling of pace in workouts would be a major feature of brain training. The new Garmin device would make pace-based training far more practicable than it had ever been before. The timing of its launch could not have been better.

Most runners pay attention to pace to some degree in training, but my analysis of the new brain-centered model of running performance led me to the conclusion that runners should consciously pursue a performance-based target pace in every key workout. There are three brain-centered rationales for this approach. First, objective performance goals stimulate the brain to allow a higher level of muscle work output than either running by feel or using non-performance-based goals, such as staying within a particular heart rate zone. In other words, pace targets make you run harder so you get more out of your key workouts. Second, gathering objective feedback in the form of pace information from workouts helps the brain calibrate maximum performance over various distances, thus improving the runner's chances of actually giving a maximal performance in races. And third, establishing and pursuing key workout pace targets that move incrementally closer to peak race goal pace over the course of a training cycle ensures that the training process is progressive, systematic, and specific to the runner's overall goal.

One of the biggest influences on my approach to training runners is Jack Daniels, Ph.D., a legendary running coach, exercise physiologist, and author of the classic book *Daniels' Running Formula*. The "formula" referred to in the title of this book is a sophisticated pace-based training system that Daniels developed over the course of his brilliant career. But at the time I received Donavon's call, my recent exposure to the new brain-centered model of running performance had led me to believe that certain modifications to Daniels's formula were necessary. Training Peaks was now presenting me with a perfect occasion to make this evolutionary step. The result of this process was what I call the target pace method, which now serves as the basis of the brain training approach to controlling running pace and intensity in workouts. Because the target pace method could not exist if Jack Daniels's running formula had not existed first, I will explain them both.

FROM INTENSITY TO PERFORMANCE

Decades of trial and error undertaken by runners around the world have produced a bunch of classic workout formats that are proven to reliably produce optimal race fitness when done correctly and in the appropriate combination and sequence. These workouts include tempo runs, long runs, recovery runs, intervals, and hill repetitions. When Daniels began coaching runners in the late 1960s, he relied on these tried-and-true workouts to develop peak fitness in his athletes.

At the same time, Daniels was engaged in research that focused on the physiology of running intensity. Specifically, he studied the relationships among various intensity variables, including oxygen consumption, lactate production, heart rate, and so forth. Daniels believed that each type of workout was most effective if performed at the correct physiological intensity, or the correct fraction of a given runner's maximum running intensity. But because there was no practical way to use any direct measurement of physiological intensity to guide one's training efforts in real time (for example, monitoring oxygen consumption requires that the runner breathe through a tube attached to a cumbersome machine), Daniels sought to create a reliable system to link physiological intensity to running pace, which was relatively easy to monitor in real time as long as one ran on a measured course.

Daniels found an ingeniously straightforward way to achieve this objective. First, based on extensive physiological testing of runners, he created his own set of parameters for the various classic workout formats (interval lengths, recovery period durations, and so forth) that virtually ensured his runners performed each workout at the appropriate physiological intensity level. Then he simply recorded how fast his athletes tended to run in each type of workout. Through this process he was able to make two important observations: (1) that runners who performed at the same level in races also performed at roughly the same level in all of the classic workout formats; and (2) that the pace ranges that seemed most effective for each level of runner in each workout type demonstrated a consistent mathematical relationship across all levels.

The first observation allowed Daniels to create a table that runners could employ to find their current performance level using the result of a recent race or time trial at any distance from one mile to a marathon. The second observation allowed Daniels to create another table that showed runners of every level precisely which pace to target in each type of workout to achieve the appropriate physiological intensity level. Runners could move back and forth between the two tables using a unique number (called a VDOT ranking) that was associated with each performance level. I've used both tables in my own training and in coaching other runners, and they work very well. Now, however, I use a modified pair of tables that I created after partnering with Training Peaks and in response to the new brain-centered model of running performance.

Daniels's tables are based on the catastrophe theory of fatigue, which is grounded in the belief that running performance is limited by the body's ability to maintain certain types of homeostasis (such as low blood lactate levels) while a given running pace is sustained. The top priority of training, therefore, is to push back these physiological limiters by performing work-outs at pace levels where these particular causes of fatigue come into play. Thus, in Daniels's system, tempo runs are performed at anaerobic threshold intensity, longer intervals are performed at VO_2max intensity, and so forth.

According to the brain-centered model, however, fatigue is not caused by any hard physiological limit but is instead a sensory manifestation of a pacing strategy (teleoanticipation) that the brain adopts when presented with a particular running challenge, whether in a workout or in a race. The goal of training, then, is not to push back particular physiological causes of fa-tigue. Rather, the goal of training is simply to gradually increase the speed you can sustain over race distance and the duration you can sustain race speed (or faster) until you are able to sustain your goal pace over the full peak race distance. There's no need to focus on training at specific physio-logical thresholds, because the causes of fatigue are far too complex for such a thing to be possible. You're not really doing it even when you think you are.

This shift in mind-set does not necessitate a wholesale transformation of Daniels's system, but it does suggest a few key modifications. All of the tried-and-true workout formats still stand—because they're tried and true, after all. The intensity-based pace levels that Daniels prescribes for each workout type, however, go out the window and are replaced with performance-based target pace levels. So tempo runs are performed at the individual runner's current or estimated half-marathon or 10K race pace, longer intervals are usually performed at the individual runner's current or estimated 5K race pace, and so forth.

The actual difference between the target pace you'll find yourself run-ning in, say, a Jack Daniels tempo run performed at anaerobic threshold pace and the target pace called for in a brain training tempo run at half-marathon or 10K pace is not large. (Half-marathon pace happens to be slightly slower than anaerobic threshold pace for most runners, while 10K pace is slightly faster.) The real differences lie in the *meaning* of these targets—in *knowing* you're training at your current race pace for a particular event—and also in the way workouts emphasizing various target pace levels are arranged in the training cycle. In brain training, everything is oriented toward performing highly race-specific workouts at your peak race goal pace in the final weeks of training. Doing these workouts precisely at your peak race goal pace—rather than at some physiologically based "threshold" pace that approximates it—makes a big difference, I believe, in giving your brain and body experience in doing what they will be expected to do in the peak race itself.

TARGET PACE LEVELS

In the target pace method, Daniels's VDOT ranking system is replaced with a target pace level (TPL) ranking system. In the TPL system, a unique number between fifty and one is assigned to each running performance level, from back of the pack (TPL 50) to world class (TPL 1). The first step in using this system is to go to Table 4.1 on page 71 and find your current TPL level by looking up a recent race time at the 5K, 10K, half-marathon, or marathon distance that equates to your *current* fitness level, or by estimating your finishing time at one of these distances given your *current* fitness level. *Note: This process is different from that of choosing a peak race goal time, as described in the previous chapter. A peak race goal time is an endpoint. The purpose of determining your present TPL is to establish a* starting *point for your training.*

If you choose to use a performance estimate instead of an actual race time, I recommend that you use an estimated finishing time for 5K or 10K, unless you're currently near peak half-marathon or marathon shape. Due to the special endurance requirements of longer races, you could be in great 5K shape yet unable to even finish a marathon. Therefore, your current performance level at shorter distances will give you a better indication of your proper training pace levels when your extensive endurance fitness level is not especially high.

Once you have determined your current TPL number, go to Table 4.2 on page 74 to find the workout target pace levels associated with it. Let's say you ran a 10K as a tune-up race in your previous training cycle, when your fitness level was roughly where it is now, and your finishing time was 47:11. This time falls between TPL 38 and TPL 37 on the table. Since it's closer to TPL 37, it is probably most sensible to use the TPL 37 workout target pace levels initially in your next training cycle. In the case of TPL 37, these are as follows:

Recovery: 10:57–9:42/mile
Base: 9:41–8:47
Marathon Pace: 8:15
Half-Marathon Pace: 7:57
10K Pace: 7:34

5K Pace: 7:18/mile; 1:48/400m
3K Pace: 7:04/mile; 1:45/400m
1-Mile Pace: 6:41/mile; 1:40/400m

These are the pace levels you should target in your workouts. Table 4.3 on page 78 provides a summary of the types of workouts in which each target pace is used, and the key workout training effect (extensive endurance, intensive endurance, and speed) that each target pace is used to achieve. Use recovery pace in your recovery workouts. Use base pace in base runs and in most endurance runs. Use marathon pace in marathon-pace endurance runs and progression runs. Use half-marathon pace and 10K pace in tempo runs and cruise intervals. Use 5K pace and 3,000m pace in interval workouts, including some fartlek workouts. And use one-mile pace in short interval workouts. Naturally, it would be impossible for you to run at exactly your target pace throughout every workout, nor should you even try. These numbers are merely targets. Ultimately it is the afferent feedback your brain receives from your body that must tell you whether it is best to run slightly faster or slightly slower than your target pace at any given moment of a workout.

You will also need to adjust your TPL number as you build fitness over the course of a training cycle. As your running fitness goes up, your TPL number will go down and your target pace levels will become faster. There are two ways you can go about making these adjustments. The formal way is to run a race or time trial once every four weeks or so and use the result to adjust your TPL. A less formal and no less effective way is to let your workout performances—and especially your key workout performances—guide you. For example, suppose you're currently training at TPL 37 and you perform a 10K-pace tempo workout. Your target pace for this workout is 7:34 per mile. You start the tempo segment of the workout at this pace, but once you get into it you decide that the pace feels too easy and you increase it to 7:25 per mile. Based on this performance you should consider increasing all of your workout target pace levels to TPL 36. Don't lower your TPL number every time you have one great workout. Do so only when you notice a consistent trend of outperforming your targets.

Be careful to avoid the pitfall of trying to "demolish" your target pace in key workouts—of turning key workouts into quasi races, in other words. Target paces are intended not only to help you run hard enough but also to help you avoid running too hard. Except in breakthrough workouts, it's important to avoid running to absolute exhaustion in training, because doing so will very likely sabotage your performance in subsequent workouts. On those special days when you find that you are able to blow your target pace out of the water *without* running to complete exhaustion, however, go right ahead and do it. Taking advantage of your best days by running faster than planned is as important a part of training responsively as cutting back on planned training when you feel lousy.

Over the course of a sixteen- or twenty-four-week training cycle you can expect to lower your TPL number four to six times. In the final few weeks of the Peak phase you should be able to do all of your workouts at the target pace levels associated with the TPL number corresponding to your peak race goal time. Going back to our example in which we imagine you are a runner with a current TPL of 37, let's now say that your peak race goal is to break 43:00 for 10K. This goal time corresponds to a TPL of 32. So you should aim to perform all of your workouts at the target pace levels associated with TPL 32 in the final three or four weeks before your scheduled peak race.

All of the workouts prescribed in the brain training plans presented in Part II use the training pace levels shown in Table 4.2. In following one or more of these plans, you will not only enjoy the benefits of target pace training but will also learn how to most effectively use target pace training to build your fitness toward the goal of sustaining your peak race goal pace over race distance. This will enable you to do the same if you choose to modify any of the plans for better customization in the future.

MONITORING YOUR PACE

There are four ways to monitor your pace during workouts: by running on a treadmill, by running on a 400-meter track, by running on another measured course (such as a bike path with markers at every quarter mile), and by wearing a speed and distance device, such as a Garmin Forerunner 305. Each method has advantages and disadvantages.

Treadmill

Advantages: Treadmills provide accurate real-time pace information (assuming they are properly calibrated, which is not a given) and a controlled environment (no hills, stops, turns, or bad weather).

Disadvantages: Don't expect to achieve the same performance level on a treadmill as you can on, say, a track. While treadmill running is physio-

TABLE 4.1 ◆ Target Pace Levels Associated with Race Performances

Although the training required for optimal performance at various race distances is different, the basic physiological requirements are the same for every race distance from 5K to the marathon. Any runner who is capable of running a world-class time for 5K is also capable of running a world-class time for the marathon. What's more, any two runners who, following optimal training, run the same time in a 5K race are very likely to run similar times at the marathon distance, following optimal training for that event. These patterns hold for middle- and back-of-the-pack runners as well as elite runners.

Therefore it's possible to establish performance equivalences at various race distances. Performance equivalence formulas enable runners to estimate how fast they could run a race of distance Y based on a past performance at distance X.

Jack Daniels established one of the first and best performance equivalence formulas for runners. The following table, based on the original table Daniels produced from his formula, presents target pace levels associated with four popular race distances: 5K, 10K, half marathon, and marathon. Just look up a recent race time at any distance, locate the corresponding TPL value, and use it to determine your initial workout target pace levels.

TPL	5K TIME	10K TIME	HALF-MARATHON TIME	MARATHON TIME
50	30:40	1:03:46	2:21:04	4:49:17
49	29:51	1:02:03	2:17:21	4:41:57
48	29:05	1:00:26	2:13:49	4:34:59
47	28:21	58:54	2:10:27	4:28:22
46	27:39	57:26	2:07:16	4:22:03
45	27:00	56:03	2:04:13	4:16:03
44	26:22	54:44	2:01:19	4:10:19
43	25:46	53:29	1:58:34	4:04:50
42	25:12	52:17	1:55:55	3:59:35
41	24:39	51:09	1:53:24	3:54:34
40	24:08	50:03	1:50:59	3:49:45

(continued)

TABLE 4.1 ◆ Target Pace Levels Associated with Race Performances (continued)

TPL	5K TIME	10K TIME	HALF-MARATHON TIME	MARATHON TIME
39	23:38	49:01	1:48:40	3:45:09
38	23:09	48:01	1:46:27	3:40:43
37	22:41	47:04	1:44:20	3:36:28
36	22:15	46:09	1:42:17	3:32:23
35	21:50	45:16	1:40:20	3:28:26
34	21:25	44:25	1:38:27	3:24:39
33	21:02	43:36	1:36:38	3:21:00
32	20:39	42:50	1:34:53	3:17:29
31	20:18	42:04	1:33:12	3:14:06
30	19:57	41:21	1:31:35	3:10:49
29	19:36	40:39	1:30:02	3:07:39
28	19:17	39:59	1:28:31	3:04:36
27	18:58	39:20	1:27:04	3:01:39
26	18:40	38:42	1:25:40	2:58:47
25	18:22	38:06	1:24:18	2:56:01
24	18:05	37:31	1:23:00	2:53:20
23	17:49	36:57	1:21:43	2:50:45
22	17:33	36:24	1:20:30	2:48:14
21	17:17	35:52	1:19:18	2:45:47
20	17:03	35:22	1:18:09	2:43:25
19	16:48	34:52	1:17:02	2:41:08
18	16:34	34:23	1:15:57	2:38:54
17	16:20	33:55	1:14:54	2:36:44
16	16:07	33:28	1:13:53	2:34:38

TPL	5K TIME	10K TIME	HALF-MARATHON TIME	MARATHON TIME
15	15:54	33:01	1:12:53	2:32:35
14	15:42	32:35	1:11:56	2:30:36
13	15:29	32:11	1:11:00	2:28:40
12	15:18	31:46	1:10:05	2:26:47
11	15:06	31:23	1:09:12	2:24:57
10	14:55	31:00	1:08:21	2:23:10
9	14:44	30:38	1:07:31	2:21:26
8	14:33	30:16	1:06:42	2:19:44
7	14:23	29:55	1:05:54	2:18:05
6	14:13	29:34	1:05:08	2:16:29
5	14:03	29:14	1:04:23	2:14:55
4	13:54	28:55	1:03:39	2:13:23
3	13:44	28:36	1:02:56	2:11:54
2	13:35	28:17	1:02:15	2:10:27
1	13:26	27:59	1:01:34	2:09:02

logically less demanding than outdoor running, I believe it's more challenging to the nervous system, due to the fact that it takes away the ability to make constant micro-adjustments in pace and stride dynamics. In addition, treadmill running is much more boring than running outdoors.

Running Track

Advantages: The fact that a running track is a precisely measured course makes it suitable for monitoring your pace, but not in real time. You can only get splits every 200 to 400 meters and use them to calculate your

---

TABLE 4.2 ◆ Target Pace Level Workout Table

The table below provides target workout pace levels for various workout types and for every fitness level from TPL 50 to TPL 1. All pace numbers represent minutes and seconds per mile except those in parentheses, which represent minutes and seconds per 400 meters (or one lap around a standard outdoor running track).

Notice that each target pace is prescribed as a precise pace number except for recovery pace and base pace, which are prescribed as fairly broad pace ranges. The reason is that recovery- and base-pace workouts are not intended to increase the speed you can sustain over distance or the duration you can sustain a higher speed. Therefore there's no need to reach for a challenging target pace. You can get the full benefit from these slower workouts by letting perceived effort guide your pace within the ranges provided.

I will present more detailed recovery-run pacing guidelines in chapter 7. The long and short of it is that you should always do your recovery runs at a pace that does not interfere with your recovery from your most recent key workout or sabotage your performance in the next key workout. Base pace is more or less the running pace you adopt naturally when going for a training run of a particular distance. I believe that a runner's natural "jogging" pace represents a subconscious compromise between the desire to cover the designated workout distance as quickly as possible (that is, to complete the task) and a competing desire to perform the run without discomfort. Indeed, research has shown that runners of all ability levels tend to naturally adopt a running pace that is associated with a moderate level of perceived exertion—neither low nor high. (Obviously, this pace increases as the individual runner gains fitness.) I see no reason to interfere with this mind-body wisdom by prescribing base-pace guidelines other than the following: Do your base-pace runs at the pace that feels right relative to the prescribed distance.

The base ranges in the table below are therefore really more diagnostic than prescriptive. In other words, use them mainly to monitor your target pace level, not to establish pace targets for individual workouts. For example, if you feel generally uncomfortable when running at a pace corresponding to the middle of the base-pace range associated with what you believe is your current TPL, take it as a sign that you are not, in fact, ready to train at that TPL just yet.

TPL ↓	TARGET PACE →	RECOVERY PACE	BASE PACE	MARATHON PACE	HALF-MARATHON PACE	10K PACE	5K PACE	3K PACE	1-MILE PACE
50		14:03–12:43	12:42–11:39	11:02	10:45	10:15	9:52 (2:27)	9:37 (2:23)	9:11 (2:17)
49		13:45–12:25	12:24–11:22	10:45	10:28	9:59	9:36 (2:23)	9:21 (2:19)	8:55 (2:13)
48		13:27–12:07	12:06–11:05	10:29	10:12	9:43	9:21 (2:19)	9:06 (2:15)	8:41 (2:10)
47		13:11–11:51	11:50–10:50	10:14	9:57	9:28	9:07 (2:15)	8:52 (2:12)	8:27 (2:06)
46		12:50–11:30	11:29–10:34	10:00	9:42	9:14	8:53 (2:12)	8:39 (2:09)	8:14 (2:03)
45		12:41–11:21	11:20–10:21	9:45	9:28	9:01	8:41 (2:09)	8:26 (2:06)	8:01 (2:00)
44		12:25–11:05	11:04–10:07	9:33	9:15	8:48	8:29 (2:06)	8:15 (2:03)	7:49 (1:57)
43		12:12–10:52	10:51–9:54	9:20	9:02	8:36	8:17 (2:03)	8:03 (2:00)	7:38 (1:54)
42		11:59–10:39	10:38–9:41	9:08	8:50	8:24	8:06 (2:00)	7:52 (1:57)	7:27 (1:51)
41		11:47–10:27	10:26–9:30	8:56	8:39	8:13	7:56 (1:58)	7:41 (1:54)	7:17 (1:49)
40		11:30–10:15	10:14–9:18	8:46	8:27	8:03	7:46 (1:55)	7:32 (1:52)	7:07 (1:46)
39		11:19–10:04	10:03–9:08	8:35	8:17	7:53	7:36 (1:53)	7:22 (1:50)	6:58 (1:44)
38		11:07–9:52	9:51–8:57	8:25	8:07	7:43	7:27 (1:51)	7:13 (1:47)	6:49 (1:42)
37		10:57–9:42	9:43–8:47	8:15	7:57	7:34	7:18 (1:48)	7:04 (1:45)	6:41 (1:40)

(continued)

TABLE 4.2 ♦ Target Pace Level Workout Table
(continued)

TPL ↓	TARGET PACE →	RECOVERY PACE	BASE PACE	MARATHON PACE	HALF-MARATHON PACE	10K PACE	5K PACE	3K PACE	1-MILE PACE
36		10:46–9:31	9:30–8:37	8:06	7:48	7:25	7:09 (1:46)	6:55 (1:43)	6:32 (1:38)
35		10:37–9:22	9:21–8:28	7:57	7:39	7:17	7:01 (1:44)	6:47 (1:41)	6:25 (1:36)
34		10:27–9:12	9:11–8:18	7:48	7:30	7:08	6:53 (1:42)	6:40 (1:39)	6:17 (1:34)
33		10:17–9:02	9:01–8:10	7:40	7:22	7:01	6:46 (1:40)	6:32 (1:37)	6:10 (1:32)
32		10:08–8:53	8:52–8:02	7:32	7:14	6:53	6:38 (1:38)	6:25 (1:35)	6:03 (1:30)
31		10:00–8:45	8:44–7:53	7:24	7:06	6:46	6:32 (1:37)	6:18 (1:34)	5:56 (1:29)
30		9:47–8:37	8:36–7:46	7:17	6:59	6:39	6:25 (1:35)	6:11 (1:32)	5:50 (1:27)
29		9:40–8:30	8:29–7:38	7:09	6:52	6:32	6:18 (1:33)	6:05 (1:30)	5:44 (1:26)
28		9:31–8:21	8:20–7:31	7:02	6:45	6:26	6:12 (1:32)	5:58 (1:29)	5:38 (1:24)
27		9:24–8:14	8:13–7:24	6:56	6:38	6:19	6:06 (1:31)	5:52 (1:27)	5:32 (1:23)
26		9:17–8:07	8:06–7:17	6:49	6:32	6:13	6:00 (1:30)	5:47 (1:26)	5:27 (1:21)
25		9:10–8:00	7:59–7:11	6:43	6:25	6:07	5:54 (1:28)	5:41 (1:24)	5:21 (1:20)
24		9:03–7:53	7:52–7:04	6:37	6:19	6:02	5:49 (1:26)	5:36 (1:23)	5:16 (1:19)
23		8:56–7:46	7:45–6:58	6:31	6:14	5:56	5:44 (1:25)	5:31 (1:22)	5:11 (1:17)
22		8:50–7:40	7:39–6:52	6:25	6:08	5:51	5:38 (1:24)	5:26 (1:21)	5:06 (1:16)

TPL ↓	TARGET PACE →	RECOVERY PACE	BASE PACE	MARATHON PACE	HALF-MARATHON PACE	10K PACE	5K PACE	3K PACE	1-MILE PACE
21		8:44–7:34	7:33–6:44	6:19	6:02	5:46	5:33 (1:22)	5:20 (1:19)	5:02 (1:15)
20		8:33–7:28	7:27–6:39	6:14	5:57	5:41	5:29 (1:21)	5:16 (1:18)	4:57 (1:14)
19		8:26–7:21	7:20–6:35	6:09	5:52	5:36	5:24 (1:20)	5:11 (1:17)	4:53 (1:13)
18		8:21–7:16	7:15–6:30	6:04	5:47	5:32	5:19 (1:19)	5:07 (1:16)	4:49 (1:12)
17		8:15–7:10	7:09–6:25	5:59	5:42	5:27	5:15 (1:18)	5:03 (1:15)	4:45 (1:11)
16		8:10–7:05	7:04–6:20	5:54	5:38	5:23	5:11 (1:17)	4:58 (1:14)	4:41 (1:10)
15		8:04–6:59	6:58–6:15	5:49	5:33	5:18	5:07 (1:16)	4:54 (1:13)	4:37 (1:09)
14		7:59–6:54	6:53–6:10	5:45	5:29	5:14	5:03 (1:15)	4:50 (1:12)	4:33 (1:08)
13		7:53–6:48	6:47–6:05	5:40	5:24	5:10	4:59 (1:14)	4:47 (1:11)	4:30 (1:07)
12		7:49–6:44	6:43–6:01	5:36	5:20	5:06	4:55 (1:13)	4:43 (1:10)	4:26 (1:06)
11		7:44–6:39	6:38–5:57	5:32	5:16	5:03	4:51 (1:12)	4:39 (1:09)	4:23 (1:05)
10		7:35–6:35	6:34–5:53	5:28	5:12	4:59	4:48 (1:12)	4:35 (1:08)	4:19 (1:04)
9		7:29–6:29	6:28–5:48	5:24	5:09	4:55	4:44 (1:10)	4:32 (1:07)	4:16 (1:04)
8		7:25–6:25	6:24–6:44	5:20	5:05	4:52	4:40 (1:09)	4:29 (1:06)	4:13 (1:03)
7		7:21–6:21	6:20–5:40	5:16	5:01	4:48	4:37 (1:09)	4:26 (1:06)	4:10 (1:02)

(continued)

TABLE 4.2 ◆ Target Pace Level Workout Table (continued)

TPL ↓	TARGET PACE →	RECOVERY PACE	BASE PACE	MARATHON PACE	HALF-MARATHON PACE	10K PACE	5K PACE	3K PACE	1-MILE PACE
6		7:16–6:16	6:15–5:36	5:12	4:58	4:45	4:34 (1:08)	4:22 (1:05)	4:07 (1:01)
5		7:12–6:12	6:11–5:33	5:09	4:54	4:42	4:31 (1:07)	4:19 (1:04)	4:04 (1:01)
4		7:08–6:08	6:07–5:29	5:05	4:51	4:39	4:28 (1:06)	4:16 (1:03)	4:02 (1:00)
3		7:03–6:03	6:02–5:25	5:01	4:48	4:36	4:25 (1:05)	4:13 (1:03)	3:58 (0:59)
2		7:00–6:00	5:59–5:22	4:58	4:44	4:33	4:22 (1:05)	4:11 (1:02)	3:56 (0:59)
1		6:57–5:57	5:56–5:19	4:55	4:41	4:30	4:19 (1:04)	4:08 (1:01)	3:53 (0:58)

TABLE 4.3 ◆ TPL, Workout Types, and Key Workout Categories

The following table shows you how the various pace targets are used in training. Each pace target is appropriate in one or two types of workout and is used to stimulate one or two key workout training effects, or fitness benefits.

TARGET PACE	WORKOUTS USED IN	KEY WORKOUT TRAINING EFFECT
Recovery	Recovery Runs	N/A
Base	Base and Endurance Runs	Extensive Endurance
Marathon	Endurance Runs	
Half Marathon	Tempo Runs and Cruise Intervals	Intensive Endurance
10K		
5K		Intensive Endurance/Speed
3K	Intervals	Speed
1 Mile		

pace. The track is the best venue for fast running, so you can expect your performance level to be higher on a good track than anywhere else.

Disadvantages: Accessibility can be an issue for some runners. I have to drive half an hour to reach the closest nondirt track that doesn't have a fence and locked gate around it. Also, it's difficult or impossible to use the track in certain foul-weather conditions.

Measured Course

Advantages: Any measured course provides the track's advantage of enabling you to calculate your pace from split times. Most measured courses on roads and paths provide a more interesting route than the track. In San Diego I used to run on a bike path that wrapped around a beautiful bay and featured markers every quarter mile.

Disadvantages: Some measured courses don't provide frequent enough landmarks to be useful for monitoring pace, especially in faster workouts. A course that is marked only once per mile is fine for an endurance run, but it is useless for pace monitoring in an interval workout. You can always make a measured course that suits your needs by covering it in a car or on a bike with a bike computer and placing or noting landmarks at appropriate distance intervals.

Another potential disadvantage of measured courses is that they usually provide a less controlled environment. I always had to dodge all kinds of joggers, walkers, cyclists, skateboarders, and pets on that path in San Diego. A measured course that's hilly won't be suitable for most interval workouts.

Speed and Distance Device

Advantages: Speed and distance devices, such as the Garmin Forerunner 305 and the Timex Bodylink, provide accurate real-time pace and distance information anywhere on earth. I use a Forerunner in every key workout and I consider it a godsend.

Disadvantages: These devices are not cheap. The Garmin Forerunner 305 retails for $350. In addition, they are as much as 2.5 percent inaccurate, in my experience, which is problematic when the devices are being used to gauge performance in key workouts and provide split information in races.

CHAPTER ◆ 5

PURSUING THE PERFECT STRIDE

In the sport of running, the stride is everything. That's all there is to it: stride after stride after stride. In light of this fact, it's truly amazing how little attention has traditionally been given to stride development in the training of distance runners. Most running coaches have few ideas about the character-istics that define good running form and do nothing to actively improve the stride of their runners other than prescribe a few technique drills that are jus-tified by tradition more than by any sound biomechanical rationale.

Brain training takes a different approach to stride development. In fact, in the brain training system, stride development is actively pursued in every single step of every run, as well as in cross-training workouts (the topic of chapter 6) and, yes, technique drills. The reason stride development saturates the brain training system is that the new, brain-centered model of running performance that has emerged over the last decade more or less demands it. According to this model, there is simply no way to improve as a runner that is independent of direct or indirect changes to the running stride, which, of course, is completely governed by the brain.

Direct changes to the stride include improvements in the power-to-weight ratio, which enable the runner to take longer strides; reductions in coactivation (or tension in the muscles opposing the working muscles), which enhances stride efficiency by decreasing the amount of internal resis-tance in the stride; increases in preactivation, or stiffening of the leg prior to footstrike, which reduces ground contact time and increases elastic energy conservation; and enhancement of motor unit cycling, or the sequential resting of select motor units within the working muscles during prolonged running, which increases endurance.

Indirect changes to the stride are those that impact on fatigue. In chapter 3 I defined running as an effort to delay and resist fatigue. And how does fatigue affect performance? By changing the stride! Fatigue-related deceleration is almost always caused by a reduction in motor unit recruitment and loss of neuromuscular coordination that results in declining stride length and/or stride frequency and increased ground contact time. (The only other cause of fatigue-related slowing is voluntary speed reduction resulting from suffering and loss of motivation.) Simply put: to fatigue is to have your stride fall apart.

Studies have shown that individual muscles approach homeostatic limits, such as glycogen depletion, acidosis, and muscle cell depolarization, at different rates during running. To protect these muscles from catastrophic damage, the brain reduces motor output to them. If running were controlled by the muscles instead of the brain, the exhaustion of any single running muscle would result in a spastic and even grotesque distortion of the running stride as the first muscle to fatigue became totally unusable. But since the brain is in control, it responds to fatigue in one muscle by changing the entire stride pattern so that some semblance of a normal running stride can be maintained despite local muscle fatigue.

Nevertheless, there is a subtle loss of muscle coordination and timing that follows local muscle fatigue and has a major spoiling effect on stride efficiency and power. Efficient running requires very precise timing of muscle contractions and relaxations. As fatigue sets in, the muscle actions become less synchronized. As a result, the entire stride pattern changes. The stride loses stiffness, ground contact time increases, and the stride rate decreases. This loss of coordination is believed to be the reason middle distance runners sometimes hit the wall and slow down precipitously, instead of gradually losing momentum, in the final lap of a track race. This phenomenon is similar to the way a juggler's loss of timing causes him to drop all five balls instead of just one or two.

Highly fit runners are able to delay stride deterioration because of superior local muscular endurance in the active muscles. They are also able to maintain a more consistent stride even at the point of exhaustion, most likely because of neuromuscular adaptations that have more to do with running experience than with running fitness per se. The photograph below illustrates this point. It pictures the American runner Dathan "Ritz" Ritzenhein in the last mile of the New York City Marathon, which he ran a full minute

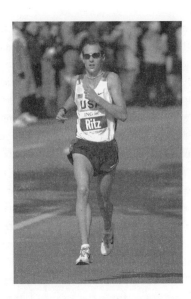

slower than his average pace for the race. Despite feeling horribly fatigued and slowing down inexorably, Ritz maintains a stride pattern that looks relaxed, fluid, and powerful.

Fatigue-related stride changes not only ruin performance but also contribute to overuse injuries. The joints slip away from preferred movement patterns into abnormal patterns that cause tissue damage and ultimately dysfunction. Stride form in general is closely connected to injury risk. Nearly every running injury that occurs has a stride flaw or abnormality as its root cause. For example, a tendency for the thigh to rotate internally during the stance phase is a common cause of patellofemoral pain syndrome (runner's knee) and iliotibial band friction syndrome. Any stride flaw that increases injury risk is likely to limit running performance even in the absence of injury. This is almost certainly why elite runners, who have the most efficient strides, are also typically able to handle much higher training volumes than average runners (well in excess of one hundred miles a week for many) without injury.

Recent years have brought numerous discoveries concerning the stride-related causes of particular running injuries. These discoveries have led to the development of a new physical therapy subdiscipline called gait retraining, which entails systematic efforts to reprogram the motor patterns governing the injured runner's stride in a way that eliminates the stride flaw suspected of causing the injury. Among the experts who practice gait retraining, there is something of a consensus that runners should not try to change their stride until and unless they are injured, because ill-advised changes can cause injuries that might not happen otherwise. In other words, if it ain't broke, don't fix it. Nearly every runner experiences at least one running-related injury sooner or later, however, so practicing this advice usually amounts to simply waiting for an injury to suggest the right stride correction to make.

Those who come at the issue of stride development from a physical therapy perspective also tend to believe that runners should not try to modify their gait on their own. They should leave it to an expert to determine what is wrong with their stride and oversee the process of correcting the flaws.

Injured runners certainly should seek the help of medical professionals with knowledge of running injuries and gait retraining techniques, if possible. But I believe the risks associated with meddling with one's own stride are greatly overstated. There is evidence that regularly fiddling and playing around with one's stride technique in sensible ways actually *reduces* injury risk by distributing the trauma of running more evenly across the bones, muscles, and joint tissues, so that no particular area suffers too much damage. (It's sort of like rotating your car's tires periodically for more even tread wear.) There are some simple means of improving stride form that any runner can implement without supervision and that are far more likely to prevent injuries than cause them, while also enhancing stride efficiency and power.

I began experimenting with gait retraining a few years ago while trying to overcome a frustrating series of injuries. Based on what I had learned from leading gait-retraining researchers in my work as a journalist, I concluded that stride flaws were probably contributing to my susceptibility to breakdowns. I knew of no qualified professionals in my area who practiced gait retraining in a clinical environment, however, nor did I have access to high-tech equipment such as force plates, accelerometers, and video cameras with high-resolution frame-by-frame replay capability. So I came up with my own method of gait retraining. This method not only helped me break free of the injury bug but also greatly improved my overall running performance. So, naturally, this method is now the brain training approach to stride development.

THE BRAIN TRAINING APPROACH
TO STRIDE DEVELOPMENT

The brain training approach to stride development has three components: emulation, proprioceptive cues, and technique drills. The techniques of emulation and proprioceptive cues, while common in some sports, are almost totally unique to the brain training system in the sport of running. Additionally, most of the specific technique drills used in the brain training system are rare. Cross-training is also used for stride development in my system, but it has other benefits, too. Thus, it is addressed separately in the next chapter.

Emulation

Athletes in many sports work to improve their technique by emulating that of the very best athletes in that particular sport. For example, baseball players study the swings of great hitters and then try to copy them. There's no reason runners can't do the same thing. While differences in body structure limit the degree to which any runner can copy the form of another, there are certain universal characteristics of good running form that all runners can enhance in their own stride.

The first step I took in my efforts to better my own running form was to develop a vision of the perfect stride using resources that included studies by leading researchers in the field of gait retraining, such as Irene Davis, Ph.D., of the University of Delaware, and a wonderful book called *Running: Biomechanics and Exercise Physiology Applied in Practice*, by Frans Bosch and Ronald Klomp, who place a heavy emphasis on stride development in their training of elite European runners. I also began an ongoing practice of closely studying the stride form of elite runners at every opportunity. The result was a list of five key characteristics of good running form, which I will describe in detail momentarily.

My next challenge was to find a way to enhance the key characteristics of good running form in my own stride. This effort led to the second component of my stride development method.

Proprioceptive Cues

Proprioceptive cues are used to improve technique in a number of sports, including swimming, which I took up many years ago in branching out from running to triathlon. Proprioceptive cues are particular thoughts and sensations that athletes focus on while performing a sports movement to help them control that movement in a desired way. They worked very well for me in swimming, so I decided to give them a try in running. The only trouble was that I had to make them up, because the use of proprioceptive cues in running is almost unheard-of.

In the end I came up with a dozen cues that I found effective in improving my stride. I'll describe them for you later in this chapter. I found the use of proprioceptive cues in general to be so effective that I now use them constantly throughout every run, and I will recommend that you do the same.

Technique Drills

The use of technique drills in run training is not nearly as radical as the constant use of proprioceptive cues, but even so, technique drills are underutilized by most runners. The six drills I have settled on as my favorites are those that specifically enhance each of the five key characteristics of good running form. I will show you these drills in the final section of the chapter.

THE FIVE CHARACTERISTICS OF GOOD RUNNING TECHNIQUE

There is no single, unified standard that defines "correct" running technique. Individual runners achieve success in running with disparate strides, just as individual baseball players achieve success as batters with distinctive swings. But there is a core set of stride characteristics that are common to all of the best distance runners—that is, all of the fastest and least injury-prone runners. These characteristics are seen in tall elite runners, such as the marathon world record holder Paul Tergat; in short elite runners, such as Kenenisa Bekele (the world record holder at 5,000m and 10,000m); and in both male elites and female elites, such as Meseret Defar (the women's world record holder at 5,000m). They represent one of the major factors that makes elite runners elite runners. And the absence of these characteristics (or an insufficiency thereof) is a major factor that makes the rest of us nonelite.

The five core characteristics of a world-class stride are stiffness, ballistic action, compactness, stability, and symmetry. Let's take a closer look at each of the five characteristics of the world-class running stride, and at the common deviations from these characteristics that the rest of us need to work on.

Stiffness

When you watch world-class runners like Kenenisa Bekele and Meseret Defar in action, the last word you might think of using to describe their running style is "stiff." These runners look smooth and fluid, not stiff. It's the back-of-the-pack runners shuffling along in their lock-kneed manner who look stiff.

Nevertheless, a certain type of stiffness is actually a hallmark characteristic of the best runners' strides. Elite runners have the most stiffness, while lesser runners like us could use a lot more of it. The type of stiffness I am referring to is the type that physicists talk about in relation to springs. The human body does in fact function as a sort of spring during running, and just as a spring with adequate stiffness will bounce more efficiently than a spring that's too loose, a runner who exhibits sufficient muscular stiffness when his or her foot strikes the ground will run more efficiently than a runner whose muscles are too loose on impact.

A spring works by reusing energy. When it falls to the ground from a given height it compresses, which converts the "kinetic" energy of the fall into "potential" energy stored in the form of tension in the spring. As the spring returns to its natural length it converts this potential energy back into kinetic energy in the form of a vector force directed into the ground. As a result, the spring bounces back up into the air.

Something very similar happens when we run. The difference is that whereas a spring-powered device such as a pogo stick achieves movement with energy that is released when its spring is *compressed* on impact and then *expands* back to its natural length, a runner's legs do the opposite. As the runner's foot makes contact with the ground, tendons and elastic components of certain muscles stretch beyond their natural length, thereby capturing and storing energy from the impact. As these tissues return to their natural length, this energy is released. Precisely timed and intricately coordinated muscle actions direct the energy back into the ground, sending the runner's body upward and forward.

Few runners realize just how much energy they are able to reuse thanks to this spring effect. Research has shown that runners consume oxygen at a rate that is sufficient to produce only about half of the energy needed to run at any given speed. The other half is provided by the spring effect.

A stiffer spring is able to reuse more energy than a looser spring because it returns energy to the ground faster. A looser spring stretches and compresses too slowly, allowing more stored energy to dissipate as heat or friction. Top runners spend less time with each foot on the ground than average runners, in part because their superior stride stiffness allows them to return more energy to the ground faster. Ironically, this is one reason why the elite runner's stride looks smoother and more fluid. These runners spend more time "floating" in the air and get more of their energy for free, so they don't have to produce as much energy through muscle contractions to propel forward movement.

What contributes to stride stiffness? Part of it comes from the actual elastic properties of the muscles and tendons themselves. These properties can be enhanced through proper training. The other part comes from running technique. A runner with excellent technique is able to coordinate his or her muscle actions in a way that increases the amount of energy that is reused for forward thrust. For example, top runners do a better job of prestretching and stiffening certain muscles (particularly the hamstrings) just before the foot makes contact with the ground, which enables the runner to capture more energy in the muscles and tendons, return it to the ground more quickly, and direct more energy backward, resulting in more forward thrust.

Compactness

There are two variables that determine running speed: stride length and stride rate. The longer your stride is at any given stride rate, or cadence, the faster you run. Likewise, the higher your cadence is at any given stride length, the faster you run. The best runners tend to make shorter strides (and hence have a higher stride rate) at any given speed than average runners. This style of running is often referred to as a "compact" stride.

The compactness of a stride is determined primarily by where the foot lands (or, more precisely, by the placement of the foot when the support leg becomes fully weighted). If the foot is directly underneath the hips, the stride is compact. If the foot is in front of the hips, the runner is overstriding.

When the foot lands in front of the body there is a lack of stability. To understand why, perform the following test. Stand normally, and then lift one foot off the ground. Is it difficult to balance in this position? Not terribly. Now stand in a split stance with one foot half a pace in front of the other. Lift your rear foot off the floor. Can you balance in this position? Impossible. Your point of support is not aligned with your center of gravity.

This is essentially the problem faced by runners whose feet land ahead of their hips. Due to the difficulty of balancing in this position, runners who overstride have to put a lot of energy into stabilizing the body against impact forces and gravity before they can begin to generate thrust. Consequently, the foot must remain in contact with the ground longer. The thrust phase will not really begin until the foot is behind the body's center of gravity, which is bad, because in this position the support leg's joint angles and muscle lengths are not optimal for generating power.

Overstriding also produces a braking effect that kills forward momentum and increases the amount of thrust energy that is required to sustain any given running speed. When your forward leg is reaching ahead on footstrike, the impact forces that travel up your leg move *backward*, against your direction of travel. By contrast, when your foot lands underneath your hips, the impact forces that travel up your leg move more or less straight up, neutral to your direction of travel. To minimize the braking effect of overstriding, runners who possess this particular stride flaw unconsciously try to land softly. Unfortunately, the softer you land, the more "free" elastic energy you waste, because it dissipates before you can reuse it. You transform yourself into a loose spring.

When your foot touches down beneath your body, you can begin to generate thrust immediately. In fact, the best runners begin to generate backward thrust *before* their foot even touches the ground. As a result, they are able to minimize the amount of energy they put into stabilization, use more free elastic energy provided by muscle and tendon prestretch and by ground impact forces, minimize ground impact time, and push off with more force. Because they begin to generate thrust when the foot is directly underneath the hips, they are able to create more power because their joints are at the optimal angles and their muscles are at the optimal lengths for power production. They are also able to push off sooner, with the foot not as far behind the body, thus enhancing the stride's compactness.

It's important to note that while compact runners tend to make shorter strides than overstriders at any given running speed, compact runners are generally *able* to run with much longer strides than overstriders. This is just another way of saying that compact runners are able to run faster. As runners increase their speed, their stride length changes much more than their stride rate. The stability and power of a compact stride enable a compact runner to cover huge distances in the air between footstrikes compared to overstriders.

Ballistic Action

Ballistic muscle actions are short and fast rather than sustained and gentle. Many distance runners believe that the ideal pattern of muscle action during running is sustained and gentle. The idea is to use energy evenly throughout the stride, landing softly, staying relaxed, and avoiding wasteful "peaks" and lazy "valleys" in muscle work. In reality, the best runners have a ballistic style of running. They contract their muscles extremely forcefully— much more forcefully than average runners do—during a small slice of the overall stride that begins in the moment of bracing for impact, continues through a very brief ground contact phase, and terminates at push-off. (This anticipatory tensing of the muscles is a major factor in creating the stiffness that enables particular leg muscles and tendons to capture more elastic energy when they are forced to stretch on footstrike.) They then relax their muscles as they float in the air between footstrikes—and they spend much more time floating between footstrikes than average runners do.

Ballistic runners use more energy during that sliver of the stride when their muscles are working the hardest, but they use less energy overall, because they get more free elastic energy and they spend more time floating and relaxing. If you closely watch elite runners in competition this ballistic pattern will be quite evident. You will see them stiffen their leg before footstrike and then drive their foot into the ground, almost seeming to bounce off it. A noticeable relaxation of the muscles follows as the runner floats airborne before stiffening once more in anticipation of the next footstrike.

Stability

Running subjects the joints of the body to tremendous downward-pulling forces. Half of the energy we use to run goes toward simply preventing our bodies from collapsing to the ground each time our feet make contact with it. The best runners are able to prevent joint collapse better than average runners. If you watch average runners in action you will see that they tend to bend the knee of their support leg more on impact and also that the hip of the unsupported (swing) leg dips toward the ground while the support foot is planted. And if you're really observant, you'll notice that the pelvis tips forward more on impact in average runners. These excessive joint movements waste a lot of energy and put extra strain on the joints that can lead to injuries.

Joint collapse is a type of stride flaw that tends to result from other stride flaws. Overstriding is the big one. When your foot lands out in front of your body, your muscles are not in a good position to absorb the impact forces that the ground sends shooting up your legs. By the time your body has caught up to your foot, these forces will have had time to pull you toward the ground at your most susceptible points: the knees, pelvis, and hips.

Symmetry

No runner runs with perfect left-right symmetry, but the best runners tend to run more symmetrically than others. All kinds of different asymmetries may crop up in a runner's stride, from the shoulders all the way down to the feet. One foot usually lands harder than the other and one foot usually pronates more than the other. The angles of the knee and hip on impact are different in the right leg than they are in the left. One leg produces more thrust than the other and the same muscles are activated to different degrees on either side of the body to produce this thrust. As long as such discrepancies are small, they are nothing to worry about. But large asymmetries are always wasteful and also tend to increase injury risk.

One of the most problematic asymmetries is long axis rotation, or twisting of the spine. Long axis rotation tends to develop in runners who are not able to begin the thrusting phase of the stride until late in the stance phase, when the body has already passed ahead of the foot. To make up for the inability of the muscles to develop adequate force in this position, the runner must keep the foot in contact with the ground longer for an extra last-moment push-off. And to keep the foot on the ground longer, the runner must rotate the pelvis in the direction of the trailing leg, which in effect makes this leg longer. Finally, to compensate for this movement, the runner must throw the opposite shoulder forward. As a result the lower (lumbar) spine twists in one direction and the upper (thoracic) spine twists in the opposite direction.

These rotational movements are very wasteful. In most runners who exhibit them, they are more pronounced on one side of the body than on the other. Top runners typically run with their hips and shoulders more square to their direction of travel. They are able to keep their pelvis fairly neutral by generating thrust early, when the foot is still underneath the body.

As you have probably noticed, the five characteristics of good running form are interconnected. Any specific movement pattern that enhances one characteristic is likely to affect most if not all of them. On the other hand, any specific deviation from good form that affects one characteristic is likely to affect most if not all of them.

For example, suppose you change your stride by stiffening your leg more in the moment preceding impact. This one change will enhance the stability of your joints in absorbing impact, reducing energy waste and increasing the amount of free elastic energy you are able to reuse for thrust. Due to greater stiffness and stability, you will be able to generate thrust earlier, thus reducing ground contact time and increasing float. The ability to generate thrust more quickly will also reduce tendencies toward asymmetrical torso rotations and overstriding. Your stride is also now inherently more ballistic, because you are concentrating more muscle work within smaller slices of the overall stride.

Some experts in the biomechanics of running now view the stride as a *complex dynamical system*, much like climatic systems and market economies, where one small change can have system-wide effects. From our perspective as runners trying to improve our stride this is a good thing, because it means we can improve our entire stride by working on one aspect of it at a time.

PROPRIOCEPTIVE CUES

Proprioceptive cues are images and other sensory cues that enable you to modify your stride for the better as you think about them while running. For example, by thinking about actively driving your feet into the ground instead of passively allowing them to drop to the ground while running, you can increase your leg stiffness on impact and your ability to generate thrust quickly and efficiently with minimal ground contact time. I have used proprioceptive cues in my training for the past four years and have found that they really work.

Using proprioceptive cues effectively requires concentration and discipline. Our natural tendency is to let our thoughts wander aimlessly while we run. If you're serious about improving your stride you must fight this tendency by forcing yourself to concentrate on and execute a particular proprioceptive cue for hundreds, even thousands, of consecutive strides. The stride improvements that proprioceptive cues facilitate do not happen overnight, because the motor patterns that underlie your current stride habits are deeply ingrained, to the point of being almost completely automatic.

You'll get the best results from proprioceptive cues if you use one at a time throughout the entire length of every run you do. At first you might find it difficult to keep your mind on your stride from start to finish in your runs, but eventually you will develop the ability to divide your awareness, so that one part of your attentional focus is always on the feel of your stride even as your thoughts wander.

It's not necessary to "master" the stride change associated with any given cue before moving on to other cues. In fact, no matter how perfect your stride becomes, you can still benefit from using each cue regularly as a reminder to keep your form sharp, especially when you're fatigued. Therefore,

I recommend that you cycle through the following cues in an endless rotation, never neglecting any of them for long. The brain training plans in Part II will give you a single cue to focus on each week.

The twelve cues described below are my personal favorites, which I've created and retained over the past four years of working to run more and more like Kenenisa Bekele.

Falling Forward

Tilt your whole body slightly forward as you run. Don't bend at the waist! Tilt your entire body from the *ankles*. When you're first getting a feel for this proprioceptive cue, feel free to exaggerate your lean to the point where you feel you're about to fall on your face. Then ease back to a point where you feel comfortable and in control, but where gravity still seems to be pulling you forward. This cue will help you correct overstriding, because when you're running with a slight forward tilt in your body, your feet will naturally land close to your center of gravity.

Navel to Spine

Concentrate on pulling your belly button inward toward your spine while running. Using this cue will activate the deep abdominal muscles that serve as important stabilizers of the pelvis and lower spine during running. In runners who do not properly contract the deep abdominals during running, the pelvis tilts forward excessively as the thigh pulls backward during the thrust phase. When the deep abs are kept tight, most of the force generated by the buttocks and hamstrings is transferred to the ground, hence into forward movement. But when the deep abs are not kept tight, some of the force generated by the buttocks and hamstrings is wasted in stretching the deep abs, causing the pelvis to tip forward, and consequently never reaches the ground.

Note that this proprioceptive cue requires an especially high degree of focus to sustain throughout a run. According to Michael Frederickson, Ph.D., a running biomechanics expert at Stanford University, more than nine in ten runners fail to engage their deep abdominal muscles properly during running. We're simply not accustomed to using these muscles, so if you let your thoughts wander away from them for even a moment, you will unconsciously relax them. The core muscle training exercises described in the next chapter are a good complement to this proprioceptive cue. They will teach you to "find" and engage these muscles in simpler movements, making it easier to do the same when running.

Running on Water

Imagine you're running on water, and your goal is to not fall through the surface. To do this, you must overcome the squishiness of your running surface by applying maximum force to the water in minimum contact time, like a skipping stone. Try to make your feet skip across your running surface in a similar way: quickly, lightly, yet forcefully. This proprioceptive cue will teach you to stiffen your stride, minimize ground contact time, and begin the thrust phase earlier.

Pulling the Road

Imagine that your running route is like a giant nonmotorized treadmill. On a nonmotorized treadmill, you are able to run in place by pulling the treadmill belt backward with your feet. Envision yourself doing the same thing with the road as you run outdoors. You're not actually moving forward—you're simulating forward movement by pulling the road behind you with each foot. This proprioceptive cue will teach you to begin generating thrust earlier, stiffen your stride, and minimize ground contact time.

Scooting

Run in a "scooting" manner by actively minimizing vertical oscillation. Don't exaggerate this action to the point where you are reducing your stride rate or increasing ground contact time. Just think about thrusting your body forward instead of upward while running. If it helps, imagine you're running beneath a ceiling just two inches above your head that will leave you with a terrible headache if you smack into it repeatedly throughout a run. This proprioceptive cue will enable you to run with greater stability by reducing vertical impact forces.

Pounding the Ground

Most runners are taught to run as softly as possible. In fact, running speed is almost entirely a function of how forcefully you hit the ground with your feet. The typical runner—especially the typical overstriding runner—allows his or her foot to fall passively to the ground with each stride. Instead, practice actively driving your foot into the ground. Be sure to give a somewhat backward pull to this driving movement rather than a completely vertical movement. Also, if you are currently a heel striker (overstrider), work on shortening your stride and landing flat-footed before using this proprioceptive cue, which teaches you to stiffen your stride, thrust earlier, and minimize ground contact time.

Driving the Thigh

Concentrate on driving the thigh of your swing leg forward a little more forcefully than you normally do. A more forceful forward-upward movement of this leg will create a counterbalancing downward-backward action in your opposite leg as it comes into contact with the ground. (Think of the way your free arm moves in opposition to your throwing arm when you throw a ball hard.) This cue will enhance your stride symmetry and stiffness.

Floppy Feet

The human foot contains twenty-seven bones and dozens of muscles and ligaments. This complex structure enables the foot to deform in an intricate, wavelike pattern while it is in contact with the ground during running. Unfortunately, shoes greatly restrict this natural movement. You can get a lot of it back by wearing a running shoe that allows greater freedom of foot movement, such as the Nike Free. You can get even more back by concentrating on running with relaxed, "floppy" feet while running. When practicing this cue, continue to strike the ground forcefully with your feet, but use the muscles of your upper leg to generate this force while keeping your foot relaxed, enabling it to absorb and transfer impact forces in a way that will minimize stress on specific tissues and increase the amount of free elastic energy you are able to store and reuse.

Butt Squeeze

In the instant before your foot makes contact with the ground, contract the muscles in the hip and buttock on that side of your body and keep them engaged throughout the ground contact phase of the stride. This proprioceptive cue will enable you to maintain greater stability in the hips, pelvis, lower spine, and perhaps even the knees as you run, and will minimize wasteful (asymmetrical) long axis rotations.

Feeling Symmetry

Focus your attention on a specific part of your body, or stride, on both the left side and the right side. Concentrate on the feel of your arm swing, the forward movement of your swing leg, the moment of footstrike, push-off, or something else. Compare the feeling on the left side of your body to that on your right side. If there is a discrepancy, adjust your stride in a way that eliminates the discrepancy, if possible, or at least reduces it. Specifically, alter your stride on the side that feels less comfortable, natural, or "right" to make it feel more like the side that feels better. Obviously, this proprioceptive cue helps you reduce asymmetries in your stride.

Axle Between the Knees

Imagine there is an axle, dowel, post, or something else of the sort that is positioned between your knees and pushes your knees half an inch farther apart than they would normally be while you run. This proprioceptive cue helps you engage the hip flexors and hip external rotators and prevent internal rotation of the thigh—a common cause of injuries.

Running Against a Wall

Imagine there's a wall right in front of your nose that moves forward with you as you run. Your knees or feet will repeatedly knock into this wall unless you shorten your stride and place your feet underneath your hips instead of out ahead of your body. Leaning slightly forward at the ankles will also create a little more room to drive your thighs forward without banging your knees. This proprioceptive cue facilitates a more compact stride by correcting overstriding.

TECHNIQUE DRILLS

Technique drills enable you to work on improving a particular facet of your stride outside the context of normal running. An easy and effective way to integrate technique drills into your training is to do two or three of them immediately after a base or recovery run once a week.

Running No Arms

Lace the fingers of your two hands together and make a big circle with your arms at shoulder level, as though you're making a simulated basketball hoop for someone else to toss a ball through. Run 100 yards at a moderately fast tempo with your arms in this position. Jog slowly and normally back to your starting point and repeat the drill. This drill will force you to activate your deep abdominal muscles to maintain an upright posture and thereby teach you how to activate these muscles while running. It will also help eliminate rotational asymmetries by taking away your ability to compensate for these rotations with shoulder movements.

Steep Hill Sprints

Find the steepest hill that's available to you and sprint up it for 20 seconds. Walk back down the hill and repeat the drill. This drill will develop your ability to run ballistically, applying great force to the ground on footstrike and driving your swing leg forward to assist in this effort.

One-Leg Hop

Run (or hop) as fast as you can on one leg for 20 seconds. Jog back to your starting point and repeat the drill. In addition to increasing your push-off power, this drill enhances the stability of the hips, pelvis, lower spine, and knees on impact by challenging the muscles that stabilize these joints with extreme impact forces for a short period of time.

High Knees

Run with a fast cadence and highly exaggerated knee lift, bringing your thighs up parallel to the ground with each stride. Continue for 30 seconds. Jog back to your starting point and repeat the drill. This drill teaches you to drive your swing leg and couple the movement of your thighs to strike the ground with greater force.

Bounding

Run with long, leaping strides (like the first two jumps in a track and field triple jump). Continue for 30 seconds. Jog back to your starting point and repeat the drill. This drill enhances push-off power and stability on impact. It also helps teach you to begin retracting your leading leg before impact, because the braking effect of overstriding is greatly exaggerated when you're bounding.

Stiff-Legged Running

Run briskly for 20 seconds with your knees locked as much as possible. This drill greatly increases reliance on the buttock muscles and decreases use of the hamstrings for forward propulsion. It will help you increase the stiffness of your stride and also boost its compactness by teaching you to begin thrusting earlier.

CHAPTER ♦ 6

CROSS-TRAINING AS BRAIN TRAINING

Several years ago I wrote an entire book on cross-training for runners. I did so because I saw cross-training as the next big revolution in the art of training for distance running. The subject first caught my interest when, as an athlete, I branched out from running into triathlon and was surprised to find that adding swimming, cycling, and resistance training to my workout regimen actually made me a stronger runner. Subsequently I began to notice a trend toward increased reliance on cross-training and the use of more sophisticated cross-training methods among America's new generation of elite runners. The Olympic miler Alan Webb is the poster boy for this trend. Less than half of his total training time is spent running.

My growing interest in cross-training led me to explore the recent scientific research on the effects of various types of cross-training on running performance, and I was impressed by the findings I uncovered. In a large and growing number of studies, particular cross-training methods were credited with significantly increasing running economy, boosting stride power, elevating aerobic fitness, reducing injury risk, and aiding injury rehabilitation. My growing excitement about cross-training led me to pick the brains of the pioneering coaches, trainers, physical therapists, and others who had developed some of the latest cross-training methods. I took the best of what I learned, mixed it with some ideas of my own, and wrote my book.

And nobody bought it. The problem was that I had naively assumed runners would find my pitch for cross-training irresistible, given all of the benefits

98

it promised, the big-name elite runners who had already hopped on the cross-training bandwagon, and the science that supported its benefits. But I was wrong. The average competitive runner simply has little interest in doing any form of exercise besides running, no matter how great the benefits are. Runners are runners because they love running, not resistance training, bicycling, and inline skating.

If this description fits you, I have good news and bad news. The bad news is that cross-training is an important component of the brain training system. It is truly effective, and its benefits are all brain-mediated. The good news is that a little cross-training goes a long way, and the brain training programs presented in chapters 11–14 won't require you to do too much of it.

A HARD SELL FOR CROSS-TRAINING

Without a doubt, running should be your primary training focus. But it's equally certain that you'll get better results when your running is properly supplemented with cross-training, which I define as any type of exercise besides running that is done for the sake of improving one's running. In fact, I don't believe any runner can achieve his or her full potential without cross-training.

The rationale for cross-training is simple. Running is a complex, whole-body movement that is cobbled together from simpler movements affecting particular parts of the body. Cross-training improves the overall running movement by enhancing the strength, power, and efficiency of the parts that make up the stride in ways that running itself does not. For example, the Single-Leg Box Jump (described and pictured on page 124) simulates one component of the running stride (thrust and push-off) but exaggerates the power challenge of this movement more than running itself does. As a result, if you do this exercise consistently while continuing to do your normal run workouts, you will increase your stride power, which in turn will have a direct impact on your race performances.

The three basic categories of cross-training are resistance training, flexibility training, and nonimpact cardiovascular training. Each improves the stride by modifying brain-muscle communications. The brain stores motor programs for the stride action and its various movement components in the motor centers and selects and executes each program as necessary. Cross-training refines these programs by forcing you to perform movements that are similar but hardly identical to running and exaggerated with added resistance, extra range of motion, or some other factor. Such exaggeration challenges your brain and muscles to find new patterns of communication that alter your brain's overall running program for the better.

Strength and power training improve communication between the brain and muscles in ways that enable you to run more efficiently and with less chance of injury. Flexibility training enhances running efficiency by training you to run in a more relaxed manner that minimizes energy waste in muscles that oppose working muscles (called antagonists) at various moments of the stride. Nonimpact cardiovascular training increases running efficiency and fatigue resistance by training neuromuscular patterns that are similar to but slightly different from those used in running. Your brain then transfers some of these patterns back to running in a manner that boosts efficiency and fatigue resistance.

In recognition of the fact that cross-training offers tremendous benefits to runners, my brain training system incorporates all three types of cross-training. In recognition of the fact that most runners would rather eat paint chips than lift weights, however, cross-training is incorporated in a minimalist and flexible way. The brain training programs presented in chapters 11–14 prescribe only two resistance training sessions per week (involving minimal equipment). Flexibility training is limited to dynamic warm-up exercises on high-intensity running days. Targeted static stretches and corrective strengthening exercises for problem areas are performed on an as-needed basis only. (I present my recommended static stretches and corrective strengthening exercises in chapter 9, which covers the topic of injury prevention and rehabilitation. Runners need not do any static stretches or corrective strengthening exercises except to prevent or rehabilitate specific injuries.) Finally, nonimpact cardiovascular cross-training is entirely optional. My Level 1 (beginner) and Level 2 (intermediate) brain training plans offer one optional nonimpact endurance cross-training workout per week. My Level 3 (advanced) plans allow you to do as many as four.

RESISTANCE TRAINING

There are three types of resistance exercises featured in the cross-training component of the brain training system: core conditioning exercises, power exercises, and corrective strength exercises addressing common muscle imbalances in runners that often contribute to running-related injuries. As just mentioned, I will show you some corrective strength exercises—which only runners with muscle imbalances need to do—in chapter 9. Here I will focus on the two *mandatory* types of resistance training: core conditioning and power development.

CORE CONDITIONING

Core conditioning is perhaps the trendiest form of cross-training among runners these days. But even though we're all talking about core conditioning, and some of us are actually doing it, many of us misunderstand its purpose and practice it incorrectly.

The most common misconception about core conditioning is that its main purpose is to strengthen the muscles of the trunk. In reality, developing strength is only a secondary purpose of core conditioning. Its primary objective is to teach your brain how to activate important stabilizing muscles and coordinate the use of these muscles with that of other muscles in sport-specific movements. The reason this objective is so important is that most of us are unable to functionally activate some of our most important stabilizing muscles during running, and this problem reduces our efficiency of movement and contributes to overuse injuries. It doesn't take any special strength to use the key stabilizers correctly. It merely takes good communication between the brain and muscles.

Consider the example of the deepest muscles of the abdominal wall (the transversus abdominis and internal obliques). These muscles are vital to proper stabilization of the pelvis during running. Yet the vast majority of runners (including most elite runners) are unable to activate these muscles functionally to maintain pelvic stability on the run. The results are energy waste and increased risk of certain overuse injuries.

Again, weakness is not the issue. It only takes a 10 percent contraction of the deep abs to do the job. Rather, the problem is a lack of neuromuscular communication. Our brains literally cannot find these muscles, probably because of the absurd amount of time we spend slouching in chairs and seats— a posture that certainly requires no use of the deep abs. So correcting the problem does not require that we increase the maximum force-generating capacity of the deep abs. Instead it requires that we learn how to use them, especially in sport-specific movements.

One of the most common errors made in the practice of core conditioning is failing to train progressively. In order to enhance the stabilizing capacity of your core muscles, you have to bring them along step by step. Too many runners fail to divide their core training into properly ordered stages, beginning with very basic exercises that help them to simply find the right muscles and advancing a step at a time toward sport-specific movements centered on activation of targeted stabilizing muscles. Leaping straight into advanced core conditioning exercises makes about as much sense as running 22 miles on the very first day of training for your first marathon. Sure, you may build some strength by doing these advanced exercises, but there will be little or no functional carryover to your running, hence little or no benefit. The strongest abs in the world are useless if you can't activate them functionally.

Conditioning your core properly requires patience and a willingness to spend a fair amount of time working on exercises that might not look like they're doing much. The brain training approach to core conditioning proceeds in four phases. In the first phase, you will do basic isolation exercises that train the connection between your brain and the targeted muscles with little or no requirement to coordinate this action with other muscle actions. Once you are able to consistently and easily activate your stabilizers, you will begin to do exercises in Phase 2 that involve core activation in coordination with other muscle movements. And in the third phase, you will move to exercises in which core activation is incorporated into movements similar to those involved in running, at least some of which include a balance requirement (as running also does). The fourth and final phase is a maintenance phase.

CORE CONDITIONING WORKOUTS

The most important stabilizing muscle groups in runners are the aforementioned deep abdominals and the hip stabilizers—namely, the hip abductors and external rotators on the outside of the hips and buttocks. The core-conditioning program I'm presenting here is a bare-bones program that focuses on just these two muscle areas with only four exercises per workout.

Start your core-conditioning program when you begin formal training for a peak running race. In the brain training plans presented in chapters 11–14, the start of the core-conditioning program coincides with Week 1 of each training plan. The first three phases last three weeks apiece. The final, maintenance phase lasts until the week of your peak race.

PHASE 1 CORE WORKOUT: FINDING YOUR STABILIZERS

Do these exercises twice per week for three weeks. In the first week, do each exercise once. In the second week, do each exercise twice. And in the third week, do each three times.

Lying Hip Abduction

Conditions the hip abductors and hip external rotators, enhancing hip stability

There are two versions of this exercise. First, lie on your right side with your legs bent ninety degrees and your knees together. Prop up your head on the palm of your right hand. Now rotate your left leg upward and backward, keeping the foot of this leg in contact with the other foot. Repeat this movement twelve to fifteen times or until you feel fatigue in your buttock, then switch sides. To make this exercise more challenging, perform it with a resistance band tied around your lower thighs.

To do the second version, straighten your legs and repeatedly lift the top leg toward the ceiling (toes pointing forward) as high as you can. Repeat the movement twelve to fifteen times and then switch sides. To make this exercise more challenging, do it with an ankle weight strapped to the ankle of your working leg.

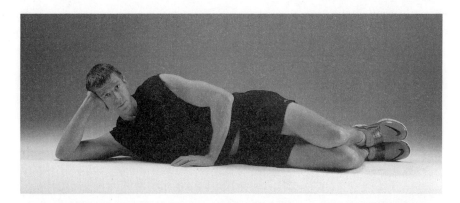

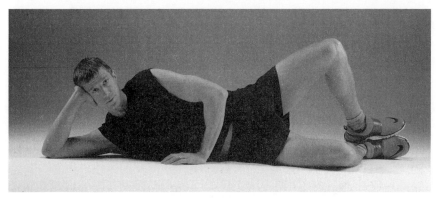

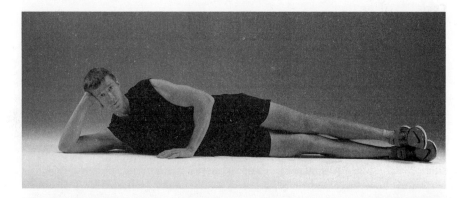

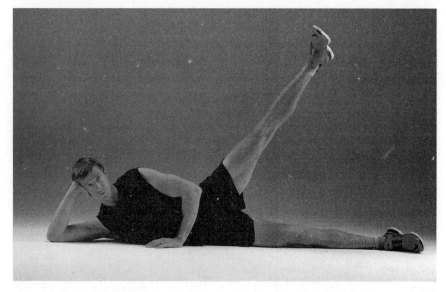

Cook Hip Lift

Trains the deep abs to stabilize the lower spine and pelvis while the buttocks and hamstrings generate backward thrust

Lie faceup with your legs sharply bent. Place your left foot flat on the floor and draw the right leg up against your torso, holding it in place with pressure from your hands. Now contract the hamstrings and buttocks of the left leg to lift your butt off the floor two or three inches. Concentrate hard on keeping your deep abs contracted and your pelvis neutral. Hold this position for five seconds and relax. Repeat five times and then switch legs.

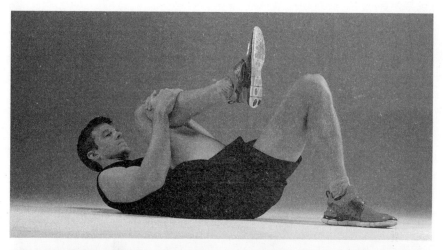

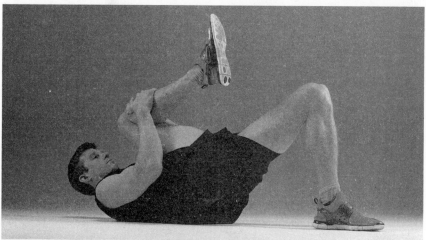

Kneeling Overhead Draw-In

Teaches you how it feels to contract the deep abs for stabilization in an upright position

Kneel on both knees and raise your arms straight overhead. Draw your navel toward your spine and try to lift your fingertips another inch or so toward the ceiling, as though you're reaching to place an object on a high shelf. Hold the contraction for five seconds and relax. Repeat a total of five times. Progress by adding repetitions and/or holding the contractions longer (up to 10 seconds). To make this exercise more challenging, do it while holding dumbbells or a weight plate in your hands.

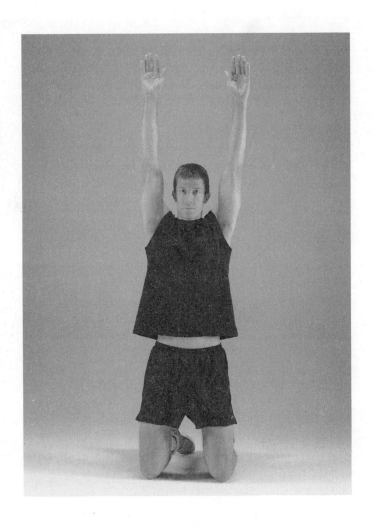

Knee Fall-Out

Teaches you to sustain activation of the deep abs as your hips rotate

Lie faceup with your legs sharply bent, knees together, and feet placed flat on the floor. Contract your deep abdominal muscles by drawing your navel toward your spine and trying to flatten your lower back against the floor. Now slowly let your knees fall outward toward the floor without relaxing your deep abs. (This is very difficult at first. If it feels easy, you're letting your deep abs relax!) Once your legs are splayed as wide as you can get them, pause briefly and return to the start position. Repeat a total of ten times.

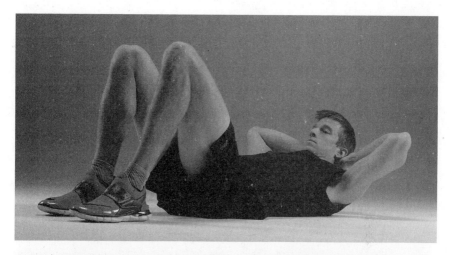

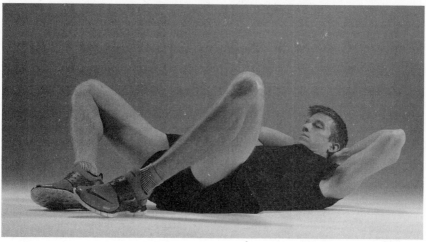

PHASE 2 CORE WORKOUT: STABILIZATION AND COORDINATION

This phase of your core-conditioning program should also last three weeks. Continue training your core twice per week. In the first week of this phase, do each of the four exercises described below just once and do the exercises of the previous phase twice per core session. In the second week, reverse this ratio. And in the third week, do only the four exercises presented below, three times apiece.

Single-Leg Squat

Trains the hip abductors and external rotators to maintain hip stability during a single-leg movement similar to running

Stand on your right foot and bend the left leg slightly to elevate the left foot a few inches above the floor. Lower your butt slowly toward the floor, keeping most of your weight on the heel of your support foot. Reach the left leg either behind your body (easier) or in front of your body (harder) to keep it out of the way and to help maintain balance. Squat as low as you can go without your butt swinging outward (a sign that the targeted muscles have become overwhelmed and that other muscles have been activated to take up the slack). Return to the start position. Do eight to ten squats on each foot.

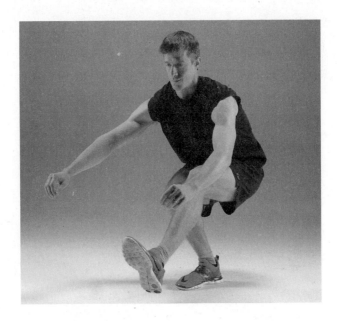

Oblique Bridge

Trains all of the muscles involved in maintaining lateral stability at the hips, pelvis, and spine

Lie on your side with your ankles together and your torso propped up by your forearm. Lift your hips upward until your body forms a diagonal plank from ankles to neck. Hold this position for 20 seconds, concentrating on not allowing your hips to sag toward the floor. (You may watch yourself in a mirror to make sure you're not sagging.) Reverse your position and repeat the exercise. To increase the challenge, perform several Straight-Leg Hip Abductions from the bridge position.

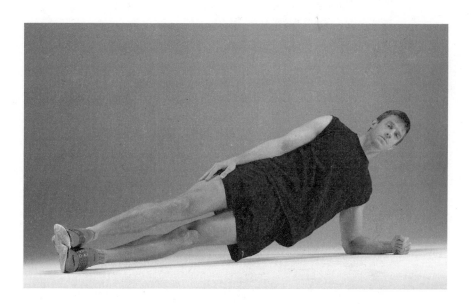

Lying Draw-In with Hip Flexion

Teaches your deep abs to stabilize the pelvis during alternating leg movements

Lie faceup with your head supported by a large pillow or foam roller. Begin with your legs bent ninety degrees and your thighs perpendicular to the floor, feet together. Engage your deep abs by drawing your navel toward your spine and trying to flatten your lower back against the floor. While holding this contraction, slowly lower your right foot to the floor. Return immediately to the start position, and then lower the left foot. If you find this movement easy, you are failing to hold the contraction of your deep abs. Lower each foot to the floor eight to ten times.

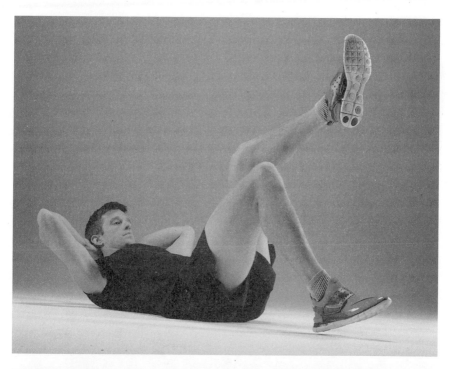

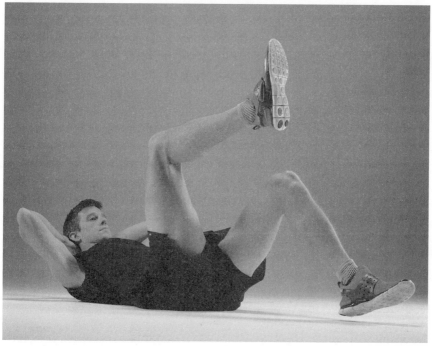

Quadruped

Teaches your deep abs to stay active against a balancing challenge while you perform alternating limb movements

Kneel on all fours with a broomstick, cue stick, or dowel rod balanced along your spine. Engage your deep abs by drawing your navel toward your spine. Holding this contraction, extend your right leg until it forms a straight line with your torso. Do this without rotating your hips. If you cheat and allow your hips to rotate (a movement that would permit your deep abs to work less), the broomstick will roll off your back to the left. Hold this position for 10 seconds, return to the start position, and then extend the left leg, making sure the stick doesn't fall to the right. Repeat on both sides. To make this exercise more challenging, extend your left arm forward as you extend your right leg backward, and then extend your right arm and left leg together.

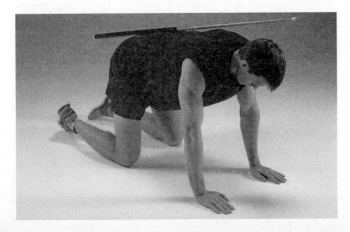

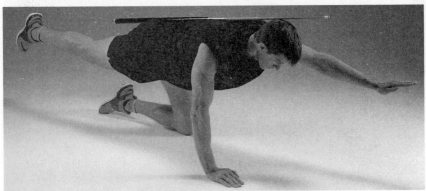

PHASE 3 CORE WORKOUT: FUNCTIONAL STABILITY

Continue training your core twice per week throughout this third phase of your core-conditioning program. In the first week, do each of these exercises just once and do the exercises of the second phase twice per core session. In the second week, reverse this ratio. And in the third week, do only the four exercises presented below, three times apiece.

Box Lunge

Trains the hip abductors and external rotators to maintain hip stability during a single-leg power movement similar to running, with impact

Stand atop a box, step, or other sturdy platform that's six to twelve inches high. Take a large step forward with your right leg, plant your right foot on the floor, and bend your right knee to ninety degrees. Now reverse this movement with a powerful upward and backward thrust off the right foot and return to the start position. Complete eight to twelve repetitions and then work the left leg. To increase the challenge level of this exercise, do it while holding dumbbells at your sides.

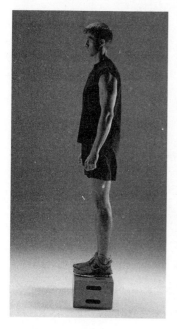 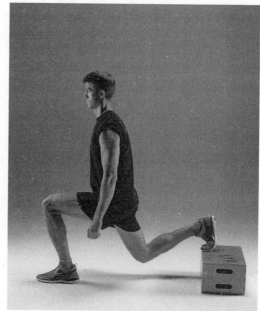

Stability Ball Leg Curl

Trains your deep abs to maintain pelvic stability against a balance challenge while the buttocks and hamstrings generate backward thrust

Lie faceup and place your heels together on top of a stability ball. Raise your pelvis so that your body forms a straight plank from head to toes. Contract your buttocks and hamstrings and roll the ball toward your buttocks. Pause briefly and return to the start position. Focus on keeping your pelvis from sagging toward the floor throughout this movement. Do eight to twelve repetitions.

For a greater challenge, do a single-leg stability ball leg curl. Elevate your left leg above the ball and keep it straight while using the right foot to roll the ball. Complete eight to twelve repetitions and switch legs.

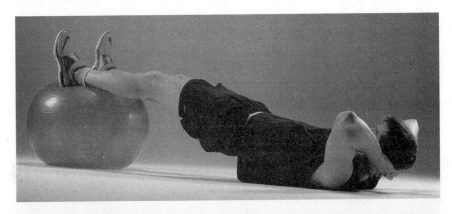

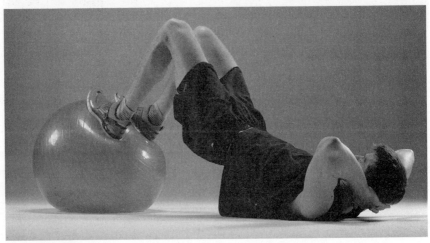

Forearms to Palms Bridge

Trains your deep abs to maintain stability in the pelvis and lower spine against a balance challenge while performing alternating arm movements

Start in a modified push-up position with your forearms flat on the floor. Now move into a standard push-up position by putting your left palm flat on the floor and then your right palm and extending your elbows. Concentrate on contracting your deep abs and keeping your torso and legs in a straight line. Now reverse what you just did, putting your left forearm back to the floor and then your right forearm. When you repeat the exercise, put your right palm down first and then your left, and then return your right forearm to the floor, followed by your left. Continue alternating which palm you put down first. Complete four to ten total repetitions.

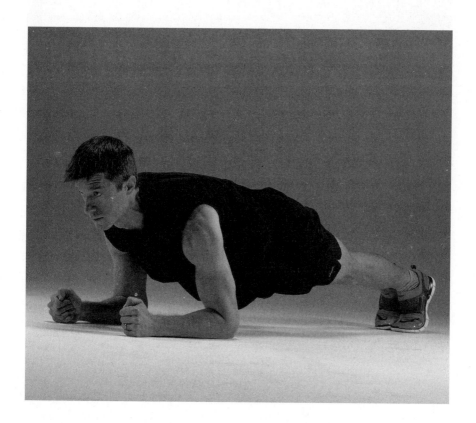

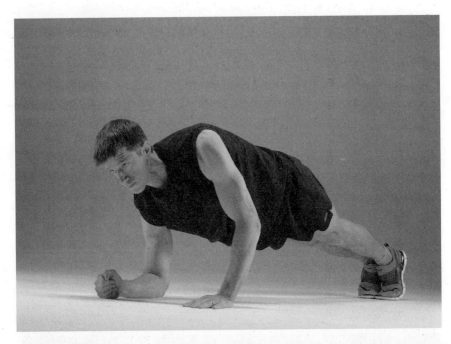

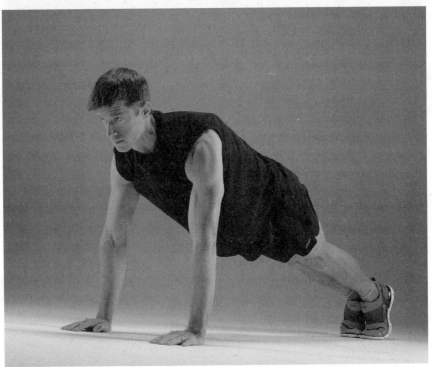

Dead Bug

Trains your deep abs to maintain stability during alternating arm and leg movements

Lie faceup with your head slightly elevated above the floor and engage your deep abs by drawing your navel toward your spine. Begin with your right leg fully extended and elevated a few inches off the floor, your right arm reaching toward your right foot, your left leg sharply bent with the knee drawn toward your chest, and your left arm extended straight behind your head, roughly parallel to the floor. Keeping your navel drawn toward your spine, slowly reverse the position of your arms and legs, and continue alternating arm and leg positions for 20 to 30 seconds.

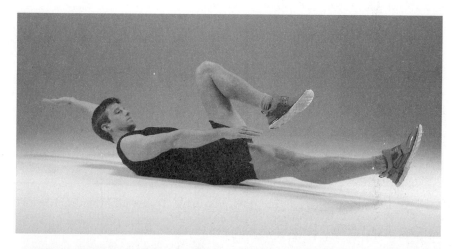

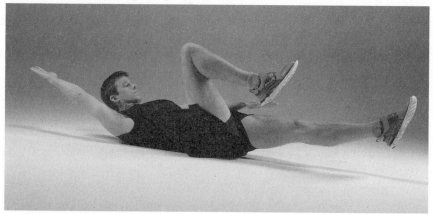

PHASE 4 CORE WORKOUT: MAINTENANCE

The maintenance phase of your core-conditioning program picks up at the end of phase three and continues until the week of your peak race. Throughout phase four, do two core-conditioning sessions per week. In each session, do one exercise from phase one, one exercise from phase two, and two exercises from phase three. Complete each exercise one to three times per session. Mix up the exercises from one session to the next and feel free to incorporate new core-conditioning exercises that provide similar benefits. You can learn new exercises from a personal trainer or from a book such as *Core Performance* by Mark Verstegen.

POWER TRAINING

Distance running is not often thought of as a power sport, but it is. As a competitive runner your goal is to increase your speed, and speed comes directly from stride power. Stride power is measured as the amount of force a runner's foot applies to the ground *and* the speed of its application in the push-off phase of the stride. The more force your foot applies, and the more quickly it is applied, the longer your stride will be, and the longer your strides are, the faster you run. (Remember, a stride can be both long *and* compact.)

Running alone won't maximize your stride power. You have to supplement your running with specific power training. This was shown in a recent Australian study. A group of runners that replaced some of their running workouts with power training for six weeks improved their three-kilometer race time by 2.7 percent, compared to no improvement for a control group that only ran. This study and others like it have determined that power training improves running performance by increasing running economy—that is, by reducing the energy required to run at a given speed. And power training appears to increase running economy by increasing the stiffness of the stride. Runners who engage in power training are better able to preactivate their muscles before footstrike, resulting in shorter ground contact time and more floating.

Since power is essentially a combination of speed and strength, to increase your power you need to do explosive movements against resistance. Power is also movement-specific. Therefore, if you want to increase your stride power you need to do power exercises that mimic specific components of the running stride. Running is a whole-body, multijoint jumping action in which the hip extensors (buttocks and hamstrings) are the primary movers. Your power training routine should also include whole-body, multijoint movements, jumps, and exercises for the hip extensors.

A little power training goes a long way. You can get significant benefits from doing just one or two power exercises at a time, twice a week. In the resistance workouts prescribed in my brain training programs, one or two of the following power exercises are included in each resistance workout along with the core exercises described in the previous section.

Squat Jump

Stand normally. Squat down deeply and then leap upward as high as you can. Use your arms to create prestretch and upward momentum. When you land, immediately sink back down into another squat. Complete twelve to twenty repetitions.

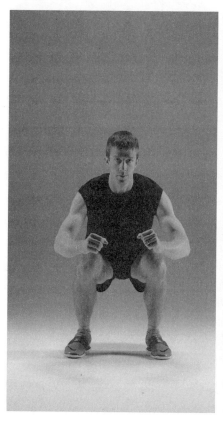
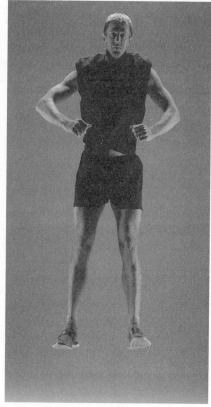

Split Squat Jump

Start in a split stance with your right foot flat on the ground and your left leg slightly bent, with only the forefoot of your left foot touching the ground a half step behind the right. Lower yourself down into a deep squat and then leap upward as high as possible. In midair, reverse the position of your legs. When you land, sink down immediately into another squat and then leap again. Use your arms for balance and to generate extra upward thrust with each leap. Complete ten to twenty jumps with each leg.

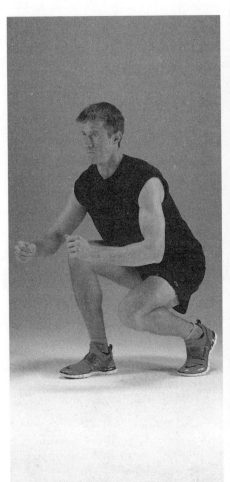
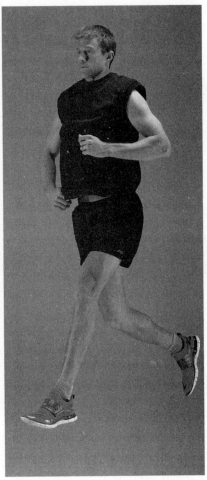

Single-Leg Squat Jump

Stand on your right foot with your left leg slightly bent and your left foot held a few inches above the floor. Bend your right knee thirty to sixty degrees and then leap upward as high as possible. Use your arms for balance and to generate extra upward thrust. Land on your right foot only and bend your right knee again to prepare for the next jump. Complete ten to twenty jumps and then repeat the exercise with your left leg.

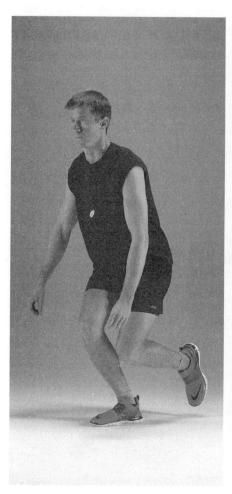
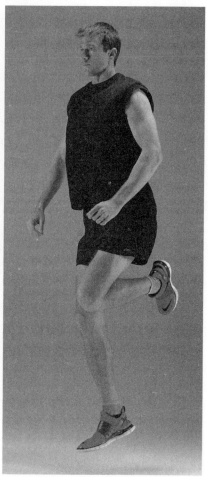

Broad Jump

Stand with your feet slightly farther than shoulder-width apart and your knees slightly bent. Swing your arms backward and bend your knees slightly more to create prestretch tension, and then swing your arms forward to create momentum and leap forward as far as you can. Push off with both feet and land on both feet. Pause briefly, stand upright, and jump again. Complete ten to twenty jumps.

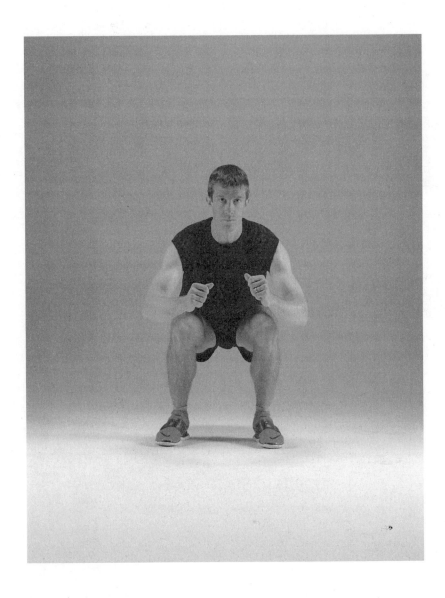

Wall Jump

Stand facing a wall with your feet close together and your arms extended overhead. Bending your knees minimally, jump upward with maximum force and touch your hands as high up on the wall as you can reach. Land and immediately jump again. Continue jumping at a rapid tempo, like a human pogo stick.

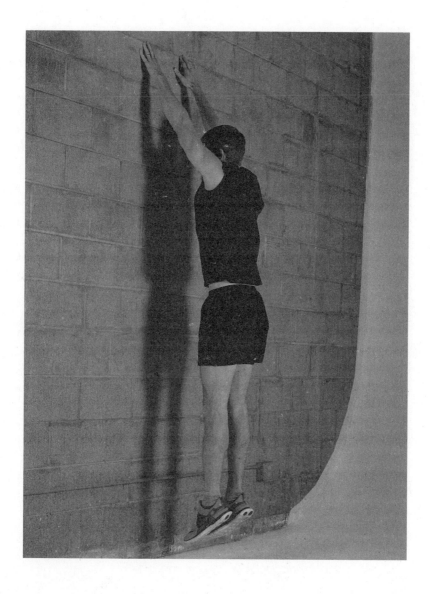

Single-Leg Box Jump

Stand on your right foot facing a sturdy platform eight to sixteen inches in height (such as stacked aerobics steps). Bend your left leg, swing your arms back and then forward to generate momentum, and then leap up onto the support. Do not allow your left foot to touch down. Immediately jump back down to the floor, again landing on the right foot only. Continue jumping for 30 seconds and then switch to the other leg.

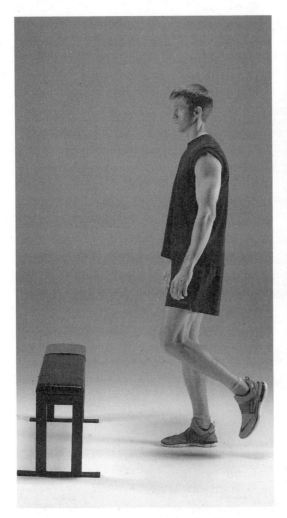
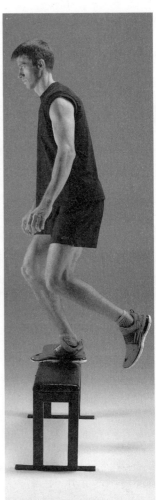

DYNAMIC FLEXIBILITY EXERCISES

Whenever you perform a sports action such as running, your working muscles (called agonists) have to overcome a certain amount of resistance from other, nonactive muscles (called antagonists). Dynamic flexibility is the ability of nonactive muscles to relax and stretch during sports actions so they present minimal resistance to the working muscles, thereby enhancing the efficiency of the movement. The more tension is held in your antagonists during running, the more resistance your agonists will have to overcome in contracting, and the worse your running economy will be.

Contrary to popular wisdom, muscle tension is not a structural problem—namely, "tightness"—within the muscles. Rather, it comes from motor signals from the brain that tell the fibers in that muscle to hold tension. Therefore, the secret to improving your dynamic flexibility in running is to train your brain to tell your antagonists to relax and stretch when required to during running.

For runners, dynamic flexibility is much more important than passive flexibility, or simple range of motion in particular joints. Studies have shown that elite runners have normal flexibility in most joints. But they have a high degree of dynamic flexibility in running-specific movements. For example, during the swing phase of the stride action the hip flexors act as agonists, shortening to pull the thigh forward, while the hamstrings and glutes act as antagonists, relaxing and lengthening to allow the thigh to swing forward easily. In more efficient runners, less tension is held in the hamstrings and glutes during the swing phase, enabling the thigh to swing forward faster and farther with less force application from the hip flexors.

The best method to increase dynamic flexibility is dynamic stretches, which are sometimes also referred to as mobility exercises. Dynamic stretches are movements that mimic the way your muscles and connective tissues actually stretch during running, but with an exaggerated range of motion that increases the cost of holding tension in the antagonists and thus challenges these muscles to "learn" to relax.

I recommend that you do dynamic stretches as a warm-up, particularly before high-intensity runs. Dynamically stretching your muscles before running will gently warm, loosen, and lubricate your muscles, preparing them to perform better in the workout that follows. A second advantage of doing your dynamic stretches as a warm-up—especially in workouts involving faster running—is that it reduces the likelihood of muscle strains. These injuries tend to occur when the muscles are required to contract from a stretched position. Including dynamic stretches in the warm-up allows the muscles to perform these "eccentric contractions" with less strain.

The following dynamic stretching warm-up routine takes only five minutes to complete. Always do it before training at 10K race pace or faster to reduce the likelihood of muscle strains. The long-term benefits you'll derive from regularly doing these stretches are increased dynamic flexibility and a more economical stride.

Tilt Walk

From a standing position, take one step forward with the left foot and balance on the forward foot. Keeping a very slight bend in your left knee, tilt your torso forward at the waist until your trunk is parallel to the floor. At the same time, extend your right leg behind you for balance. Return to an upright position and then step forward with the right foot and tilt once more. Continue for thirty seconds.

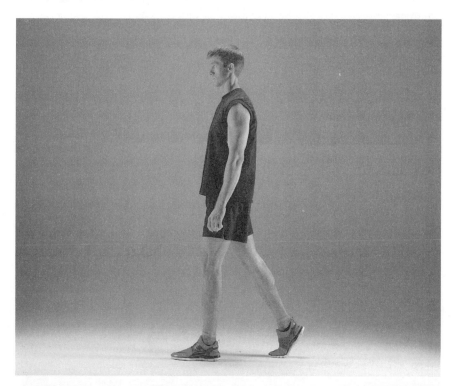

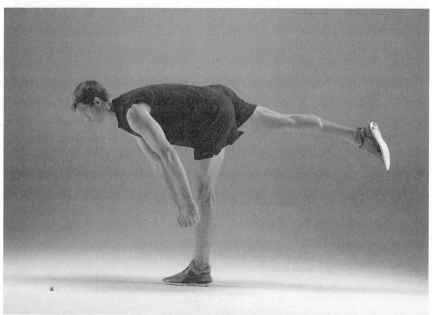

Zombies

Begin in a standing position with both arms extended straight in front of you like a cartoon zombie. Begin walking slowly forward by kicking each leg forward as high as possible, aiming to touch your right toe to your right palm and your left toe to your left palm. Keep your legs as straight as possible and don't let your trunk flex forward. Continue for 20 to 30 seconds.

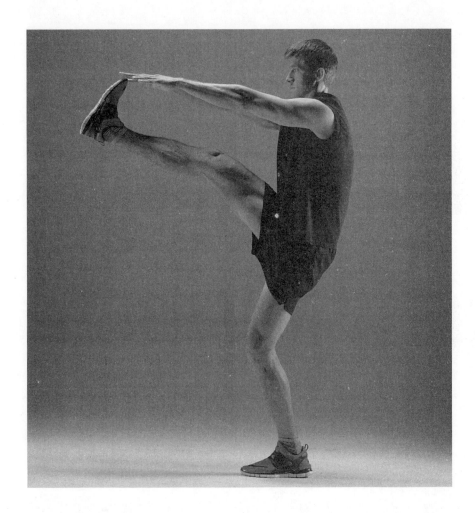

Trunk Rotation

Raise your arms straight out to the sides. Twist your torso as far as you can to the right. Without pausing, reverse direction and twist over to the left. Repeat ten times.

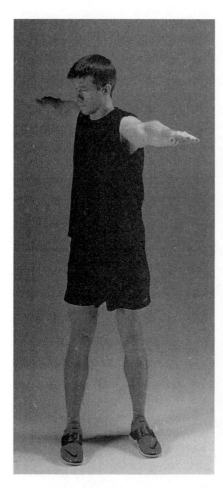 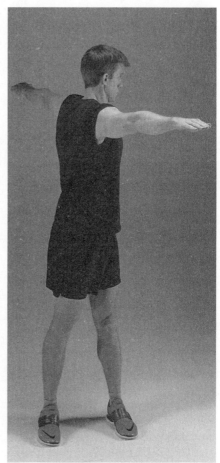

Lunge Walk

Take ten giant steps forward with each foot, lunging as far forward as you can each time.

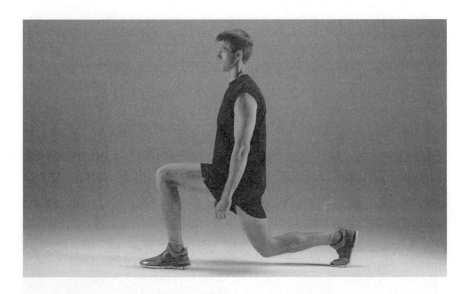

Lateral Lunge

From a standing position, take a large step to the left with your left foot and lower yourself into a deep squat. Return immediately to a standing position and lunge to the right. Lunge five times to each side.

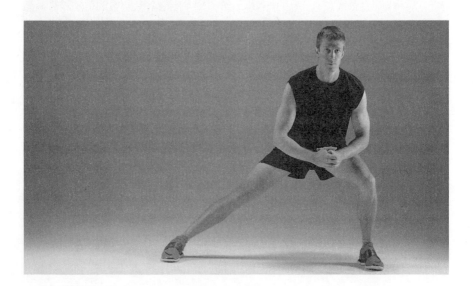

Forward Leg Swing

Stand on your right foot and swing your left leg backward and forward in an exaggerated kicking motion. Complete ten swings and repeat with the right leg.

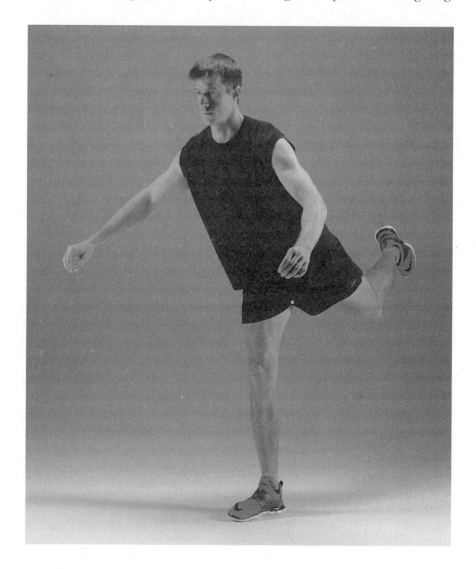

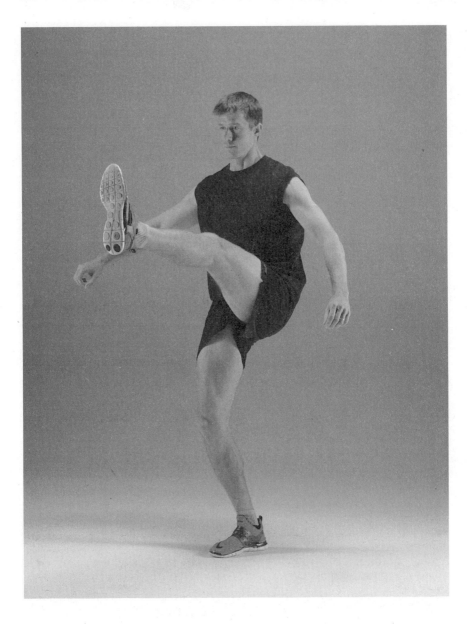

Lateral Leg Swing

Stand facing a wall, lean toward it slightly from the waist, and brace both palms against it. Swing your fully extended left leg right to left in wide arcs between your body and the wall. After completing ten swings, swing your right leg.

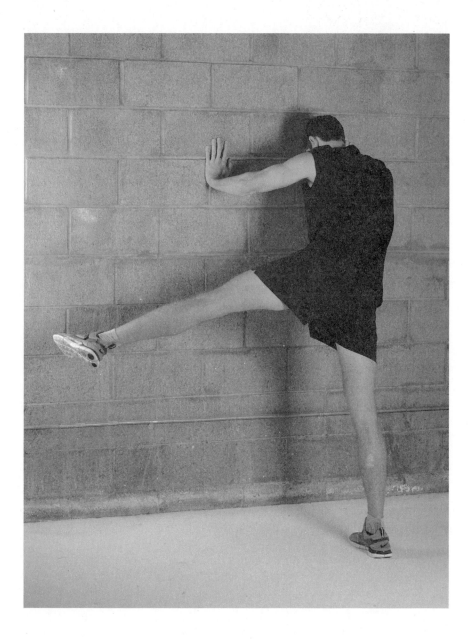

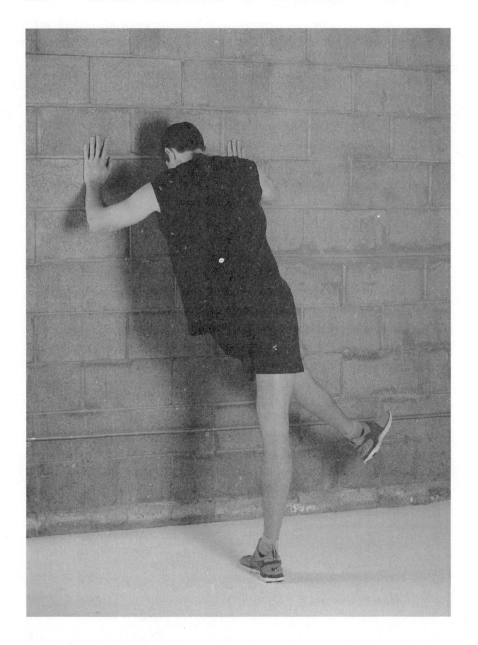

Heel Bounce

Assume a modified push-up position, with your legs as close to your hands as you can get them without bending your knees, and your butt in the air. Lift your left foot off the ground, bend your left leg slightly, and rest the top of your left foot against the back of your lower right leg. Lift your right heel as high off the floor as you can. Without pausing, lower your heel back to the floor and "bounce" it off the floor, back into another heel raise. Bounce your right heel twenty times and then repeat with the left leg.

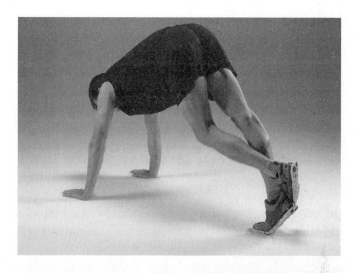

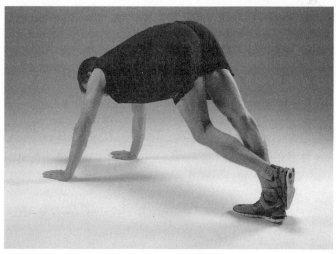

NONIMPACT CARDIOVASCULAR EXERCISE

Runners have long used low- and nonimpact forms of cardiovascular exercise to keep in shape when unable to run due to injury. But today many elite runners perform cardiovascular cross-training workouts throughout the training cycle to facilitate recovery from hard runs and to provide an additional aerobic training stimulus without the increased risk of injury that would come with additional high-impact running. The current standard among the elite runners who take this approach is one active recovery workout per week in a nonimpact cardiovascular modality such as pool running. But a few trailblazing runners do a lot more cardio cross-training—sometimes as much as they do running—because they experience a significant crossover fitness benefit alongside substantially reduced injury risk. Olympic marathon silver medalist Mebrahtom Keflezighi of the United States, who rides a bike as often as he runs, is one such runner.

It makes sense. The pounding that running inflicts on the body causes it to break down through injury well before its fitness potential is tapped out. Adding an activity like pool running, bicycling, or walking to your running allows you to realize more of this fitness potential without additional pounding.

The more similar to running your chosen cardio cross-training modality is, the more benefit you'll get from it. Forms of exercise that require your brain to activate your muscles in ways similar to running have the greatest potential to create new efficiencies in the motor programs used in running. In order of decreasing specificity to running, I recommend underwater treadmill running (not an option for most of us), inline skating, slide boarding (a slide board is a slippery platform that allows you to simulate a side-to-side skating action indoors), elliptical training, and bicycling.

Following are basic guidelines for the three uses of endurance cross-training: active recovery, fitness maintenance during injury rehabilitation, and performance enhancement.

Active recovery: As a baseline, do one workout per week in your modality of choice within twenty-four hours after completing a key running workout. The nonimpact nature of the workout will enable your muscles to recover faster than they would if you ran, but the fact that the workout elevates oxygen consumption and muscle activation as much as running does means you get a greater training stimulus than you would if you took the day off.

Because the purpose of these workouts is to provide a training stimulus without interfering with muscle recovery, these cross-training workouts should not be terribly long or intense. But you should feel free to work out as long and intensely as you are able to without affecting your performance in your next key running workout. In addition to doing one scheduled active recovery cross-training workout per week, replace planned runs with additional cardio cross-training workouts when you are feeling especially sore or are experiencing warning signs of a potential running-related injury (pain felt in a specific area during and/or following runs).

Injury rehabilitation: When you have an injury that limits your running or makes running impossible but allows you to safely perform at least one type of nonimpact alternative to running, simply maintain the structure of your running program but replace runs with pool runs, bike rides, or other such workouts. Perform cardio cross-training workouts that imitate as closely as possible the duration, intensity, and structure of the land running workouts you would perform if you were healthy. For example, if you were scheduled to do a dozen 400-meter intervals on the track at 90 seconds per interval, then do a dozen hard 90-second intervals in the pool or on the bike, separated by rest intervals that also match what you normally do on the track. Be sure to warm up and cool down as normal, too.

Performance enhancement: If you wish to use endurance cross-training to enhance your running performance, you'll need to experiment a little. The core of your training program will remain your key running workouts. There is no substitute for these. How much more additional running you do depends on how much more you feel you need, but it should remain well within the range of what you know you can handle. At first, add just one easy cardio cross-training workout to your schedule of run workouts. When you've adjusted to this one, add another, and so on.

If you're highly competitive and seem to derive a lot of benefit from cardio cross-training, you can do as many as six such workouts per week. Most or all of these workouts should be recovery or base-type workouts, but you can experiment with some high-intensity work if you wish, as long as it does not interfere with your key running workouts.

CHAPTER ◆ 7

STRESS AND RECOVERY

As a runner, you not only fight individual battles against fatigue within workouts and races, but you also wage an ongoing war against fatigue throughout the training process. As we've already discussed, the faster and farther you can run without experiencing acute fatigue in a workout or race, the better your performance will be. But the same principle also applies on a broader scale, in the sense that the more total running—and especially the more race-specific running—you are able to do from week to week without succumbing to persistent or chronic fatigue (or injury), the more your running performance will improve.

In most hard workouts and races, you start off feeling fresh and finish feeling fatigued. But sometimes you feel fatigued from the very first step of a run. If this happens only once or twice a week, it's nothing to worry about, especially if it happens on days when you do not have a key workout scheduled. If you begin to feel "prefatigued" on a regular basis, however, even on key workout days, you have a problem: Your body is not fully recovering from the stress of your workouts and, as a result, you're not building fitness as quickly as you should be, if at all. In a word, you are overtraining.

Most runners think of acute fatigue (the kind of fatigue you feel at the end of a good run) and overtraining fatigue (the kind you feel at the beginning of a bad run) as being completely different, but in fact they are very much the same. Both types of fatigue are brain-centered ways of forcing you to slow down or stop so you don't harm yourself.

As we've seen, during any given workout or race, fatigue is the performance limiter. You can run only so fast for so long before your brain begins to receive warning signals of impending health risks through afferent feedback from the body. For example, during a short, fast race, rising muscle lactate levels might trigger pain receptors that warn your brain of increasing muscle acidity, which could cause muscle damage if allowed to go too far. Your brain responds to these signals by creating feelings of discomfort and inhibiting motor output to the working muscles, causing you to slow down and avert the health risk.

A similar system operates at the level of long-term training. Sometimes, as runners increase their training workload in preparation for a peak race, they cross a threshold beyond which body tissues, organs, and systems are no longer able to properly recover from the previous workout stress before the next is administered. Thus, as the training workload increases, tissue damage caused by running begins to accumulate, threatening not only these tissues themselves but also the immune and neuroendocrine systems, which are responsible for repairing tissue damage and enabling tissues to adapt to the stressors (in this case running) that are causing it. At some point it becomes a losing battle, and the body sends signals to the brain conveying this message. The brain responds by producing symptoms to discourage continued training at the present workload. The runner begins to feel flat, tired, and heavy in the majority of his or her workouts. Post-workout muscle soreness becomes almost constant. Motivation plummets.

One of the main concerns of every runner should be to avoid the downward spiral of accumulating muscular, immune system, and neuroendocrine system stress that characterizes overtraining. Of course, the easiest way to avoid overtraining is to train very lightly, or not at all. The problem with this approach is—quite obviously—that running performance is closely correlated with training workload. In other words, the harder you train within the limits of your body's recovery capacity, the fitter you become. So your true objective in relation to the danger of overtraining is to consistently train as hard as you can without exceeding your recovery capacity, and in ways that increase your maximum training limit.

In the following sections I will show you how to strike this balance using the brain training system of integrating subjective feedback (how your body feels), objective feedback (your training numbers), and collective feedback (the latest scientific knowledge of what's really going on when you are experiencing overtraining fatigue). My brain training methods of balancing training stress and recovery are somewhat different from conventional methods, primarily because they are based on the new, brain-centered conception of overtraining fatigue. Before I share these methods, let me first say a little more about the brain's role in overtraining fatigue.

STRESSED OUT AND INFLAMED

The word "stress" is given a variety of meanings in everyday speech, but its scientific meaning is very precise. Stress is a specific set of physiological reactions to perceived threats to the organism. A good example of a threat most runners can relate to is a growling dog. Such threats are perceived by the hypothalamus gland deep inside the brain, which initiates a cascade of nervous system and hormonal events that focus attention on the threat, increase fuel breakdown (to provide energy for fighting or running away), stimulate the immune system (in case an injury occurs), and reduce noncritical functions, such as digestion (to spare energy).

The stress response is an indispensable asset for handling threats, but when threats occur too frequently or persistently, the organs and systems involved can be thrown off balance and break down. For example, one of the most important stress hormones is cortisol, which is produced by the adrenal glands. When the adrenal glands are forced to produce too much cortisol too often, they may wear out and become unable to produce sufficient cortisol to handle future threats. But before that happens, chronically high cortisol levels are likely to suppress the immune system, cause weight gain, and even cause the brain to deteriorate.

We are accustomed to thinking of stress as beginning with information that reaches the brain through the senses. Examples include an argument with one's spouse and a near accident on the freeway. But the stress response may also be triggered by physical events, such as a bacterial infection or injury. Exercise is another physical stressor. A hard run triggers the release of stress hormones, stimulates the immune system, and so forth. The stress response to exercise not only enables the body to better meet the challenge of a hard run, but it also causes many of the positive physiological adaptations to training, such as increased resistance to exercise-induced muscle damage. But as with other stressors, if exercise is too extreme, such that it outstrips the capacity of the stress response to consistently restore homeostasis to the body between workouts, a loss of balance may occur.

Both psychological and physical stressors cause immune cells to produce cytokines, which are chemical messengers that provide two-way communication between the brain and the body. Cytokines released from peripheral organs and tissues provide information concerning a threat, injury, or infection to the brain. In turn, the brain responds by initiating appropriate reactions in the nervous, endocrine, and immune systems, again using cytokines to coordinate the reactions. In the case of injuries and infections, the brain uses cytokines to produce an inflammation response.

Inflammation is a key player in overtraining fatigue. Tissue damage that occurs during and after running triggers the inflammation response, an immune system process whose purpose is to remove cellular debris from the site of damage and initiate repair. There are three phases of the inflammation response. First, blood vessels upstream from the site of damage dilate, increasing blood flow to the area. At the same time, blood vessels downstream from the site of damage constrict, causing blood to accumulate there. This flooding effect causes the classic symptoms of swelling, heat, and stiffness that are associated with inflammation. Next, specialized white blood cells called neutrophils migrate to the injured area and absorb the debris of damaged cells. Finally, other cells known as macrophages accumulate at the site of damage to complete the cleanup process and stimulate tissue regeneration.

Inflammation does several important things for runners. First, as mentioned, when a significant injury occurs, inflammation heals it and also produces symptoms of pain and stiffness that discourage activity during the healing process. If inflammation did not produce these symptoms, we would probably continue training as normal despite our injuries and make them continually worse until total dysfunction forced us to stop.

Most of us associate inflammation with acute injuries such as ankle sprains. But a much milder inflammation response occurs after normal workouts in which we do not suffer any serious injuries. Every workout causes microscopic damage to muscle fibers, which are repaired with the aid of inflammation during the following recovery period. The main cause of muscle damage during exercise is eccentric (pronounced "ee-centric") muscle contractions, which are also known as lengthening contractions. An example of an eccentric contraction is the lowering phase of a biceps curl. During this action the active muscle fibers are essentially pulled in two directions as they resist the force of gravity, but not enough to overcome gravity and shorten, so they actually lengthen while "trying" to shorten. Eccentric contractions occur at various moments in the running stride—most notably at footstrike, when the quadriceps and other muscles are forced to lengthen by ground impact forces but contract to absorb these forces and prevent the collapse of the joints they attach to. The strain of these lengthening contractions results in damage to some of the sarcomeres that are linked together like a chain to form a muscle fiber. Sarcomere damage produces chemical signals that trigger the process of inflammation, which begins about two hours after a workout and typically resolves after 48 hours.

In addition to repairing everyday muscle damage from exercise, inflammation promotes training adaptations such as satellite cell proliferation, an essential step in the development of bigger, stronger muscle fibers. Inflammation even makes the athlete more resistant to muscle damage in the future—a phenomenon known as the repeated bout effect. Studies have shown that untrained individuals become more resistant to exercise-induced muscle damage after just a single workout. It appears that the inflammation response triggered by the first workout increases the activity of neutrophils in the next workout, protecting the muscle fibers from some of the damage that would otherwise occur.

There is a negative side to inflammation, however. Ironically, although inflammation repairs tissue damage caused during exercise, it also causes further damage, known as secondary muscle damage, between workouts. Secondary muscle damage is believed to be caused at least in part by the release of free radicals from active neutrophils. Secondary muscle damage is the main reason you feel sorer the morning after a particularly hard workout or race than you do right afterward, and why you sometimes feel sorest two days after the workout or race. This phenomenon is aptly referred to as delayed-onset muscle soreness (DOMS).

More than an unpleasant feeling, DOMS is a symptom of muscle tissue damage that can seriously compromise the quality of your training while it persists. A recent Spanish university study found that DOMS reduced running economy in a group of trained runners by more than 3 percent (which is a significant amount, considering the fact that a lifetime of training may only increase running economy by 10 percent). The loss of efficiency seen in athletes experiencing DOMS stems from changes in their normal movement patterns. These changes also place unaccustomed stress on the joints, increasing injury risk. In another study, cyclists with DOMS exhibited higher than normal heart rates, blood lactate levels, and cortisol levels during a workout, indicating that when lingering muscle damage exists, normal training becomes more stressful to the body. DOMS has even been shown to delay muscle glycogen replenishment (that is, muscle refueling) after workouts, leaving less energy available for the next session.

In runners who train hard every day, inflammation may not be entirely resolved and muscle damage may not heal adequately between workouts. When runners persist in training too hard and resting too little, they risk entering a cycle of persistent tissue trauma and chronic inflammation. Some exercise scientists believe that this cycle is at the heart of overtraining syndrome, a disorder that is characterized by loss of performance, low motivation, compromised immune function, disturbed sleep, and other symptoms. Athletes suffering from overtraining syndrome exhibit abnormal concentrations of cytokines, which are responsible for transforming the localized inflammation response at the site of damage into chronic, whole-body (or systemic) inflammation. Overtraining syndrome is a serious condition that sometimes requires months of recovery time. It is somewhat rare, but a less severe pattern of compromised training and recovery that results from exercise-related tissue damage and inflammation is common among competitive runners.

Joint tissues (tendons, ligaments, and cartilage) also suffer damage during exercise (especially when there are biomechanical irregularities) and undergo a subsequent inflammation response. When joint tissues fail to regenerate fully between workouts, they may become chronically inflamed and/or degenerate to the point of serious injury. Some overuse injuries that are all too familiar to runners—including runner's knee and Achilles tendinosis—develop in this manner.

In summary, inflammation is a double-edged sword. Without it, our bodies could not heal tissue damage incurred during exercise, or gain fitness in response to workouts, or develop greater resistance to muscle damage in subsequent workouts. In competitive runners who train hard, however, inflammation can become a problem unto itself, causing secondary muscle damage between workouts that compromises our recovery and performance and may even lead to injuries.

TRAIN TO RECOVER, RECOVER TO TRAIN

Most runners become injured before they are able to train hard enough for a long enough period of time to develop full-blown overtraining syndrome, which is seen almost exclusively in elite athletes. Garden-variety overtraining, or training staleness, is a phenomenon that most competitive runners experience now and again, however, and the fitness development of all competitive runners is limited by their capacity to recover from the stress of training. The secret to maximizing your fitness development, therefore, is to enhance your recovery from workouts and to increase the training workload that you are able to adequately recover from between workouts. There are two general strategies you can use to achieve these objectives. The first strategy involves finding better ways to balance training stress and recovery—that is, to apply the right types and degrees of training stress at just the right times. The second is to facilitate recovery by getting the most out of three lifestyle factors that promote recovery: nutrition, sleep, and stress management. Following are some specific methods you can use to prevent overtraining fatigue from hampering your running.

Know Your Limits

Your running fitness will reach the highest level for a peak race if, throughout the training cycle that precedes it, your training workload is just slightly less than the most you can handle without experiencing overtraining fatigue. There is extreme variability in the amount of training stress individual runners can handle. Nevertheless, all runners can increase their training capacity over time.

The only way to know your training workload limit is to exceed it every once in a while. As long as it doesn't happen too often (more than once or twice over the course of a training cycle), and the transgression is slight, such that you never experience anything worse than a brief stale patch in your training, and you reduce your training workload quickly in response to this experience, you will be okay—better off, in fact, than if you trained very conservatively and never neared your limit.

To begin, follow a training plan that you expect to keep you just on the safe side of overtraining, based on past experience. If, at any point in your execution of this plan, you encounter a period in which you feel lousy in several consecutive workouts, give yourself a chance to recover by taking a day off and doing only recovery workouts for the next few days. When you resume normal training, reduce your overall workload slightly (5–15 percent) for the remainder of the training cycle.

If you feel far from overtrained as you move through your planned training, feel free to experiment with efforts to increase your training workload a little more than planned. Proceed cautiously, by adding just a few minutes to key workouts or by adding one additional recovery running or cross-training workout to your weekly schedule at a time. Again, if you hit a stale patch, pull back slightly and wait until the next training cycle to increase your training workload further. If you train well and feel good all the way to your peak race, you can increase your training workload somewhat more aggressively in the next training cycle.

The bottom line is that it's good to overtrain very slightly and very briefly every once in a while, because it provides useful information about your current limit that you can use to your benefit going forward. This cautious, conscious way of overtraining is sometimes referred to as "overreaching" to distinguish it from the more careless and thoughtless way of overtraining.

Learn Your Recovery Profile

All runners are unique in terms of how they recover from training. Some runners recover faster from long runs than from high-intensity runs, while other runners do the opposite. Some runners experience big fluctuations in their recovery speed as their fitness level changes, while others are more consistent in their recovery. There are many other examples of differences in individual recovery profiles I could list. By paying attention to and learning how your body recovers from training—your personal recovery profile—you can adjust your training in ways that enable you to perform most of your key workouts at a high level and minimize overtraining fatigue.

For example, in paying attention to my own recovery, I discovered that I tend to get stronger and stronger as the week progresses. I responded to this observation by tweaking my training schedule so that I train very lightly on Monday and Tuesday, waiting until Wednesday to do my first key workout, and I do my hardest workouts on Friday and Sunday. Back-loading my weekly training schedule in this manner leaves me feeling even more of a wreck on Monday and Tuesday, but it works out for the best because it also enables me to do my hardest workouts when I feel strongest.

Nothing is off limits when it comes to adjusting your training patterns to maximize your key workout performances and minimize overtraining fatigue, as long as each adjustment is a sensible response to a consistent self-observation. You can run twice a day three days a week instead of once a day six times a week if the former pattern seems to work better for you. Or you can do key workouts on back-to-back days and wait three days to do your third weekly key workout. The worst that can happen is that you try a new training pattern based on a hunch and find that it doesn't work out, so you go back to your old pattern.

Train Responsively

In chapter 1 I defined responsive training as modifying your planned workout as necessary depending on how you feel immediately before or after you start running. Responsive training is most crucial in key workouts. If you're too fatigued from previous training (or whatever else) to perform adequately in a key workout, you're better off doing an easier alternative workout instead.

In my experience, it is seldom possible to anticipate ahead of time whether you are going to perform well or poorly in a key workout. You just have to start running and then make a judgment about whether to continue based on how you feel. Here are some responsive training guidelines.

- Always complete your planned workout if you are hitting your target pace and feel at least "fair" on a scale of great–good–fair–bad–terrible.
- If you are failing to hit your target pace and you feel fair, cut the planned workout in half. For example, instead of doing 20 minutes of tempo running at 10K pace, do 10 minutes.
- If you are failing to hit your target pace and you feel bad, switch to an easier key workout featuring short intervals at a high intensity. Runners usually feel and perform better on their flat days when they shorten and speed up their high-intensity efforts. I have no idea what the neurophysiological mechanism behind this phenomenon may be, but that doesn't make it any less real. So, for example, if you start a 20-minute tempo run at 10K pace and feel bad, try switching to 5×400m at 5K pace. You'll probably feel better and you'll get more out of the workout than you would if you had to resort to the next option, which is this:
- If you are failing to hit your target pace and you feel terrible, switch to a recovery run. Make the run as short and slow as necessary to feel at least "fair" (you probably won't feel any better than fair on such days).

Practice Recovery Nutrition

Nutrition is one of the most important influences on the body's ability to absorb and adapt to training stress. In particular, the right nutrition habits will strengthen your immune system, accelerate postrun muscle tissue repair, and minimize inflammation. The two most effective nutritional means to enhance muscle recovery are maintaining a diet that's high in antioxidants and consuming fluids, carbohydrates, and proteins within the first hour after completing exercise.

Antioxidants are nutrients that neutralize the free radicals that are released from damaged muscle cells. Vitamins C and E are perhaps the best-known antioxidant nutrients. Many runners try to boost their levels of antioxidants with supplements, but ingesting these free radical fighters in natural foods is the best way to get the volume and variety of antioxidants needed to maximize recovery. Many antioxidants work synergistically, so it's preferable to get a balance of different antioxidants, as in natural foods, rather than taking just one or two antioxidants, as in supplements.

All foods contain antioxidants, but the best sources are fresh fruits and vegetables. Fruits and vegetables have not only vitamins C and E in them, but also dozens of other antioxidants, such as isoflavones, catechins, and carotenoids. For optimal muscle protection, consume seven to nine servings of fresh fruits and veggies per day.

Free radicals aren't the only culprits that cause muscle damage long after you've completed a run. Stress hormones, particularly cortisol, tend to stay elevated for some time after exercise. Cortisol breaks down muscle proteins to release energy—which helps you function and refuel after a run, but also causes the damage that leads to sore legs.

You can counteract cortisol by eating and drinking as soon after a run as possible. By bringing hydration and blood sugar back to a normal state you limit stress hormone production and therefore limit the amount of muscle damage that can occur.

In addition to water, which increases blood flow to the muscles, the most important nutrients for quick muscle repair are carbohydrates to turn off the cortisol switch, and proteins, which provide the amino acids your muscles need to rebuild. Timing is all-important. In a study by Vanderbilt University, subjects were given a carbohydrate-and-protein supplement either immediately after a cycling workout or three hours later. The first group experienced a net gain in muscle protein, while the second group experienced a net loss, indicating they did not fully repair the muscle damage incurred in the workout. You don't have to use a commercial recovery drink—although they work. A real-food mix of carbs and protein, such as a piece of chicken with pasta, or peanut butter on a bagel, is also effective. The important thing is to be fanatical about refueling immediately after a run.

Get Plenty of Sleep

Lack of adequate sleep is itself a stressor, so if you consistently undersleep, you will not recover from workouts as quickly and you will also be unable to handle as much training as you could handle if you did sleep adequately. As few as four nights of partial sleep deprivation result in skyrocketing levels of circulating cortisol. In addition, research in nonathletes has shown that short-term partial sleep deprivation increases circulating levels of C-reactive protein, a biomarker of inflammation. Therefore muscle damage–related inflammation is likely to be exacerbated by inadequate sleep.

How much sleep is enough? Sleep experts believe that there is a high degree of variation in sleep needs among individuals. It's best to sleep until you are "slept out," regardless of how much time it takes. In other words, you should sleep long enough so that you awaken spontaneously in the morning and couldn't sleep more if you tried.

Sleep also benefits runners in ways that are more strictly brain-centered. For example, recent neuroscientific research has found that the brain actually practices motor skills (everything from running to playing video games) during sleep. In a study performed at Harvard Medical School, two groups of right-handed subjects practiced a rapid typing task with their left hand, at the end of which time they were tested for improvement in the skill. Then they waited 12 hours and were tested for further improvement in the task. One group was tested at ten a.m., following a practice session, and was retested at ten p.m. the same day without any additional practice. The other group was tested at ten p.m. and was retested at ten a.m. the next morning, after sleeping, and without additional practice. Members of the first group showed a 2 percent improvement when they were retested. Members of the second group, who slept between tests, showed a 20 percent improvement the next morning without any additional practice of the skill.

The lesson is plain: Much of the improvement in our ability to perform motor tasks, such as running, occurs within the brain during sleep. So if you want to get the most out of your workouts, get plenty of sleep!

Manage Your Life Stressors

Remember, the body does not distinguish among causes of stress. Any influence that triggers the physiological stress response will affect your body in more or less the same way; hence, the concept of the "total stress load" (also known as allostatic load), which refers to the total physiological effect of all the stressors in your life. There is a limit to the amount of stress anyone can handle, so the more non-running-related stress there is in your life, the less running you will be able to handle without experiencing overtraining fatigue. For the sake of your running and your overall health and well-being, you should make stress management a daily priority in your life.

Among the major sources of psychological stress in modern life are family and relationship conflicts, overworking, feelings of lack of control at work, commuting, and financial concerns. Among the most effective stress relievers are exercise, spending time with friends, laughter, practicing hobbies, meditation—and sex!

Get the Most out of Recovery Runs

If you asked a stadium-size crowd of other runners to name the most important type of running workout, some would say tempo runs, others would say long runs, and still others would say intervals of one kind or another. None would mention recovery runs. Unless I happened to be in that stadium.

Now, I won't go quite so far as to say that recovery runs are more important than tempo runs, long runs, and intervals, but I do believe they are no less important. Why? Because recovery runs, if properly integrated into your training regimen, will do just as much to enhance your race performances as any other type of workout. Seriously.

It is widely assumed that the purpose of recovery runs—which we may define as relatively short, slow runs undertaken four to 24 hours after a harder run—is to facilitate recovery from preceding hard training. You hear coaches talk about how recovery runs increase blood flow to the legs, clearing away lactic acid, and so forth. The truth is that lactic acid levels return to normal within an hour after even the most brutal workouts. Nor does lactic acid cause muscle fatigue in the first place. Nor is there any evidence that the sort of light activity that a recovery run entails promotes muscle tissue repair, glycogen replenishment, or any other physiological response that actually is relevant to muscle recovery.

In short, recovery runs do not enhance recovery. Nevertheless, recovery runs are almost universally practiced by top runners. That would not be the case if this type of workout weren't beneficial. So what are the real benefits of recovery runs? The conventional, muscle-based and energy-focused models of running performance cannot account for the effectiveness of recovery runs. But the new, brain-centered theory can. Here's how.

There's a cytokine called interleukin-6 (IL-6) that plays a variety of crucial roles in coordinating the body's response to tissue trauma and stress, including the stress and trauma of exercise. Large amounts of IL-6 are released into the bloodstream by the muscles during exercise and travel to organs throughout the body, including the brain. Exercise scientists have recently discovered that increasing levels of IL-6 in the brain are a major cause of fatigue during exercise. In a South African study, runners injected with interleukin-6 before a 10K time trial ran a full minute slower than they did when given a placebo. Inside the brain, IL-6 causes feelings of fatigue and inhibits motor impulses sent from the brain to the muscles.

In addition to causing fatigue during running, IL-6 is believed to facilitate many of the body's adaptations to exercise training, ranging from increased fat burning to greater resistance to muscle damage to improved cognitive function. So the very molecule that causes fatigue during exercise helps you become fitter after exercise.

The primary trigger for IL-6 release during exercise is glycogen depletion. Glycogen consists of long chains of glucose molecules stored in the muscles and liver. It is the muscles' primary fuel during moderate-to-high-intensity running. Glycogen is also the muscles' limiting fuel, because it is stored in relatively small amounts, and when its supply runs too low, running performance drops precipitously. Because glycogen depletion produces high levels of IL-6, and because IL-6 coordinates many fitness adaptations to training, it follows that training in a glycogen-depleted state will tend to produce stronger training adaptations (of certain kinds, anyway) than training in a glycogen-replete state.

Recovery runs are exactly that. They occur within 24 hours of hard training, when muscle glycogen is not fully replenished and there is still lingering muscle damage (which is another cause of IL-6 release). Instead of promoting recovery from previous exercise, recovery runs actually enhance running fitness by challenging the runner to perform in a glycogen-depleted state. The notion that relatively short, slow runs can increase the fitness of a runner who also does longer and faster workouts is counterintuitive, but it's true, thanks to IL-6.

A study from the University of Copenhagen, Denmark, provided some validation for the hypothesis that recovery workouts enhance fitness. Subjects exercised one leg once daily and the other leg twice every other day throughout the study period. The total amount of training was equal for both legs, but the leg that was trained twice every other day was forced to train in a glycogen-depleted state in the afternoon (recovery) workouts. After several weeks of training in this split manner, the subjects engaged in an endurance test with both legs. The researchers found that the leg trained twice every other day increased its endurance 90 percent more than the other leg.

The release of interleukin-6 is probably not the only mechanism by which recovery runs enhance fitness. Research has shown that when athletes begin a workout with glycogen-depleted muscle fibers and lingering muscle damage from previous training, the brain alters the muscle recruitment patterns used to produce movement. Essentially, the brain tries to avoid using the worn-out muscle fibers and instead involve fresher muscle fibers that are less worn-out precisely because they are less preferred under normal conditions. When your brain is forced out of its normal muscle recruitment patterns in this manner, it finds neuromuscular "shortcuts" that enable you to run more efficiently (using less energy at any given speed) in the future. Prefatigued running is sort of like a flash flood that forces you to alter your normal morning commute route. The detour seems like a setback at first, but in searching for an alternative way to reach the office you might find a faster way—or at least a way that's faster under conditions that negatively affect your normal route.

Another benefit of involving less-used muscle fibers during recovery runs is that these muscle fibers become conditioned to prolonged running. They adapt to the demands placed on them in recovery runs by producing more mitochondria (intracellular aerobic "factories"), capillaries, and aerobic enzymes, so they can be more helpful whenever called upon again.

Finally, recovery runs help you become fitter simply by adding volume to your training without spoiling your key workouts. While hard key workouts boost running fitness more than easier runs individually, high overall running volume is also a powerful fitness booster. The most effective way to enjoy the benefits of key workouts and high running volume simultaneously is to supplement your three weekly key workouts with one or more recovery runs.

The reason high running volume is beneficial is that increases in running economy are very closely correlated with increases in running mileage. Research by Tim Noakes and others suggests that while improvement in other performance-related factors such as VO_2max ceases before runners achieve their volume limit, running economy continues to improve as running mileage increases, all the way to the limit. For example, if the highest running volume your body can handle is 50 miles per week, you are all but certain to achieve greater running economy at 50 miles per week than at 40 miles per week, even though your VO_2max may stop increasing at 40 miles.

The explanation for this linear relationship between running volume and running economy goes back to neuromuscular coordination. Running is a bit like juggling. It is a motor skill that requires communication between your brain and your muscles. Great jugglers have developed highly refined communication between their brain and muscles during the act of juggling, which enables them to juggle three plates with one hand while blindfolded. Well-trained runners have developed super-efficient communication between their brain and muscles during the act of running, allowing them to run at a high, sustained speed with a remarkably low rate of energy expenditure. Sure, the improvements that a runner makes in neuromuscular coordination are less visible than those made by a juggler, but they are no less real.

For both the juggler and the runner, it is time spent simply practicing the relevant action that improves communication between the brain and the muscles. It's not a matter of testing physiological limits, but of developing a skill through repetition. Thus, the juggler who juggles an hour a day will improve faster than the juggler who juggles five minutes a day, even if the former practices in a dozen separate five-minute sessions and therefore never gets tired. And the same is true for the runner.

The analogy only goes so far, however, because the primary goal of every runner is to push back the wall of fatigue. This requires that runners frequently complete workouts that leave them seriously fatigued. But recovery workouts, which you should always finish feeling no more fatigued than when you started, also help to push back the wall of fatigue by enhancing economy of movement.

Now that I've sold you on the benefits of recovery runs, let's look at how to do them so that they most effectively serve their purpose of balancing training stress and running volume in your training. There are six specific guidelines I suggest you follow.

1. Recovery runs are only necessary if you run four times a week or more. If you run just three times per week, each run should be a key workout followed by a day off. If you run four times a week, you will also do three key workouts, and your fourth workout only needs to be a recovery run if it is done the day after a key workout instead of the day after a rest day. If you run five times a week, at least one run should be a recovery run, and if you run six or more times a week, at least two runs should be recovery runs.

2. Whenever you run again within 24 hours of completing a key workout (or any run that has left you severely fatigued or exhausted), the follow-up run should usually be a recovery run.

3. There's seldom a need to insert two easy runs between hard runs, and it's seldom advisable to do two consecutive hard runs within 24 hours.

4. Recovery runs are largely unnecessary during base training, when most of your workouts are moderate in both intensity and duration. When you begin doing formal high-intensity workouts and exhaustive long runs, it's time to begin doing recovery runs in roughly a one-to-one ratio with these key workouts.

5. There are no absolute rules governing the appropriate duration and pace of recovery runs. A recovery run can be as long and fast as you want, provided it does not affect your performance in your next scheduled key workout (which is not particularly long or fast, in most cases). Indeed, because one purpose of recovery runs is to maximize running volume without sacrificing training stress, your recovery runs should generally be as long and fast as you can make them without affecting your next key workout. A little experimentation will be needed to find the recovery run formula that works best for you.

6. Don't be too proud to run very slowly in your recovery runs, as Kenya's runners are famous for doing. Even very slow running counts as practice of the running stride that will yield improvements in your running economy, and running very slowly allows you to run longer (that is, to maximize volume) without sabotaging your next key workout.

The following tables show how key workouts and recovery workouts are typically scheduled in the Level 1, Level 2, and Level 3 training plans for all peak race distances in Part II of this book. These general templates show only running workouts and do not include cross-training workouts. The Level 2 and Level 3 plans appear identical because the Level 3 plans include more cross-training workouts that aren't shown here (as well as more challenging key workouts).

TABLE 7.1 ◆ Weekly Workout Template for Level 1 Brain Training Plans

Monday	Tuesday	Wednesday	Thursday	Friday	Saturday	Sunday
Off	Base Run	Key Workout	No Run	Key Workout	No Run	Key Workout

TABLE 7.2 ◆ Weekly Workout Template for Level 2 and Level 3 Brain Training Plans

Monday	Tuesday	Wednesday	Thursday	Friday	Saturday	Sunday
Off	Base Run	Key Workout	Recovery Run	Key Workout	Recovery Run	Key Workout

CHAPTER ◆ 8

MASTERING THE EXPERIENCE

Discomfort is a big part of competitive distance running. When you run at maximum effort over a given distance, whether it's a mile or a marathon, you cannot avoid experiencing the unpleasant sensations associated with extreme exercise fatigue—not always the whole way through, but at least near the end. Your legs become increasingly sore and heavy, energy drains from your body like water from a leaky cup, your windpipe burns, and you may even feel light-headed or dizzy. As we've seen, the brain produces these sensory symptoms of fatigue to reinforce a "decision" to reduce motor drive to the muscles. I use scare quotes around "decision" because the reduction in motor output from the brain to the muscles that causes you to slow down usually occurs without conscious intention, in response to afferent feedback from the body telling the brain that a loss of homeostasis is imminent. But the conscious mind seems to have some leeway to override this automatic mechanism, and the experience of fatigue, the acute pain and suffering of nearing the limit, serves to discourage the conscious mind from doing so.

In previous chapters of this book I have focused on showing you how to combat fatigue primarily by developing your fitness in ways that allow you to run faster and farther before fatigue-causing afferent feedback is sent from the body to the brain. But it is also possible to combat fatigue at the conscious, or experiential, level—for example, by learning and practicing techniques that enable you to override the automatic fatigue mechanism. A risky but instructive analogy can be made between the two ways of battling race fatigue—physical and experiential—and the two ways of treating depression: medication and therapy. Depression usually occurs when, for one reason or another, an imbalance of neurotransmitters (usually low levels of serotonin) develops in the brain. Certain drugs effectively treat depression by helping to restore the normal balance of neurotransmitters. Psychotherapy is also effective in treating depression, but it works in a completely different way. Depression is characterized by symptomatic ways of thinking and behaving (defeatist thoughts, inactivity, and so on). Through psychotherapy, depression sufferers can learn to think and act in ways that are more consistent with their normal selves, which may in turn normalize the balance of neurotransmitters in the brain, making it easier to think and act normally.

The training methods discussed in previous chapters are like the drugs that treat depression: They combat fatigue on the physical level. The mental training strategies presented in this chapter—for example, race prioritization (discussed on page 164)—are like psychotherapy: They combat fatigue on the conscious, experiential level. But the distinction between physical and experiential levels is really a false one. These two levels merely represent different pathways to affect the physical. The sensations of fatigue are always associated with specific chemical events in the brain. There is no way to prevent, delay, or reduce fatigue and race pain and suffering that does not entail preventing, delaying, or attenuating these chemical events. But both physical influences (such as a good prerace taper) and experiential influences (such as achieving an optimal state of prerace emotional arousal) are capable of affecting the neural basis of fatigue-related performance decline and the experience of fatigue.

MASTERING THE EXPERIENCE OF FATIGUE

I have just explained that there are two overlapping ways to combat running fatigue: physical and experiential. There are also two distinct and complementary ways to combat, or master, the experience of fatigue. They are as follows:

1. Increase your tolerance for the pain and suffering of fatigue.
2. Reduce the amount of fatigue-related suffering you experience at maximum running effort.

In my early years as a runner I had poor mastery of the experience of fatigue. My stomach was always tied up in knots from homeroom all the way through the final bell on the Friday before a Saturday cross-country or track meet. I was one of the better runners in my state, so some of the butterflies came from the pressure to win, but most of them came from fear of suffering. I became quite a head case as a result of this fear, and did some shameful things. In one track race I pretended to accidentally step on the inside curb and twist my ankle. I fell to the track and writhed in phony agony as the other competitors ran on. Another time I pretended to unintentionally miss the start of a track race. I wallowed in shame through the entire bus ride home, but I still preferred this shame to the race discomfort I had spared myself.

Shortly before my high school graduation I burned out and quit competitive running for a number of years. When I made my comeback at age twenty-six, I vowed that I would not become a head case again. I would learn how to master the pain and suffering of racing so that I might realize my full potential as an athlete, which I clearly had not done back in high school. I'm happy to say that I had good success in boosting my ability to tolerate race pain and suffering and to experience less suffering in races. The solution was not any single magic bullet, but was instead a collection of useful strategies and methods that I picked up one by one. Collectively, these strategies and methods now represent the brain training approach to pushing back the wall of fatigue on the experiential level. In the next section, I will share with you those strategies and methods that raised my tolerance for race pain and suffering. Then I will share those techniques that enabled me to experience less suffering at maximum effort.

First, however, allow me to draw a quick distinction between pain and suffering. If you reread my descriptions of the two ways of mastering the experience of fatigue closely, you might notice that while the first method refers to pain *and* suffering (specifically, increasing one's tolerance for both), the second method refers to suffering only (in the context of reducing the amount of suffering one experiences while running at maximum effort). This is because there's an important difference between pain and suffering.

Pain encompasses the raw sensations of discomfort associated with fatigue: screaming muscles, burning windpipe, and so forth. Suffering, on the other hand, is a layer of emotional unpleasantness that emerges from the runner's conscious reaction to pain. Specifically, suffering is a conscious rejection of pain—a way of saying, "I hate this pain!" Indeed, it's not too much of a stretch to describe suffering as fear of pain. A given amount of pain *bothers* some runners more than others. In other words, the same amount of pain causes different amounts of suffering in different runners. Those who suffer more can be said to fear pain more.

There's nothing we can do about the pain of racing, but we do have some control over how much suffering our fatigue-related pain causes. You'll learn how to turn this control to your advantage later in the chapter.

INCREASE YOUR TOLERANCE

The late, great Steve Prefontaine, who was well on his way to becoming the finest American runner who ever lived when he died in a car accident at age twenty-four, once said, "I can endure more pain than anyone you've ever met. That's why I can beat anyone I've ever met." Pre's performance in the 5,000-meter run at the 1972 Olympic Games provides solid evidence that his pain tolerance was indeed beyond extraordinary. Just twenty-one years old at the time, Pre made three separate "last-ditch" surges for the lead in the race's final lap (something I've never seen happen in any other elite-level race) before finally relinquishing the bronze medal position at the finish line.

Only one runner at a time can have the world's highest tolerance for pain and suffering, but all runners can increase their capacity to endure the experience of fatigue and improve their performance as a direct result. Here are the two strategies that have worked for me.

Embrace Your Pain

Fatigue-related pain is the subconscious brain's way of trying to convince the brain's conscious decision-making center to voluntarily slow the pace of running or stop entirely. The conscious mind has some leeway to reject this message and keep the proverbial pedal to the metal. But the only way your conscious mind can really reject pain's message ("Slow down!") is to accept the pain itself, because more pain is the inevitable price paid for not slowing down. All available evidence suggests that "mentally tough" runners accept race pain—to the point of even welcoming and embracing it—more than other runners, and that this acceptance enables them to run harder.

The meaning of "accepting pain" is quite literal. When it comes, you don't wish it away, but instead welcome it as an indication that you are working as hard as you should be. How can you do something as counterintuitive as learning to accept fatigue-related pain? One answer to this question is contained in another famous quote from Steve Prefontaine: "Most people run a race to see who's the fastest," he said. "I run a race to see who has the most guts." In other words, Pre set out to prove to himself that he could tolerate great pain in every race. It was even his primary racing goal, ahead of winning. He did not just vaguely fear the pain before racing and deal with it during the race, as most runners do. Instead he consciously anticipated it and sought it out, and afterward used it to rate his performance.

I began to do something similar when I embarked on my running comeback in my mid-twenties. I was ashamed of having been mentally weak in my days as a high school runner and was determined to prove to myself that I could be mentally tough. So I started each race with a conscious goal of being willing to endure as much pain as necessary to achieve my best performance, and like Prefontaine I was more satisfied with a slower-than-expected race in which I did not shrink from pain than I was with a faster race in which I did. Without a doubt, this approach has increased my overall tolerance for fatigue-related pain, and it continues to help me perform better in every race I run.

A good first step to take on the path toward embracing pain more fully is to grade the toughness of your performance after each race. Ask yourself: "How much did I give out there today?" If the answer is anything less than 100 percent, you should not be entirely satisfied with your performance, regardless of how pleased you are with your time or placing. Vow to give a little more next time.

Practice Suffering

In the field of brain science there is a phenomenon known as habituation, or desensitization. The renowned neuroscientist Joseph LeDoux describes this phenomenon in the following terms: "Habituation is a form of learning in which repeated presentation of a stimulus leads to a weakening of a response—you jump the first time you hear a loud noise, but if it is repeated over and over, you jump less." The human brain is designed to focus attention and be most sensitive to novel stimuli, because a stimulus that is not already known to be benign may be dangerous. The habituation mechanism helps us avoid wasting attention and energy in reacting to stimuli that, however annoying or unpleasant, are not going to kill us.

It is possible to habituate oneself to fatigue-related discomfort in running, and thus to fear it less, experience at least the suffering component less acutely, and react to feelings of fatigue less strongly (by not slowing down as much, or as soon, or at all). As with every other form of habituation, the secret to desensitizing your brain to fatigue-related pain and suffering is to experience it and survive it. The most useful types of experience in this regard are tune-up races and breakthrough workouts (which can be one and the same, as they are in the brain training programs presented in Part II). Due to the motivating effect of competition, you can almost always run harder (and tolerate more fatigue) in a race than you can in any workout. Breakthrough workouts are the hardest workouts you'll ever do and therefore the best opportunities to experience the discomfort of extreme fatigue outside of racing.

Whether you're a head case as I once was or a runner who's already mentally strong and wants to become even tougher, the simplest way to achieve a greater habituation to suffering is to run as hard as you can in breakthrough workouts and tune-up races. My primary goal in the first race or two I do in each training cycle is not a time or finishing place but is literally to experience as much pain and suffering as possible, because I know that this experience, more than anything else, will set me up to achieve my time and place goals in later, more important races.

One of the most extreme examples of habituation to suffering involves the great Alberto Salazar, who almost died of heat illness in the 1978 Falmouth Road Race but survived and became mentally stronger as a result of the experience. Years later, Salazar explained this effect in an interview: "A lot of people asked, 'Well, are you going to be scared to push yourself again?' I wasn't. What happened was I finally said to myself, 'That's how hard you can push yourself if you're tough enough.' That fall, I broke through tremendously. It was completely from that race. I won the NCAA Championship and continued to improve. So that was a turning point."

I don't recommend that you emulate Salazar's method of building mental toughness *too* closely. (He was literally given his last rites after collapsing in Falmouth.) But by actively habituating yourself to the experience of fatigue you can trigger a more modest mental breakthrough of your own.

HOW TO SUFFER LESS

The most important lesson I learned from the process of learning to master suffering was that when I performed best I suffered the least, and when I suffered least I performed best. One of my finest high school performances was a two-mile track race in my sophomore season in which I broke the 10-minute barrier for the first time. Not only did I beat my previous personal best time by more than 20 seconds, but I also felt strong from start to finish.

The race was hard, a truly maximal effort, but I felt somehow in control of the effort. I felt totally equal to the challenge I was experiencing. I was "in the zone"—that is, fully absorbed in the task at hand, almost as though my entire self had become the act of running. The work was very difficult, but it felt absolutely right. When I returned to endurance sports as an adult I began to have similar experiences, not in every race, but in enough races that I came to see the achievement of this state as an objective that I should actively pursue in every race. To race in the zone is to have your best possible race.

I once asked 2:28 marathon runner Libbie Hickman to describe the zone for me. "It's a fabulous, effortless feeling," she said. "It's otherwordly— almost as if I'm watching things from outside myself. When I'm having one of those races, when I'm in that zone, it's almost like it's not me; it's just— *running*. I feel so strong, and so fluid. Every step is perfect."

There is a high degree of overlap between feeling bad during running and running badly. That's because your brain generates feelings of suffering to let you know it has decided to make your body slow down. Put another way, suffering is a sign that your brain has calculated that your body is not quite able to give you what you're asking of it. In a perfect race you experience extreme effort most of the way through, but you experience real suffering only toward the very end, because your training, goals, and race execution are well harmonized, so that you run an aggressive but steady and controlled pace that leaves you one step shy of catastrophic fatigue at the finish line. The earlier you begin to feel fatigued during a race, the more likely it is that you will fall off your pace before finishing.

The easiest way to avoid suffering during a race is, of course, to intentionally run slower than you feel you could run. As one who sandbagged a few races in the past, I can tell you that taking it easy on yourself is a thoroughly unsatisfying way to race. It is much better to race "in the zone," which is a very different feeling from taking it easy, and which is achieved only when you are running as hard as you can, in a state of peak readiness, and with confidence but not assurance of achieving a challenging goal. It's a special state in which "hard" feels "good."

Neuroscience has a long way to go before it fully explains the unique psychological state of being in the zone. But given what we already know about the experiential side of this state, and about how the brain functions, particularly with respect to endurance performance and fatigue, it's pretty clear what is going on generally in the zone state. Runners experience the zone when they are attempting to perform at a higher level than they have performed at in the past (or at least the recent past), and when feedback from the body and recent training give them reason to believe that they are ready to perform at a higher level. When you start a race in this state of being ready for and actively seeking a breakthrough performance, you choose a pace that feels appropriate. You know you have found the appropriate pace when you start to feel in the zone: totally unself-conscious, absolutely focused, giving it all you have yet feeling in control and confident.

The zone is, on the one hand, the product of a subconscious calculation that the body is performing beyond its recent limits but within its new limit, and on the other hand, a way of encouraging your conscious mind to not let up. The zone is the brain's way of saying, "Keep it right here; don't speed up, don't slow down; just push ahead."

GO WITH THE FLOW

The psychologist Mihaly Csikszentmihalyi (pronounced Chick-sent-me-high) spent his entire career studying the unique psychological state of being in the zone, which he called *flow*. Through exhaustive research, he was able to demonstrate that people in all walks of life, from every culture, and of all ages and both genders experience flow in the same general way and in the same kinds of situations. In particular, he isolated eight specific elements that together define the experience of flow, all of which are present in the runner's experience of the zone.

1. The nature of the situation is a task, which is to say it is a controlled and structured situation with well-defined parameters. In the case of running, it is a fixed race distance or workout format on a designated route.
2. The situation facilitates concentration. The primary task is the only thing happening, so there is nothing else to prevent you from immersing yourself in it. This condition is manifest to some degree in virtually every running race or challenging workout. Seldom are we distracted from our efforts to concentrate on running by things like trying to solve math problems or wondering how we look to the other runners around us. Less obvious distractions, however, such as performance-related fears and doubts, are common spoilers of concentration, hence flow, during running.
3. You have a specific goal. Having a measurable goal encourages you to push yourself to your limits. The flow (or zone) experience only happens when one is really testing a particular skill. Also, having a goal

symbolizes and reinforces the meaningfulness of the task. Flow happens exclusively when the task matters a great deal to the participant.

4. There is a balance of challenge and skills. You feel that your skills are equal to the challenge, but just barely. The task is not overwhelming, but neither is it a cakewalk.

5. The situation offers feedback, such that you can tell whether you are moving closer to achieving your goal. In running, the most important feedback with respect to flow is time and distance information, but it can also take the form of the relative position of other runners (as in, "My training partner is only five paces ahead of me").

6. The task absorbs your complete attention, so that you are conscious of nothing outside it, nor even self-conscious. In essence, in the flow state, *you become what you are doing.* As Libbie Hickman described, "It's almost like it's not me; it's just—*running.*"

7. You feel in control of your actions in relation to the task. Flow happens exclusively in those activities that we do especially well, or have a lot of experience in doing. What's more, flow does not occur except when we are performing our best in such activities. Even the most gifted runners seem to experience flow only when having a particularly good workout or race.

8. The situation is likely to yield an improvement in the skill or skills that are tested in the situation. This condition is most obvious in the case of activities involving fine dexterity, such as playing a musical instrument; musicians commonly *feel* their skills improving as they play. In running, this condition takes a slightly different form—that of experiencing a breakthrough performance, of running better than one has run recently, or perhaps ever.

Each of these eight characteristics of flow situations is interesting, but more important, some of them can be actively exploited to facilitate flow and produce maximum performance. For example, if you are prone to doubts and fears in race situations, you can improve your chances of experiencing flow more often by consciously working to overcome them.

STRATEGIES TO FACILITATE FLOW

It is not possible to experience flow every time you run as hard as you can. But it is possible to increase the frequency of the flow experience in races. Following are my eight best strategies for putting your brain into the optimal state for maximum performance.

Race When You're Ready

Flow happens when your body is ready to perform at a higher level than it has recently. There are two prerequisites for a breakthrough performance. First, your training workload must have increased in recent weeks, while staying within your recovery limits. Second, you must have fully absorbed your recent training and be well rested. You should race only when these two prerequisites for flow have been met.

Your peak race at the end of each training cycle should occur after you have gradually built your training to the highest race-specific workload you are currently capable of handling and then enjoyed a taper period of very light training. If you succeed in triggering a peak in this manner your body may be capable of performing as much as 3 percent better than at any previous point in the training cycle. The physiological changes that occur during the final weeks of training and tapering will communicate themselves to your brain during the race.

For example, tapering produces a sudden, dramatic increase in fast-twitch muscle-fiber power. The cerebellum, which is the part of the brain primarily responsible for integrating motor output with sensory feedback, will register the fact that these muscle fibers are producing greater power with equal effort, along with various other peak fitness adaptations. In the aggregate, this type of feedback will produce a general sense of readiness for a breakthrough performance that will facilitate flow.

Set Goals

Some scientists speculate that it is possible to consciously override the fatigue-exacerbating effect of suffering during exertion, and that this capacity may have evolved as a way for humans to achieve a higher level of performance in life-threatening situations. Because it is essentially a mechanism that prevents us from exercising to death, fatigue normally occurs when the body is not yet in imminent danger of suffering catastrophic damage caused by overexertion. But when you're being chased by a saber-toothed tiger, you are likely to suffer death if and when you do fatigue, so it makes sense that your brain is capable of using this objective feedback to squeeze out an extra measure of performance that is normally not possible. This extra measure of performance may come at the cost of severe muscle damage or other health effects, but it beats being eaten alive.

If these speculations are accurate, then it's also accurate to say that the immediate limit of one's running performance capacity is defined in part by the importance of the running experience one is presently engaged in. True maximum performance is probably possible only when the run is literally of life-or-death importance. But there are infinite degrees of relative importance beneath this limit. Setting race goals, and particularly peak race goals, is one way to increase the importance of a race so that you are capable of achieving something closer to a "lifesaving" performance.

Prioritize Your Races

Prioritizing your races is another way to elevate the importance of some races toward the "life-or-death" level. If every race is equally important to you, then no race can be all that important. But if you consciously designate your peak races as more important than any others, you will put yourself in the right frame of mind for optimal performance in your peak races.

It makes the most sense to give the least importance to your first race of the training cycle and increasing importance to each subsequent race throughout the training cycle, because if you train right you will be fitter for each subsequent race. So if you race four times in a training cycle, the first race should be of low importance, the second race moderately important, the third race very important, and the last (peak) race supremely important.

Prioritizing races has been one of the most effective measures I have found for overcoming my fear of race pain. There came a point when I realized that I am simply not capable of "going to the wall" and "leaving it all out there" in every race. I can run very hard in every race, but I can't dig down to the deepest level. I can always do so in a peak race, however—a race that I have been looking forward to for many weeks if not months, and that I arrive at with a good chance of achieving a lifetime best performance. Prioritizing races gives me permission to be satisfied with a 99.5 percent effort in my lower-priority races.

Keep It Fun

Setting goals and prioritizing races may be the most obvious ways to make certain races more meaningful, hence more flow-friendly, but they are not the only ways. Nurturing your love for and enjoyment of running is another way that's no less effective. In fact, if running ceases to be fun for you, no amount of goal setting or prioritizing will enable you to race in the zone. What's more, elevating the importance of particular races through goal setting and race prioritization can even take the fun out of running in some cases.

The key difference between the sport of running and running to flee a saber-toothed tiger is that the former is totally voluntary. It's a hobby. And as such, running has to be fun enough to motivate the occasional 100 percent effort and to make the pain and suffering that comes with it seem worthwhile, or else you will never achieve the performances that such an effort makes possible. Enjoyment is often underestimated as a psychological requirement for optimal athletic performance. Runners whose love of running and happiness in running are at peak levels are able to throw themselves into a running effort more completely than runners who are burned out. Indeed, flow itself is a form of enjoyment. It's impossible to achieve the enjoyment of flow in a race if you have not generally enjoyed the training leading up to it.

Having fun enhances running performance not only by boosting motivation, but also by relaxing the runner and minimizing energy waste through fear and tension. One of the risks associated with wanting to achieve specific results in races is that the fear of failing to achieve these results can become overwhelming and take the fun out of the process of pursuing them, which, ironically, sabotages the whole effort. Sports psychologists use the terms "outcome orientation" and "process orientation" to distinguish the mind-set of focusing on the results of training and competing and the mind-set of focusing on the process of training and competing. Every competitive athlete cares about outcomes, but it's process orientation that yields enjoyment. So the best mind-set is one that balances outcome orientation with process orientation. Athletes who become too outcome-focused can't help but overlook the process and stop having fun.

It's the process of running that gets us hooked on it, and the only thing that can keep our passion for running in full flame is to sustain that childlike thrill in putting one foot in front of the other. Continuing to run for the reasons we became runners in the first place also gives us our best chance of achieving whatever race outcomes we may desire.

Carry Your Successes

Flow requires confidence. The feeling emerges when integrated feedback from your body, the race environment, and relevant past experiences tell your brain that you can sustain your goal pace all the way to the finish line. If you start the race without confidence that you can achieve your race goal, it hardly matters what your body's subjective feedback or the objective feedback of your split times tells you during the race.

Confidence requires an evidential basis. You can't be confident of achieving a certain race goal unless past experiences give you good reason for this belief. Therefore, the best way to build confidence is to perform highly race-specific key workouts during the peak phase of training. If you've trained properly up to that point, and you perform those workouts in a state of high readiness, they will very likely give you a confidence-building experience.

Although confidence must be earned through achievement, naturally confident athletes tend to make more of their achievements than naturally underconfident athletes. It's one thing to have a successful workout or race. It's another to actively draw upon that experience when pursuing future successes. Two athletes may have the same race goal and may experience the same successful peak workout two weeks before the race, but if one of them is naturally confident and the other is naturally underconfident, the former will think about the successful workout more often during those last two weeks and during the race itself, and thus feel more confident and have a better chance of achieving his or her race goal.

Underconfident athletes tend to allow a natural tendency toward doubt, fear, and insecurity to steal their attention away from those experiences that provide real evidence of their true capabilities. If you have this tendency, make a conscious effort to frequently reflect on and draw confidence from experiences that give you good reason to believe you can achieve your race goals.

Tackle Your Fears

Another critical prerequisite for flow, and thus for optimal performance, is the ability to concentrate completely on the situation at hand. Self-consciousness must disappear as your attentional focus becomes fully absorbed in your senses. One of the greatest spoilers of "being in the moment" during racing is fear. The most common fears during racing are fear of failure and fear of suffering. It's perfectly normal to experience fear of failure and suffering as a race approaches, and even during a race. If your fears become too intense, however, they sabotage flow, hamper performance, and ruin the entire race experience.

Even elite runners experience performance-destroying fears. Alan Webb suffered through two years of poor performance because of excessive pre-race anxiety caused by pressure he felt to live up to the standard he set in high school by demolishing the U.S. national high school mile record. "All of that pressure, I just got so worked up about it," Webb said in an interview. "The nerves killed me. Before a race, my stomach would be a knot. I couldn't relax, because I felt like I had to win."

The key to keeping your race-related fears within manageable limits is to identify them and adopt a problem-solving attitude toward them. There is great power in naming your fears. A fear that has no name is unsolvable. But to name a fear is to give it boundaries, a beginning and an end, and then you can make efforts to move away from it or climb on top of it.

If you feel so nervous you could almost throw up on the morning of a race, don't just assume that's the way it is for you; treat this unpleasant situation as a problem that can be addressed. If, in the final days before a race, you start to question your ability to achieve a goal that you have not doubted until that point, don't just let those doubts happen. Resist them. And if, during a race, when the discomfort and mounting fatigue sets in, you begin to think such thoughts as, "I'm never doing this again. I hate this"—don't believe it. Take such thoughts for what they are: counterproductive fear-based reactions to the discomfort of fatigue.

Embracing your pain—the strategy presented above as a way to increase your pain tolerance—is also an effective way to reduce your suffering, I believe. To embrace your pain is to tackle your fear of pain—to refuse to allow pain to make you suffer. Again, the pain-embracing method I find most effective is to start each race (or at least each tune-up race) with a conscious goal of experiencing as much pain as you can tolerate during the race. This advice might sound ghastly, but it's not. The ghastly thing would be to experience *more* pain than you can tolerate—something your brain will never allow during running.

Get Aroused (but Not Too Aroused)

Your emotional state—also called your arousal state—in the hour immediately preceding a race has a major impact on your ability to achieve flow and optimal performance during the race. Conscious awareness that a major physical challenge is imminent triggers a state of sympathetic nervous system arousal that is designed to prepare the body for maximum effort. The heart rate and blood flow become elevated in anticipation of further increases once the effort begins. Feelings of nervousness and anxiety prepare your mind for the discomfort to come. You may even feel weak and lethargic—your brain's way of preventing your body from wasting energy that will soon be badly needed.

Some runners become overaroused before races. They become so tense and anxious that they wind up wasting energy instead of conserving it. Over-anxiousness is usually caused by fear, as described above. Addressing any fears that may cause you to become too tense before a race will help you stay within the arousal zone that's optimal for maximum performance.

Another good way to reliably achieve the proper level of arousal before racing is to develop a specific prerace routine that works for you. There are certain things every runner needs to do in the final hour before racing: Visiting the restroom, warming up, and taking in a final shot of carbohydrate are among them. But there is leeway for individual approaches, and you should take free advantage of this leeway to develop a custom-fitting prerace routine. For example, some runners like to listen to psych-up music, while others benefit from silence. Some runners like the distraction of talking to fellow runners or supporters, while others prefer to be alone with their thoughts. For some runners, a longer warm-up, perhaps featuring some high-speed strides, provides a productive outlet for pent-up nervous energy. Other runners fare better with a shorter, gentler warm-up.

Listen to your mind and body before races and use the feedback you receive to learn what works for you and what doesn't work. Once you have a routine that reliably puts you in the optimal state of arousal—eager, focused, and a little nervous—stick with it.

CHAPTER ◆ 9

HOW TO OUTSMART INJURIES

Back in 2002 I developed a case of patellofemoral pain syndrome, or runner's knee, that plagued me for more than three years before I was able to silence the pain it caused and return to normal training. As frustrating as it was to lose three of my prime running years (I was thirty when the injury struck), I don't regret the experience, because in overcoming the breakdown I developed the brain training method of injury prevention, which has helped me stay injury-free ever since, and will help you, too.

It began as a dull pain under my right kneecap, which first manifested itself in early November, when I was beginning to log some heavy miles in preparation for the Boston Marathon the following April. As with most overuse injuries, it introduced itself as a mild, local ache that emerged after five or ten minutes of running and went away as soon as I completed my workout. Like all too many competitive runners, I stubbornly continued to increase my running volume despite the pain, and as a result it became increasingly severe during my runs and lingered increasingly longer afterward. Eventually, even everyday activities became painful.

The wheels came off during a planned 16-mile endurance run. My right knee was tender from the first stride and became steadily worse. I kept running. By the time I reached the midpoint of my route the pain had become so intense that I began to fear I would never run again if I did not stop, so at last I pulled up. I was eight miles from my apartment in either direction. It was a long, agonizing, despondent walk home.

Running was impossible for the next few days. When mere walking was no longer painful I tried to resume running, but the pain quickly returned, so I backed off again and tried other treatments, turning to bicycling to keep fit. These other treatments included icing, which gave me only temporary relief, and acupuncture, which did as much good as lighting money on fire would have done. I persisted in believing that if I just gave the knee enough time to heal, and then eased carefully back into running, I'd be cured without ever having to know exactly what I was cured of or what had caused the injury. But after completing two full trips around the same circle of resting and then dipping my toes back into training, only to feel the knee degenerate all over again, I decided I needed to see an orthopedist.

The orthopedist first prescribed conservative measures: knee taping, anti-inflammatory medication, and physical therapy. None of these measures helped, so he scheduled me for arthroscopic surgery. During the surgery he found some fissured cartilage—a condition called chondromalacia—that might have been the cause of my pain, so he filed it down to make it smooth. When I recovered and resumed running, the knee degenerated yet again. Another magic bullet had missed its mark.

I never did find a magic-bullet cure for my injury. Instead, I pieced together a "cure puzzle" by finding individual measures that helped a little and accumulating them until, almost surprisingly, I had made a complete comeback. As I progressed through the long process of trying everything, discarding things that didn't work and retaining things that seemed to help my knee, if only a little, I began to make slow, almost imperceptible progress. At last, some forty months after that abandoned 16-miler, I was able to complete an entire marathon and declared myself officially cured.

What were the particular pieces of my cure puzzle? Strength exercises that improved the stability of my hips during running represented one piece. A few small gait modifications—including tilting forward to correct a problem of overstriding—provided another. Switching to a pair of minimalist running shoes that allowed my feet to enjoy more freedom of movement turned out to be a third piece.

These corrective measures shared one common characteristic that I only observed in retrospect, after I learned more about how the brain controls the running stride: They allowed me to run more naturally. The strength exercises corrected muscle imbalances caused by my normal but unnatural lifestyle of spending most of each day sitting in chairs. The gait modifications corrected stride flaws that are caused by the historically unnatural act of running while wearing shoes. And my change of shoes also helped me run in a more barefoot-like manner.

The final piece of my knee cure puzzle was a zero-tolerance pain policy that I adopted during the cautious, yearlong training ramp-up that culminated in my comeback marathon. The reason the injury became as severe as it did in the beginning was that I tried to run through my knee pain instead of reducing my running in response to it. And one of the main reasons it took me so long to overcome the injury was that I kept on reacting to pain too slowly in each new attempt to resume normal training. Instead of cutting back again at the first hint of soreness, I waited until the pain was at least moderate. Sure, by doing so I was able to squeeze in a few more workouts before having to take time off again, but I had to skip many more workouts than I would have missed if I had reacted to pain (by backing off my running) with a hair trigger.

In that final, successful return to full training I made a commitment to stop running as soon as I felt the least soreness in my knee (or pain anywhere else, for that matter) and to resume running only when I could at least start the workout pain-free. The plan was to run as often and as far as I could run without any pain, no matter how frequently I had to abandon workouts and take extra days off and no matter how frustrated I got by the regularity of these setbacks. When I began to execute this plan I found that the setbacks were indeed frequent and the frustration was, at times, almost unbearable, but I stayed the course. As a result, my progress was decidedly of the two-steps-forward-one-step-back variety, but it was progress nevertheless. It took many weeks to advance from 20 miles a week to 30, and from 30 to 40, and eventually I hit a hard limit at roughly 60 miles per week. As exasperating as this process often was, the only alternatives were quitting completely and the old cycle of rushing ahead and breaking down, so I celebrated it.

The journey was much longer than I would have preferred, but taking the slow route was the very thing that allowed me to eventually reach my coveted destination of being able to train for and complete marathons. Best of all, I am confident that because of everything I learned in dealing with my knee injury, I will never suffer another major overuse injury. In fact, this experience left me convinced that nearly every running injury is preventable. Behind the particulars of the methods I developed to beat my knee pain is a general injury-prevention strategy that, if practiced faithfully, can drastically reduce any runner's risk of developing any type of running-related overuse injury. The two core tenets of this strategy are as follows:

1. Run more naturally.
2. Never run in pain.

If you do these two simple things you will outsmart potential injuries virtually every time.

As you might expect, the brain is at the center of both tenets of this injury-prevention strategy. The concept of running naturally is based on the understanding that the brain's motor centers store preferred stride patterns that the body is not always able to properly execute for one reason or another; that this failure is a major cause of many running injuries; and that reactivating one's natural, preferred stride patterns will prevent injuries. And pain is your subconscious brain's way of telling your conscious mind that running is damaging tissues in a particular area of your body and therefore you need to stop running and/or change how you run. It's amazing how often we runners act as if this fact were not perfectly obvious, and how much more healthily we can run when we begin listening to our subconscious brain's warnings.

WHY RUNNING INJURIES AREN'T NATURAL

In a widely publicized article published in the journal *Nature*, Dennis Bramble of the University of Utah and Daniel Lieberman of Harvard University argued that running was a key factor in the evolution of human beings from earlier hominid species. Most discussions of early human evolution focus on the brain. The growth and development of this organ in our immediate genetic ancestors is generally considered to be the pivotal factor in the emergence of humanity. The burgeoning brainpower of the last prehumans allowed them to create better and better tools and more and more sophisticated ways of cooperating with each other to increase their chances of survival on the African plains. But according to Bramble and Lieberman, changes from the neck down were no less critical than those that happened inside the skull. And the most important factor driving these changes may have been a selective pressure toward becoming better endurance runners.

Bramble and Lieberman pointed to the many changes in physiology that made us better runners as we evolved away from the tree apes, including the development of upright posture, longer legs, more rigid feet, and bigger buttocks. In addition, our loss of body hair and the development of one of the most effective sweating mechanisms in the entire animal kingdom gave us a tremendous capacity to maintain a safe body temperature while running for long stretches on the sun-baked African savanna. These changes are believed to have given us the ability to hunt down and kill prey, such as antelope, that were much faster over short distances but tired out quickly, as all sprint specialists do.

When I read this article, I bought into the argument immediately. But almost as quickly I found myself asking an obvious question: If humans are naturally engineered to run, why are running injuries so common? Surveys estimate that more than half of runners suffer at least one injury per year that's serious enough to interrupt training—an injury rate that rivals that of tackle football. You would expect a species to demonstrate far greater durability in a pursuit for which it is genetically designed.

As a longtime student of the sport of running, and of running injuries, I was able to answer my own question. I concluded that the epidemic frequency of running injuries is due to the fact that our modern lifestyle, in relation to running, is unlike the lifestyle of our primitive ancestors in two key ways—we spend most of our nonrunning time sitting in chairs and seats, and when we do run, we wear shoes—and that these two factors cause us to run unnaturally, resulting in injuries.

HOW SITTING CAUSES RUNNING INJURIES

The average office worker spends almost nine and a half hours of each weekday sitting. The most notorious consequence of sitting too much and moving around too little is weight gain. One study found that men and women who spend more than seven hours of each day sitting are nearly 70 percent more likely to be overweight than those who spend less than five hours sitting.

There's another major health consequence of excessive sitting that you don't hear much about: muscle imbalances. Over time, spending hours of every day curled up in a seated position causes some muscles to become abnormally tight and weak and others to become just plain weak. Such imbalances are known to result in pain and dysfunction in the low back and other areas, reduced performance in sports and exercise activities, including running, and sports injuries, including runner's knee.

Muscles tend to work in pairs of agonists and antagonists. When a muscle or group of muscles shortens and moves a joint, it acts as an agonist. The muscle or group of muscles on the opposite side of the joint that stretches to allow this joint movement acts as an antagonist. When the joint is moved in the opposite direction, the roles switch: The agonist becomes the antagonist and vice versa.

The agonists and antagonists that act on each joint should have a good balance of strength. If the muscles that move a joint in one direction become significantly stronger or weaker than those that move it in the opposite direction, a muscle imbalance exists and the potential for joint breakdowns is greater. It's like a bicycle wheel that becomes "out of true," hence dysfunctional, because the spokes on one side are tighter than those on the other side.

Muscle imbalances develop when a person uses a certain muscle group much more than the opposing muscle group. During sitting, certain muscles tend to be active, while other muscles that oppose these active ones remain inactive. As a result, particular muscle imbalances are frequently seen in men and women who spend a lot of time sitting. The most prevalent ones are weak deep abdominal muscles, tight hip flexors, weak buttocks and hips, tight hamstrings, and weak quadriceps.

The deep abdominal muscles wrap like a corset around the midsection of your body. Their job is to maintain upright trunk posture and stabilize the pelvis and lumbar spine during activities. When you sit in a chair or seat, however, you don't naturally use your deep abdominal muscles unless you make a conscious effort. Consequently, these muscles tend to become weak in those who spend a lot of time sitting. It's the hip flexors, which are muscles that cross the hip joint in front of the body, that do the job of keeping the trunk upright when we sit in chairs and seats. As a result of using our hip flexors for multiple hours every day, these muscles become really tight. (Interestingly, the deep abdominals are much more active, and the hip flexors less active, when we sit cross-legged on the floor, as our ancestors probably did commonly before the La-Z-Boy was invented.)

There is a common misconception that a tight muscle is structurally shortened. In fact, a tight muscle is simply one that holds tension due to a constant low-level activation by the brain. In the case of tight hip flexors, the brain spends so much time activating these muscles during sitting that it loses the ability to fully relax them.

Tight hip flexors create problems for body alignment by causing a forward tilt of the pelvis. When you're standing, the hip joints should be in a neutral position relative to the pelvis. But due to tight hip flexors, the vast majority of us stand with the hip joints slightly flexed. When you stand with your hip joints slightly flexed, your center of mass is in front of your balance point, so the body compensates by tilting the pelvis forward and arching the lower back. This postural compensation puts a tremendous strain on the hamstrings, which become active in pulling down on the rear side of the pelvis to correct for its forward tilt. As a result of constantly holding tension when you stand, the hamstrings become relatively strong compared to their antagonists, the quadriceps.

The muscles of the buttocks and outer hips are required to relax and stretch as you sit. As a result of spending so much time relaxed and stretched, these muscles, like the deep abdominals, become weakened.

All of these imbalances have consequences for your running performance and injury risk. Running involves heavy use of the hip flexors and hamstrings, so it tends to strengthen these muscles, thus exacerbating their tightening and the strength imbalance between the hamstrings and quadriceps that sitting causes. Runners with tight hip flexors are unable to fully extend their hips in the push-off phase of the stride. You should be able to achieve a 10-degree backward extension of the hip during push-off. If, like most runners, you cannot, then you can't completely use your strong extensor muscles—your gluteus maximus and your hamstrings—to generate thrust. In addition, tendonitis of the hip flexors often develops in runners with tightness in these muscles.

Weak quadriceps muscles are commonly implicated in causing patellofemoral pain syndrome, or runner's knee—the injury I know all too well from personal experience (and the most common running injury of all). One of the four quadriceps muscles, called the vastus medialis oblique (VMO), is responsible for pulling the kneecap into alignment with the femur as the leg extends. Weakness in this muscle often results in improper tracking of the kneecap during running, meaning the kneecap fails to come fully centered as the leg extends and the foot makes ground contract, causing chafing between the kneecap and femur, like an askew door that gouges its frame every time the door is shut.

Weak buttock and outer hip muscles compromise the stability of the hips, pelvis, and even the knees. An excessive internal rotation of the thigh is often seen in runners with weakness in these areas, a compensatory movement that is known to cause iliotibial band syndrome, hip and pelvic injuries, and runner's knee.

Runners with weak deep abdominal muscles frequently exhibit an excessive forward tilt of the pelvis when running. This error may contribute to various injuries, including low back pain and hip flexor tendonitis.

ANTI-SITTING

Fortunately, what is tightened can be loosened, and what is weakened can be strengthened. There might not be much you can do about the amount of time you spend sitting each day. But by learning to sit differently, and by practicing a few simple stretches and strengthening exercises, you can reverse the imbalances that sitting causes and avoid their painful consequences.

The first thing you can do is to improve your sitting form by activating your deep abdominal muscles. As you're sitting, think about drawing your navel toward your spine. Make sure you continue breathing normally. You'll feel more stable in your sitting and you'll sit taller. When you stand up, do the same thing. For example, when you're waiting in line at the grocery store or at the bank, pull your navel toward your spine and pull your pelvis upward. It's a small enough movement that no one will notice what you're doing, but if you conscientiously counteract your automatic postural tendencies in this way whenever you think of it, you will greatly improve your posture and core stability over time.

You can get the job done a lot faster with corrective stretches and strengthening exercises, however. The following stretches and strengthening exercises will correct the underlying muscle imbalances that are caused by excessive sitting more quickly because they really challenge your tight muscles to stretch and your weak ones to work against resistance. (Not included are strengthening exercises for the deep abdominals, which are the focus of the core workouts presented in chapter 5.) Do the stretches once a day and the strengthening exercises two or three times per week. You can do them anytime; I like to perform both the stretches and strengthening exercises while watching ESPN in the evening; another option is to do the stretches immediately after your runs and the strength exercises in the context of your strength workouts.

Lunge Stretch

Loosens tight hip flexors

Kneel on your left knee and place your right foot on the floor well in front of your body. Draw your navel toward your spine and roll your pelvis backward. Now put your weight forward into the lunge until you feel a good stretch in your left hip flexors (located where your thigh joins your pelvis). You can enhance the stretch by raising your left arm over your head and actively reaching toward the ceiling. Hold the stretch for twenty seconds and then repeat on the right side.

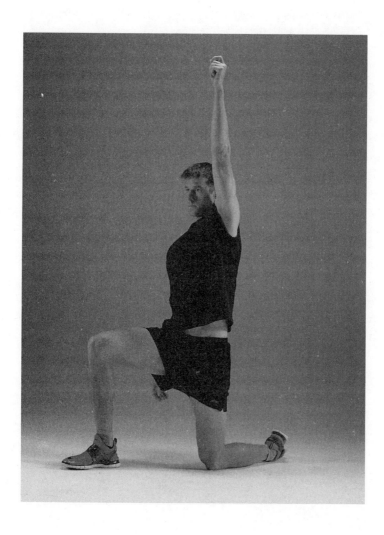

Supine Hip Extension

Strengthens weak buttocks

Lie faceup on the floor with your knees bent, both feet flat on the floor, and your arms folded on your chest. Straighten your left leg fully so that your left thigh remains in line with your right thigh. Press your right foot into the floor and contract your buttocks, causing your hips to lift until your torso comes in line with your thighs. Pause for one second and relax, keeping your left leg extended. Complete ten to twelve repetitions and then switch legs.

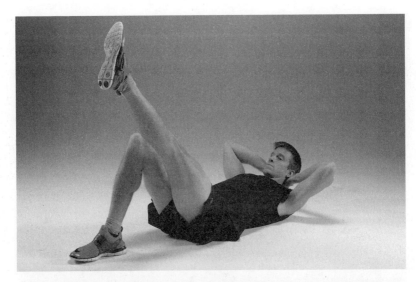

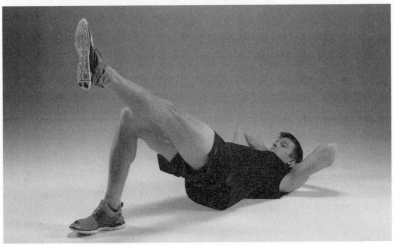

VMO Dip

Strengthens weak quadriceps

Stand on an exercise step that's eight to twelve inches high. Pick up your left foot and slowly reach it toward the floor in front of the step by bending your right knee. Allow your left heel to touch the floor but don't put any weight on it. Return to the start position. Complete eight to twelve repetitions and then switch legs.

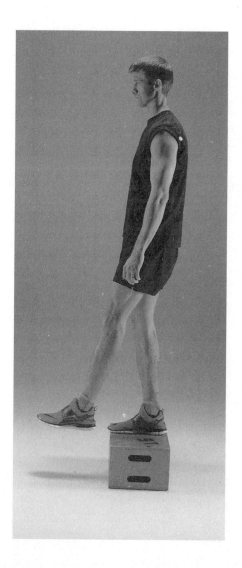
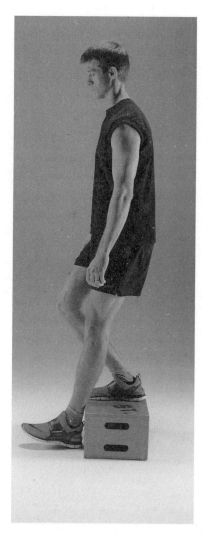

Spider Stretch

Loosens tight hamstrings

Assume a standard push-up position. Pick up your left foot, sharply bend your left knee and flex your left hip, and reposition the foot next to your left hand on the pinky side. Allow gravity to sink the weight of your body toward the floor slightly until you feel a warm stretch in your left hamstrings. Hold the stretch for 20 seconds. Now reverse your position and stretch the right hamstrings.

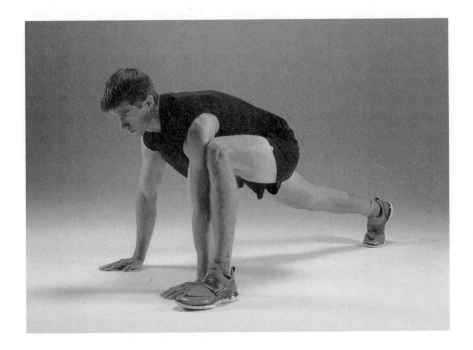

Cat Stretch

Loosens tight lower back muscles

Kneel on your hands and knees. Begin with your spine in a neutral position. Now round your back like a scared cat, pushing your mid-spine as high toward the ceiling as you can. Hold the stretch for five seconds and relax. Repeat the stretch five times.

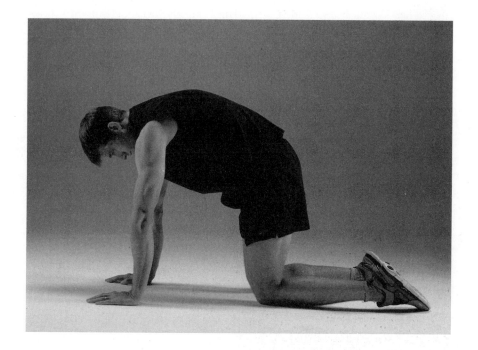

HOW SHOES CAUSE INJURIES

Until relatively recently in history, humans ran exclusively barefoot. There is a major difference between the way humans run with shoes and the way we run barefoot. Specifically, people tend to overstride when wearing shoes, but not when barefoot. Exactly zero percent of runners overstride, landing heel-first with the foot ahead of the body, when running barefoot. The reason is simple: If you land heel-first while running barefoot you will experience significant pain in your heel and quickly bruise it. But with shoes on, 80 percent of runners overstride and land heel-first.

Why does the switch from barefoot to shod running cause so many of us to change the way we run? I suspect that running shoes confuse the brain in a way that causes it to select the wrong motor pattern—namely, a motor pattern that is meant for walking, which involves a heel-first footstrike whether the foot is shod or unshod.

The heel of the foot contains proprioceptive nerves that transmit information about the hardness of the running surface and the force of impact to the brain. This information probably helps the brain decide whether to adopt a running gait or a walking gait. A slower pace results in a less forceful impact and a greater likelihood that the brain will determine a walking gait is most appropriate. But cushioned running shoes produce a softer impact at any speed. Again, the foot always lands heel-first during walking. So when we run with cushioned running shoes, the actual pace demands a running action, in which both feet lose contact with the ground at certain moments, but the softness of impact encourages a heel-first landing, as in walking. Consequently, 80 percent of us adopt a hybrid, overstriding walk-run action that increases injury risk by increasing ground contact time, reducing joint stability, and causing a more abrupt and extreme concentration of impact forces in the joints and other susceptible tissues.

This explanation is somewhat speculative. But what is certain is that shoes make most of us run unnaturally, specifically by overstriding, and this is a major cause of overuse injuries. The rigidity of shoes also prevents the foot from deforming upon ground contact in the natural wavelike pattern that the unshod foot normally uses to absorb impact. As a result, impact forces are sent shooting up the leg, concentrating in the knee, hip, pelvis, or even the lower spine.

I learned about these injury-causing effects of running shoes while researching a chapter on shoes for my book *The Cutting-Edge Runner*. From that point forward I often wished that one of the major shoe manufacturers would develop a "barefoot running shoe" that encouraged the wearer to run more naturally. Then Nike came out with a running shoe called the Free 5.0, a revolutionary piece of technical footwear for runners that fulfilled my wish exactly. Nike promoted the Free 5.0 as a foot-strengthening tool designed to be worn only once a week. But I was not fooled. Nike couldn't very well admit that the Free 5.0 was really designed to allow the wearer to run naturally, thus reducing injury risk, because in doing so they would have to admit what their other shoes were doing: *causing* injuries! Fair enough.

The Nike Free 5.0 had minimal cushioning—no more than was needed to run pain-free on asphalt, which is probably less than you think you need. It was extremely flexible, and provided no lateral stability. In other words, it had none of the features that runners have been taught to think of as virtues in a running shoe, but really aren't, because it's these very features that make wearing a running shoe unlike running barefoot. For example, the only reason conventional running shoes require stability features such as a heel counter is to overcome the instability that running shoes cause in the first place by elevating your feet above the ground on a narrow, mushy platform. If you get rid of the excessive cushioning, your running shoe has no more need for stability features than barefoot antelope hunters on the African savanna of twenty thousand years ago needed stability features added to their feet.

I bought a pair of Free 5.0s the day they became available to the public and immediately started wearing them for every run except track workouts (in which I continued to wear super-lightweight racing flats). Sure enough, I discovered that when my feet landed on the ground they were able to pronate and deform as they were evolutionarily designed to do, and as a result my feet and ankles absorbed much more impact force than they ever did in conventional running shoes, and consequently transferred less impact force to my long-suffering knees and hips. Despite Nike's dire warnings not to run more than 20 minutes in the Free 5.0s, I ran as much as 60 miles a week in them, and I even ran my comeback marathon in them, and far from creating any problems of their own, these shoes clearly helped prevent injuries that my previous shoes were contributing to.

Interestingly, when Nike came out with the Free 4.0—an even more minimalist running shoe—the company dropped the whole foot-strengthening shtick and provided guidelines for gradually making the Free 4.0 one's full-time running shoe. The latest version of the Free, the 3.0, is lighter and more flexible still. I now split time between this shoe and something called the Vibram Five Fingers (www.vibramfivefingers.com), which is not a shoe but a sort of foot glove that makes the Nike Free 3.0 seem bulky by comparison. I rave to other runners about the Five Fingers all the time, but most are afraid to run in something that allows them to literally feel the texture of the twigs, leaves, and pebbles they step on. There are, however, less-extreme options available to runners who are willing to move in the barefoot direction, but prefer to do so cautiously. Specific models include the Puma H Street (not technically a running shoe) and the Adidas ZX Racer.

While I am fully convinced that minimalist running shoes are less likely to cause injuries than conventional running shoes, this proposition has not been subjected to formal scientific evaluation. Therefore, rather than give you an unqualified recommendation to make the same transition I have made, I will leave you with the following footwear suggestions:

- If you are currently uninjured, do not have a significant injury history, and like your current running shoes, keep using them.
- If you are currently injured, have a significant injury history, or do not like your current running shoes for any reason, consider buying a pair of minimalist running shoes and wearing them once a week for a short run.
- If you find the minimalist shoes comfortable and they don't cause any problems, consider increasing the number of runs you wear them for, one by one. Don't feel compelled to wear them for every run or even for more than one run per week. Any amount of time you spend in them will likely reduce your injury risk.
- If you do not like the feel of the minimalist shoes or if wearing them does not seem to reduce your injury risk, you may need to consider going in the opposite direction: switching to a shoe with more cushioning and/or more stability, and possibly having a sports podiatrist fit you for prescription orthotics.

As a general rule, the running shoe you find most comfortable will be the one you're least likely to get injured in. The feeling of comfort in a particular running shoe represents your proprioceptive system's way of telling your brain that the shoe is allowing your muscles and connective tissues to move in more or less the way they prefer to move.

RETRAINING YOUR GAIT

Merely correcting your muscle imbalances and switching your footwear will not automatically make you run more naturally. These measures will make you better *able* to run more naturally, but in order to *actually* run more naturally you must consciously modify your stride. Because you repeat the stride action so often as a runner, the motor patterns that govern your stride are deeply ingrained within the motor centers of your brain. Correcting your muscle imbalances and changing your shoes will alter these patterns slightly by providing altered proprioceptive feedback to your brain, but the only way to make significant improvements to your stride, such as correcting overstriding and internal thigh rotation, is to proactively retrain your gait. Use the guidelines provided in chapter 5 to correct your unnatural stride patterns with proprioceptive cues and technique drills.

WHEN PAIN STRIKES

Pain is unpleasant by definition, and it is usually thought of as a negative thing. But the ability to feel pain is really a gift and an asset. Pain is almost always caused by damage to body tissues. The fact that we feel pain enables us to react in ways that help us prevent further damage.

There is a difference between feeling pain and reacting to pain. It is possible to reflexively react to pain signals without consciously feeling pain, and to feel pain without reacting to it. Simple organisms such as worms have pain receptors that enable them to shrink away from painful stimuli, such as being poked with a needle, but they do not have the mental apparatus to experience pain in a way that is even remotely similar to the way we do. The advantage that conscious awareness of pain confers is that it enables us to respond to pain in far more sophisticated ways—including ignoring pain in some instances!

The human body is filled with millions of specialized pain receptor nerves. When these nerves are activated by pressure or another such stimulus, they send an electrical signal to the brain. (Interestingly, the brain itself does not contain pain receptors, and for this reason brain surgery can be performed without anesthesia.) You might assume that these signals travel to a specific brain region that is responsible for producing the conscious feeling of pain. In fact, no such brain region exists. The conscious experience of pain appears to be produced as a result of activity in multiple brain regions.

TABLE 9.1 ◆ Common Running Injuries

The following table provides information to help you identify and over-come six of the most common running injuries.

NAME OF INJURY	WHERE THE PAIN IS	MOST COMMON CAUSES	COMMONLY EFFECTIVE CORRECTIVE MEASURES
Iliotibial (IT) Band Friction Syndrome	Just below hip bone or just above knee on outside of leg	Weak hip abductors, tight iliotibial band	Strengthening hip abductors Stretching IT band Deep tissue massage
Hip flexor tendonitis	The front of the hip or groin	Weak deep abdominals, tight hip flexors	Strengthening deep abdominals Stretching hip flexors Gait retraining
Patellofemoral pain syndrome (also called anterior knee pain and runner's knee)	Just below the kneecap	Weak hip abductors, weak quadriceps, weak deep abdominals, over-striding	Strengthening hip abductors, quadriceps, and deep abdominals Gait retraining Changing shoes
Bone strain (shin splints)	The shin, usually on the medial side (the side facing the other leg)	Increasing running mileage too quickly, overstriding	Reducing running mileage, then ramping up more slowly Gait retraining Changing shoes
Achilles tendinosis	Achilles tendon	Adding fast running too quickly Age	Eccentric strengthening exercises for calf muscles Deep tissue massage (particularly active release therapy)
Plantar fasciitis	The heel	Increasing running mileage too quickly, overstriding, poor shoe selection	Ceasing running until injury heals Wearing night splint Changing shoes Gait retraining

Much like fatigue, pain seems to represent a brain "decision" to respond to a pain stimulus. The feeling of pain lets you know that the brain has already executed some kind of reaction to it (such as pulling your hand away from a flame) and also discourages efforts to consciously override this reaction.

The fact is, however, that you *can* override pain in two ways. First, your brain can simply fail to produce a conscious feeling of pain when this feeling might do more harm than good. This is what happens in a state of shock, in which pain is delayed for several minutes or more following a grievous injury. In cases of shock, temporary numbness enables the injury sufferer to take lifesaving actions that might be impossible if a degree of pain commensurate to the injury were experienced. It is also possible to feel pain yet override the natural stimulus response to that pain in situations where the natural response might only make matters worse. The classic example is the pain felt when picking up a full pot of boiling soup by its hot iron handle. In this case, the natural stimulus response of dropping the soup pot might only make matters worse.

Competitive runners often override the pain message of injuries, as I did when my forty-month knee injury began. Competitive runners place high value on achieving race goals, are hyperaware of the fact that consistent training is required to achieve these goals, and have a high tolerance for pain, thanks to their familiarity with the discomfort of extreme exercise fatigue. These factors make the decision to ignore injury pain understandable and all too feasible, but they do not make it wise. Take it from one who learned the lesson in almost the hardest way possible: You will come out ahead in the long run (so to speak) if you adopt a zero tolerance policy toward injury pain (or localized musculoskeletal pain, which is totally distinct from fatigue-related pain), and react to it with a hair trigger by ceasing your running as soon as the pain reaches red-flag level and not running again until you can do so without pain.

Some injuries are caused by too-sudden changes in training. For example, bone strains (better known as shin splints) typically occur when running mileage is increased too quickly. Achilles tendinosis often coincides with the abrupt introduction of high-speed running. Injuries caused by doing too much too soon can be overcome easily with a reduction in training followed by a more gradual ramp-up. Let pain be your guide.

When muscle imbalances, shoes, and/or stride flaws are the major causes of an injury, simply backing off your training and easing back into it after your pain symptoms have subsided may not be adequate to overcome the injury. Traditional treatments such as icing and anti-inflammatory medications will also do you little good in this regard. Until and unless you fix the underlying cause(s) of the injury, it will probably return each time you attempt to ramp up your running workload beyond a certain level. Your first step is to identify the injury. Once you've identified the injury, a sports medicine specialist and/or sports physical therapist can help you identify muscle imbalances, stride errors, and footwear-related issues that may have caused the injury. Table 9.1 provides some very basic guidelines to identify and correct six common running injuries.

In the meantime, stay fit by replacing your running workouts with similar workouts in a nonimpact aerobic activity such as bicycling or deep water running that you can do pain-free. Doing so will not only keep you fit while your injury heals and you correct its causes, but it will also greatly reduce the temptation to resume running too quickly.

CHAPTER ◆ 10

FUELING THE RUNNING BRAIN

A few years ago an exercise scientist named Asker Jeukendrup, based at the University of Birmingham, England, performed an experiment that raised a lot of eyebrows. He recruited a group of nine competitive cyclists and asked them to complete two simulated time trials of roughly an hour's duration on stationary bikes. In one time trial the subjects rinsed their mouths with a sports drink once every seven to eight minutes. The cyclists were not permitted to swallow the drink, but had to spit it out. In the other trial they rinsed their mouths out with water.

Believe it or not, the cyclists completed the time trial almost two minutes faster, on average, when they rinsed their mouths out with the sports drink. Somehow the carbohydrate in the sports drink affected the cyclists' performance without ever reaching their bloodstream. But what other part of the body could the carbs have acted upon to achieve this benefit? The brain, of course! It so happens that there are carbohydrate receptors in the mouth that communicate with the brain. Jeukendrup hypothesized that the carbohydrate rinse activated these carbohydrate receptors, which stimulated the motor centers of the brain in a way that increased "central drive" to the working muscles, boosting muscle recruitment and performance. The presence of carbohydrate in the mouth at frequent intervals might have fooled the brain into believing an extra source of energy was available, making it safe to work a little harder.

The practical implications of this study are unclear. Obviously, merely rinsing your mouth out with a sports drink cannot provide all of the benefits that swallowing a sports drink can, but it may provide an added benefit in certain circumstances. For example, during running the body cannot tolerate a high rate of fluid consumption. Perhaps runners can perform better by supplementing a moderate rate of sports drink consumption with regular mouth rinses. More specifically, in a marathon you might drink at even-numbered mile markers and rinse your mouth out at odd-numbered mile markers. Personally, I would need to see solid research confirming that supplementing actual drinking with rinsing provides additional benefits that go beyond merely drinking before I began to practice mouth rinsing in races or advising other runners to do so.

That said, Jeukendrup's study supports the results of older studies showing that when endurance athletes are given a carbohydrate sports drink to consume throughout a long performance test, they go faster from the very start compared to when they are given plain water. This observation flies in the face of conventional exercise science wisdom, which holds that consuming carbohydrate during exercise enhances performance by delaying muscle glycogen depletion. A state of muscle glycogen depletion is extremely unlikely to exist at the very beginning of a performance test. If drinking a sports drink aided performance strictly by delaying muscle glycogen depletion, athletes would not go faster from the very beginning of performance tests in which they consumed carbohydrate—they would merely be able to continue longer. The fact that they do go faster from the very start suggests that a brain-mediated factor is indeed at work. A central mechanism involving signals sent from carbohydrate receptors in the mouth to the brain is a plausible explanation.

As these studies illustrate, the practical implications of the new, brain-centered model of exercise performance are not limited to training. There are also nutritional implications for our fueling practices during running. Clearly stated: What we now know about the brain's role in running performance changes what and how we ought to drink while running. In this chapter I will discuss three specific fueling practices that have long been supported by conventional scientific wisdom, but have been discredited by new research, and I will recommend alternative, brain-centered fueling practices that are supported by the new research.

Conventional wisdom: Drink enough fluid to completely prevent dehydration during running.

Brain training wisdom: Drink according to your thirst.

Thirst is the experience of a conscious drive to drink that is triggered by thirst-specific afferent feedback mechanisms to the brain. Nerve cells known as baroreceptors, located near your heart, sense changes in blood volume and report them to the hypothalamus, which in turn makes you feel thirsty. A decline in blood pressure indicates a decline in blood volume and dehydration, which stimulates thirst. There are also believed to be "osmoreceptors," possibly located in the liver, which sense changes in cell volume. Declining cell volume is another indication of dehydration. A third mechanism is the hormone angiotensin, which is sent from the kidneys to the brain, triggering thirst, when the water level in the kidneys drops.

The thirst mechanism works very well. Several million years of evolution went into its design. The thirst mechanism almost never fails to stimulate the drive to drink when the body becomes even slightly dehydrated, and it reliably turns off the drive to drink when the body achieves complete hydration. Yet for many years, until quite recently, there was a prevailing belief among sports nutrition researchers that the thirst mechanism was unreliable during exercise. This belief grew out of studies finding that when athletes were given free access to fluids during exercise, they seldom consumed enough to compensate for fluid losses incurred through sweating and breathing. In fact, the typical voluntary (or ad libitum) drinking rate during vigorous exercise is only 70 percent of the rate of body fluid loss. On the basis of this observation, and on the presumption that any amount of dehydration was detrimental to the health and performance of the athlete, scientists decided that athletes should "drink ahead of their thirst"—that is, force themselves to drink more than their bodies told them to—in order to completely prevent dehydration.

Biological urges that are as evolutionarily hardwired as the thirst response aren't stupid, however. If we lack the drive to drink more than we do while running, there has to be a good reason. As it turns out, an abundance of recent research has demonstrated that the negative performance and health consequences of dehydration during exercise have been greatly overblown. In fact, the negative performance effects of drinking *too much* appear to be greater, and there are serious potential health effects of over-drinking during running, as well.

THE OVERHEATING MYTH

Runners commonly assume that the reason they're supposed to drink to prevent dehydration while running is that dehydration causes heat illness.

The reality is that dehydration seldom causes runners to overheat. Instead, this problem is much more likely to be caused by simple overexertion in a hot environment.

The harder the muscles work (that is, the faster you run), the more heat they produce. In hot weather (especially hot, humid weather), this excess body heat does not dissipate well, and as a result it accumulates in the body. Heat illness occurs most often during very intense exercise, when the muscles are producing the most heat. In these cases collapse occurs relatively quickly—long before dehydration has a chance to develop. Alberto Salazar's famous heatstroke collapse in the relatively short (7-mile) Falmouth Road Race (mentioned in the previous chapter) is a classic example.

Interestingly, hot-weather racing is the only circumstance in which the brain's self-protective fatigue mechanisms sometimes fail to prevent runners from seriously harming themselves. But our susceptibility to overstepping our limits when running in the heat has nothing to do with dehydration. Research suggests that elevated core body temperature accelerates nerve impulse transmission, potentially causing the protective inhibition of muscle activation to lag behind motor signals ordering continued work at the same intensity.

Body temperature does rise as dehydration progresses during prolonged exercise. This is to be expected, since the more you sweat, the more your blood volume decreases, leaving less blood to carry excess heat away from your muscles to your skin, where it can be released into the environment. It only goes so far, however. Recent field studies have shown a much smaller correlation between dehydration and core temperature increase than previous laboratory-based studies. Even severely dehydrated runners seldom experience heat illness, and those who do are rarely more dehydrated than those who do not. There is evidence that some athletes are particularly susceptible to heat illness and therefore experience it at dehydration levels that aren't a problem for most.

This is not to suggest that dehydration is benign. Extreme dehydration can be fatal. Health emergencies requiring medical attention in running races are almost never caused by dehydration, however, which must exceed 15 percent to pose serious health risks. Very rarely do runners or other athletes reach levels of dehydration approaching even 10 percent.

A PAIN IN THE GUT

Running performance tends to decline as dehydration progresses during prolonged running. Even a 2 percent loss of body fluid lowers blood volume enough to reduce cardiac efficiency. As blood volume decreases due to sweating, the heart pumps less blood per contraction and therefore delivers less oxygen to the muscles per contraction. The result is that it takes more energy to continue running at the same pace.

Traditionally, sports nutrition scientists have taken the correlation between dehydration and performance decline as grounds to advise runners to make every effort to fully offset dehydration with fluids consumed on the run. It sounds great in theory, but in practice, drinking to fully offset dehydration during prolonged race-intensity running sabotages performance to a far greater degree than dehydration itself does.

At faster running speeds it is simply impossible to absorb enough fluid to prevent mild dehydration. Runners who try to drink as fast as they lose body fluid usually encounter gastrointestinal distress. Due primarily to the jostling of the gut that occurs during running, we can neither tolerate as much fluid in the stomach nor absorb this fluid as quickly while running as we can at rest. This is the case at any running speed, but the faster we run, the lower the tolerable stomach volume falls and the slower fluid is absorbed through the gut.

When there is too much fluid in your stomach, its jostling causes an unpleasant sloshy feeling that you've probably experienced—a feeling that becomes full-blown nausea in some cases. Stomach jostling also contributes to a reduced gastric emptying rate (that is, slower absorption of nutrition through the stomach and intestine) during running. The result, if you try to drink too much, is a nutrition backlog in the stomach, small intestine, and possibly the colon that's not unlike the damming of a river and subsequent flooding of riverfront properties. Such a backlog and the resulting accumulation of fluid in places it should not be (for example, the colon) causes a bloated feeling and leads to diarrhea in extreme cases.

In a study from the Sports Science Institute of South Africa, runners did three separate two-hour workouts in the heat while drinking a sports drink at three different rates: by thirst; at a moderate rate of 130 milliliters, or about 4 ounces, every 15 to 20 minutes; and at a high rate of 350 milliliters, or roughly 9 ounces, every 15 to 20 minutes. The study found no significant differences in core body temperature or finishing times among the three trials. During the high-drinking-rate trial, however, two of the eight subjects suffered severe gastrointestinal distress and had to stop running early.

WATERLOGGED

At very slow running speeds it is possible to absorb ingested fluid at rates equaling or exceeding the rate of fluid loss. But even under these circumstances it is best to drink according to one's thirst instead of forcing oneself to drink to completely offset fluid losses in accordance with traditional advice. The reason is that drinking too much during prolonged slow running causes blood sodium dilution. Sports drinks are always preferable to water for hydration because they contain fairly large amounts of sodium, so they are able to replace some of the sodium that is lost in sweat. But even the saltiest sports drinks have a much lower sodium concentration than sweat, so if you drink too much of either a sports drink or plain water while running, the sodium concentration of your blood will drop. This will cause your tissue cells to absorb water from your blood in an effort to restore the sodium concentration level to normal, thus lowering your blood volume (just as dehydration does).

During very prolonged running, when heavy sweat losses are combined with extreme overdrinking, a potentially deadly condition called hyponatremia may develop. As the sodium concentration of body fluids falls too low, the cells soak up so much water in their efforts to correct the imbalance that they begin to swell. This is especially problematic in the case of brain cells, because the rigidity of the skull allows for no release of the resulting pressure buildup. Symptoms of hyponatremia include stomach bloating, exhaustion, dizziness, confusion, and collapse. Severe cases can lead to seizure, coma, and even death.

At rest, your body can prevent blood dilution by shunting all of the excess water to the bladder for elimination, but during running urine production decreases by as much as 60 percent due to increased blood flow to the working muscles, trapping excess water in the body fluids and tissues. Hyponatremia is also impossible at high running speeds because the body cannot absorb enough fluid to cause the cells to swell, nor can the effort be sustained long enough.

FOLLOW THE LEADERS

When the recommendations of scientists disagree with the practices of the world's best runners, it's always best to ignore the scientists and follow the example of the race winners. In the case of hydration during running, we know that the world's best runners have never drunk to fully offset fluid losses, nor even come close. The typical elite marathon runner drinks only four hundred to six hundred milliliters of fluid per hour, while sweating at rates often exceeding two liters per hour.

In other words, elite marathon runners allow themselves to become quite dehydrated. In fact, elite runners actually tend to become more dehydrated over the course of a long race than slower runners. A classic study involving English marathon runners found that the race winner was more dehydrated and had a higher core temperature than any of the other runners tested. A later study that measured fluid loss in runners competing in 30-kilometer races found a similar pattern: The highest finishers were the most dehydrated.

One would expect top finishers to lose the most sweat, because they are running the fastest and therefore generating the most heat. But one might also expect that these runners would have to replace most of this lost fluid through heavy drinking to avoid fading in the late miles due to the efficiency-spoiling effect of dehydration. Nevertheless, the above-mentioned studies provide clear evidence that this is not the case. Elite runners appear to succeed despite modest compensation of their body fluid losses through fluid consumption during the race.

The training, nutrition, and other performance-related methods of elite runners evolve through an ongoing collective trial-and-error process. Methods that work well survive and spread, while those that do not work well die out. If most top marathon runners drink at only a quarter to a third of their sweat rate in races, you can be sure that it is because this strategy works better than the alternatives. Certainly there have been cases where elite marathon runners have tried to drink more, but apparently it has not worked out, either because drinking more led to GI distress or because they had to slow down too much in order to be able to drink more without GI distress.

The lesson we need to take from the example of the top runners is plain. If your goal is to get to the finish line as fast as possible, it's better to trust your thirst mechanism and drink only as much as you can comfortably tolerate while running as fast as you can than it is to slow your pace to a level that allows you to drink more. While performance does deteriorate as dehydration progresses, the alternatives (namely, slowing down so you can drink and absorb more fluid, or drinking more at the same pace and risking GI distress) are worse.

A SIMPLE EXPLANATION

There may be a simple explanation as to why our natural drinking rate is slower than our sweat rate during running. Scientists normally assume that all of the body weight lost during a run is accounted for by body fluid depletion. But this is not really the case. While running long distances we convert large amounts of stored fat and carbohydrate into energy. Fat and carbohydrate molecules have weight, and when we metabolize them for muscle energy that weight is lost. In addition, both fat and carbohydrate are stored with water, which is released into the bloodstream when fats and carbs are burned and then contributes to sweat losses.

Over the course of a marathon, the burning of fats and carbs and the water released in these processes could easily account for a few pounds of weight loss—weight loss that does not come from body fluid and therefore has no dehydrating effect. So a runner who voluntarily drinks at a rate that represents only 60–70 percent of his or her rate of weight loss may well be drinking at a rate that's closer to matching the actual rate of body fluid depletion.

AN EVOLUTIONARY PERSPECTIVE

To understand what truly constitutes the optimal hydration strategy during running, it helps to take an evolutionary perspective. As I mentioned in the previous chapter, evolutionary biologists have recently begun to recognize a much greater role of running in the evolution of modern humans from earlier hominid species than was previously the case. Selection pressure to become more effective hunters on the vast, hot African savanna transformed us gradually from tree climbers into endurance runners able to wear out prey that was able to run faster over short distances but also fatigued more quickly. We developed upright posture, longer legs, stronger feet, and bigger buttocks for this purpose.

We also developed one of the most effective internal cooling systems in the entire animal kingdom. In *Why We Run*, Bernd Heinrich, a biologist and former champion ultra-runner, explains the advantages of this cooling mechanism:

> Our nakedness and exceptionally numerous and well-developed sweat glands are potent features that contribute to running speed under external and internal heat. Because of sweating, we can tolerate very high heat loads derived from internal metabolism and the exterior environment. . . . Without sweating, running speed and range would be dramatically reduced. Most arid-land animals are

compromised in endurance because they are highly adapted to conserve water. The fact that we, as savannah-adapted animals, have such a hypertrophied sweating response implies that if we are naturally so profligate with water, it can only be because of some very big advantage. The most likely advantage was that it permitted us to perform prolonged exercise in the heat.

We are accustomed to thinking of the fluid losses we incur through sweating as a liability. But when we take an evolutionary perspective, we see our exceptional capacity to tolerate large fluid losses as one of the keys to our endurance running gift. Our ability to become significantly more dehydrated than other animals without becoming exhausted or sick is a key reason we're naturally among the world's greatest endurance runners.

It's important to bear in mind that early human hunters had no way to drink on the run. They had to run in the heat for long stretches of time without drinking, and when they did drink they had to stop running first. So while there was a strong selection pressure toward the ability to continue running despite heavy fluid losses, there was little or no selection pressure toward being able to drink effectively while running. Consequently, we modern endurance runners have a very limited capacity to drink on the run. On this point it's interesting to note that training has no effect on the rate at which the stomach and small intestine absorb fluid during exercise. The digestive system is one of the only parts of the human body that does *not* adapt to exercise training.

Fluid belts and race fluid stations now enable us to do what the circumstances of prehistoric desert chases did not. Unquestionably, it is beneficial to take advantage of these resources to limit dehydration on the run. By keeping your blood volume higher, you allow your heart to deliver more oxygen to your muscles per contraction, which slows the loss of running efficiency that comes with dehydration, and you are also able to maintain a higher sweat rate, which allows you to run faster in hot weather without overheating. But in taking advantage of modern opportunities to drink on the run, you must not ignore two hard evolutionary facts: Our bodies are designed to tolerate dehydration quite well, and they are not designed to tolerate any more than a modest amount of drinking while we run.

Your brain's thirst mechanism is smarter than the sports nutrition scientists who tell you to ignore it. Obey the subjective feedback that is your thirst, not the men and women in lab coats. When running, drink when you're thirsty and don't drink when you're not.

Conventional wisdom: The only nutrients that provide benefits when consumed during running are water, electrolyte minerals, and carbohydrate.

Brain training wisdom: Consuming protein during running is highly beneficial for tomorrow's workout.

In 1998 a sports nutrition company called PacificHealth Labs introduced a postworkout recovery drink mix called Endurox R[4]. It contained a patented four-to-one ratio of carbohydrate and protein. The product was a hit with endurance athletes, so the company decided to launch a sports drink containing the same four-to-one ratio, but at half the concentration of Endurox R[4] to ensure that it emptied from the intestine fast enough not to cause gastrointestinal stress during intense exercise. Brought to market in 2001 under the brand name Accelerade, it was the first sports drink containing protein in any amount.

Protein had not been added to sports drinks previously for the simple reason that there was no scientific rationale to support it—no known benefit to consuming protein during exercise. But a funny thing happened when researchers performed clinical trials comparing Accelerade to conventional sports drinks: They found huge benefits associated with the added protein. In one study, conducted by researchers at James Madison University without funding from PacificHealth Labs, fifteen male cyclists rode stationary bicycles to exhaustion while drinking either Accelerade or a conventional carbohydrate sports drink (Gatorade). The following day, the cyclists completed a second ride to exhaustion at a higher intensity. The athletes were able to ride 29 percent longer in the first workout and 40 percent longer in the second workout when given the carb-protein sports drink than when given the carb-only sports drink. The researchers also took blood samples from the cyclists and tested them for signs of muscle damage. They found that Accelerade reduced muscle damage by 83 percent compared to Gatorade.

Subsequent research by the same research group and others has failed to duplicate the massive improvements in time to exhaustion found in the first James Madison study. Nevertheless, drinking Accelerade has resulted in either equal or better endurance performance compared to carb-only sports drinks in every study—even in those funded by makers of conventional carb-only sports drinks. In addition, drinking Accelerade has drastically reduced muscle damage compared to conventional sports drinks in every study designed to test this variable. Similar results have also been observed in studies involving other, newer carb-protein sports drinks.

In one recent study, twelve male cyclists performed four rides to exhaustion on a stationary bike on separate occasions. Every 15 minutes throughout each ride subjects consumed 250 milliliters of either Accelerade, a carb-only sports drink with the same number of total calories as Accelerade, a carb-only sports drink with the same amount of carbohydrate as Accelerade but fewer calories, or a noncaloric flavored placebo. Exercise sessions were repeated every five to ten days until each cyclist had used each of the four beverages. Measurements of muscle damage were taken before and after cycling. In addition, postexercise muscle function was assessed one day after each exercise session by recording the maximum number of leg extensions the subjects could perform. On average, cyclists exhibited significantly lower levels of muscle damage and were able to perform significantly more leg extensions after riding with Accelerade than with any of the other beverages.

These benefits must have come from the protein content of Accelerade, because the other sports drinks tested were otherwise identical, except that one was matched for Accelerade's carbohydrate level and the other for Accelerade's total calorie level (meaning it had more carbohydrate than Accelerade). The advantage of reducing muscle damage during running is that it results in faster performance recovery, or better performance in the next workout, as was demonstrated by the leg extension test in this particular experiment. Although no long-term studies have yet been done, a very likely long-term implication of consuming protein during workouts is faster and greater fitness gains due to consistently better performance in workouts. It could even enable athletes to handle a greater training workload with a lower risk of injury.

Researchers are still trying to figure out exactly how protein consumption reduces muscle damage during exercise. The simplest explanation is that protein provides an extra source of direct energy that substitutes for muscle protein. Exercise scientists now recognize that the body relies far more heavily on protein for energy during intense and prolonged exercise than was previously thought. Under normal circumstances, most of this protein is taken from muscle cells, resulting in muscle damage. But it's possible that food protein consumed during exercise spares muscle protein. Another possibility is that the elevated blood amino acid levels that occur when protein is consumed during exercise act as a brain signal that reduces muscle protein breakdown.

The brain might also mediate the performance benefits associated with protein consumption during exercise. One potential mechanism involves interleukin-6 (IL-6), which, as you may recall from previous chapters, is an important cytokine, or immune system agent, that plays a variety of crucial roles in coordinating the body's response to tissue trauma and stress. IL-6 is known to leak from damaged muscle cells during exercise and circulate to the brain. Increasing IL-6 levels in the brain is also known to hasten fatigue during exercise. The pain associated with muscle damage is another possible link between reduced muscle damage and increased performance that would certainly involve the brain.

Accelerade (now owned by Cadbury Schweppes) is still the only sports drink containing a proven-beneficial amount of protein. (There's a patent on that four-to-one ratio.) Based on the existing science, I recommend that you at least try it. Not every runner reacts well to it. The whey protein content produces uncomfortable gas in a small fraction of runners. But if you like the taste and seem to react well to Accelerade, continue using it in every workout during which you would normally use a sports drink—at least until the patent expires and other, copycat carb-protein sports drinks become available!

Conventional wisdom: Consume plenty of carbohydrate during your long runs.

Brain training wisdom: Do some of your long runs without taking in energy to stimulate better training adaptations.

Consuming carbohydrate during running is proven to substantially increase the amount of time a runner can continue running before exhaustion occurs and to increase the pace a runner can sustain for a fixed distance or duration exceeding one hour. It even enhances performance in high-intensity interval workouts lasting less than an hour. These proven facts represent another reason (besides sodium content) that sports drinks, which usually contain 6–8 percent carbohydrate, are preferable fueling choices to water during running.

Given the established performance-boosting effect of carbohydrate, you might assume it would be a good idea to use a sports drink during every run lasting an hour or longer and during all high-intensity interval workouts (in which drinking should occur during the slow, active recovery periods between intervals rather than during the high-speed intervals themselves). I myself have made this very recommendation in print more than once. But I changed my mind after I encountered new research suggesting that intentionally underfueling the body during running workouts may trigger a more pronounced fitness-boosting adaptive response than heeding the traditional advice to load up on carbs.

The rationale for this approach centers on interleukin-6. Again, large amounts of IL-6 are released into the bloodstream by the muscles and the brain during exercise and travel to organs throughout the body. IL-6 is believed to facilitate many of the body's adaptations to exercise training, ranging from increased fat-burning capacity and greater resistance to muscle damage to improved cognitive function.

The primary trigger for IL-6 release during exercise is glycogen depletion. So it follows that training in a glycogen-depleted state will tend to produce stronger training adaptations (of certain kinds, anyway) than training in a glycogen-replete state. Studies have shown that the muscles produce much less IL-6 when carbohydrate is consumed during exercise. Therefore, it may be beneficial for runners and other endurance athletes to intentionally underfuel themselves in some workouts so that they produce more IL-6 and stimulate greater training adaptations. It is also known that athletes burn more fat when they do not consume carbohydrate during training, and in the long term become more efficient fat burners, thus increasing their raw endurance.

In light of these facts, it's reasonable to ask whether runners should not underfuel themselves in *every* workout. This would be going too far, I believe, because there are disadvantages associated with consistently training in a glycogen-depleted state, and there are advantages to training in a glycogen-replete state. Studies have shown that athletes who consistently consume carbohydrate during exercise are able to handle higher training loads than those who don't, due to enhanced recovery. Also, athletes are able to perform at a higher level when they consume carbohydrate during training. Going 5 percent faster or farther in carbohydrate-fueled workouts will itself trigger greater training adaptations of certain kinds than going 5 percent slower or shorter in underfueled workouts.

Consequently, the best training recipe is probably a mixture of fully fueled and underfueled workouts. What constitutes the optimal balance between these two workout types is still unknown. You may need to experiment to find out what works best for you. I now carry Accelerade, containing 6 percent carbohydrate (and 1.5 percent protein), during every other weekly long run, to maximize performance, and electrolyte-fortified water with no carbohydrate on alternate weeks, to maximize adaptations associated with IL-6 release.

One thing is certain, though: You should always *compete* in a glycogen-replete state and consume plenty of carbohydrate during longer races. In workouts it pays to often make things tough on your body by training in a low-glycogen state. But in competition you want to give your muscles every possible advantage.

A SUMMARY OF BRAIN TRAINING FUELING GUIDELINES

- Drink only when you're thirsty during running. But don't allow your thirst to build—that is, drink as soon as you feel the urge and as often as you feel the urge. Never force yourself to drink more than is comfortable.
- Drink during runs lasting longer than one hour and during the recovery periods in shorter, high-intensity interval workouts.
- When performance counts, use a sports drink instead of water. Its electrolyte content enhances hydration and its carbohydrate content provides an extra source of energy and stimulates a brain signal that boosts performance.
- Consider using a carbohydrate-protein sports drink (Accelerade) instead of a conventional sports drink to promote faster recovery from workouts and perhaps greater long-term fitness gains.
- Consider using water or an electrolyte-fortified water instead of a sports drink during some of your long runs to increase the physiological stress of these runs in ways that will enhance your body's adaptations to them.

PART ◆ II

INTRODUCTION

More than once in Part I of this book I talked about the need for runners to customize their training to their individual needs and about the importance of training responsively—that is, planning workouts "in pencil" and being willing and ready to change them on the spot based on how one feels when it comes time to do that particular workout. In light of this, it might surprise you that Part II of this book presents a selection of complete training plans, which by their very nature are neither individually customized nor planned in pencil. Have I contradicted myself? Not quite.

For two reasons, I feel quite comfortable in offering the following brain training plans and equally confident that you will benefit greatly from using them. First, a high degree of individual customization only becomes important in training after you are already taking advantage of the universal best practices that work for everyone. Most runners have a long way to go in this regard. And I can count on two hands the number of runners who are (at the time of this writing) taking full advantage of the brain training methods upon which the following training plans are based. So I'm pretty sure that whichever brain training plan you choose to follow will give you better results than your past training has, even if you have to wait until you've gathered some experience in brain training to further customize it for your individual needs.

This point brings me to the second reason I feel good about giving you the brain training plans detailed in the next three chapters. Throughout this book I have taken pains to provide the tools you will need to train responsively and customize your training, regardless of which training plan you follow. As a result, you now know all you need to know to take a responsive approach to executing my brain training plans and to modify them later based on how you respond to them—or, in other words, to effectively create your own brain training plans.

So, then: The next four chapters present twelve training plans that are based entirely on the brain training system described in the previous chapters. There are three training plans culminating in peak races at each of four distances: 5K, 10K, half marathon, and marathon. Each training plan is classified as Level 1, Level 2, or Level 3. The Level 1 plans are low-volume plans appropriate for beginning and casual runners; the Level 2 plans are moderate-volume plans that are appropriate for most competitive runners; and the Level 3 plans are high-volume plans that are appropriate for highly competitive runners who are already quite fit.

All of the detailed information you need to choose and follow one of these plans is contained in the following chapters. First I would like to highlight some of the general features that are common to every plan.

Four Phases

Each plan is divided into four phases: Base, Build 1, Build 2, and Peak. The phase durations (and total plan durations) differ by peak race distance. The 5K training plans are the shortest at sixteen weeks. The marathon plans are the longest at twenty-four weeks.

One Rest Day per Week

Workouts are planned for six days of every week in the Level 1, 2, and 3 training plans. I believe that a day of complete rest is advisable for all competitive runners, and is needed by high-volume trainers most of all. On the flipside, I believe that nobody should exercise less often than six days per week, if only for the sake of the proven health benefits that come with daily exertion.

Recovery Weeks

In each plan, the training volume is reduced every third or fourth week to facilitate the absorption of and recovery from previous training and to prevent overtraining fatigue.

Three Key Workouts per Week

The workout schedule in each plan includes three key workouts per week: a speed run on Wednesdays, an intensive endurance run on Fridays, and an extensive endurance workout on Sundays. Shaded boxes indicate key workouts.

Tune-up Races/Breakthrough Workouts

Each training plan includes at least one tune-up race that also serves as a breakthrough workout. These events serve to stimulate a big leap forward in fitness and to increase the amount of pain you can endure in your peak race.

Note: In the likely event that you cannot always find an actual road race of the appropriate distance on the day a tune-up race is scheduled in a brain training plan, perform a solo time trial of the same distance on a measured course instead.

Target Pace–Based Workout Prescriptions

All running workouts include pace prescriptions based on the target pace method described in chapter 4. The only exceptions are some hill repetition workouts in which short intervals are performed at a "relaxed sprint speed."

Cross-Training

All twelve training plans include two scheduled resistance workouts per week. The length of these workouts varies somewhat by plan level. A dynamic flexibility/mobility warm-up precedes each workout involving 10K-pace or faster running. There is one optional cardio cross-training workout per week in the Level 1 and 2 plans and four such workouts per week in the Level 3 plans.

Proprioceptive Cues

A proprioceptive cue is suggested for each week of training. The specific cue named is merely a suggestion; you are free to choose any proprioceptive cue at any time. But I strongly recommend that you use a proprioceptive cue in every run.

Technique Drills

A pair of technique drills is tacked on to the end of Tuesday's run each week throughout all twelve training plans.

Built-in Flexibility

The plans feature inherent flexibility in terms of running volume and amount of cross-training. Recovery workouts are prescribed with broad duration parameters to enable you to use subjective feedback to determine the most appropriate duration in each case. Use the recovery workout guidelines in chapter 7.

As mentioned above, there is one optional cardio cross-training workout per week in the Level 1 and 2 plans. Their duration is flexible. The Level 3 plans at all four peak race distances include four optional recovery workouts—which may be either runs or nonimpact cardio cross-training workouts—per week. These are also flexible in duration. It is up to you to decide whether and how to do the optional workouts within these parameters. Use your key workout performances to determine whether you are doing too much. If your key workout performances are not what they should be, you should probably cut back on the number of optional workouts you're doing.

Note that corrective stretches and strengthening exercises, as described in chapter 9, are not prescribed within the plans. They are entirely optional, depending on your needs. If one or more of these stretches or strengthening exercises are needed to prevent injuries, add them to your scheduled resistance workouts or find other times to do them.

Responsive Training

Remember to practice responsive training in key workouts as you proceed through any of these training plans. If on any given day you find, through subjective feedback, that your body is not prepared to handle the key workout that's scheduled, replace it with an easier alternative workout using the guidelines in chapter 7.

Some Workouts Prescribed by Duration, Others by Distance

You'll note that some running workouts (and parts thereof) are prescribed by distance, while others are prescribed by duration. This inconsistency results from the fact that it is simply more practical or sensible to prescribe workouts by one standard or the other in certain cases. As a general rule, workouts are prescribed by duration when my main concern is to provide a uniform training stimulus for all runners, regardless of their current target pace level. Distance is typically used when the workout is focused on race-specific preparation, since races are run by distance, of course, not duration.

CHAPTER 11

BRAIN TRAINING PLANS: 5K

The 5K race distance is the most popular in terms of the number of events and participants. This fact is not surprising, since the 5K is the shortest of the traditional road race distances and is therefore accessible to the largest number of runners. But while the 5K distance is ideal for beginners and casual runners, it's also a great distance for runners of higher experience levels whose gift of speed happens to be greater than their gift of endurance, and a nice change of pace—literally—for runners who normally peak for longer races.

This chapter presents three brain training plans culminating in a 5K peak race. Each plan is sixteen weeks long and includes a 5K tune-up race/breakthrough workout at the end of Week 12 in addition to the 5K peak race at the end of Week 16. The sixteen weeks are divided into four four-week phases: Base, Build 1, Build 2, and Peak. Weeks 4, 8, and 12 are reduced-volume recovery weeks, and Week 16 is a reduced-volume taper week.

There are three key workouts per week in each plan: a speed workout on Wednesdays, an intensive endurance workout on Fridays, and an extensive endurance workout on Sundays. Key workouts are indicated by shaded boxes.

LEVEL 1

Use this plan if you are most comfortable with a 5K training plan that features four runs per week and a maximum run distance of 6.5 miles. The plan also includes two resistance workouts per week and one optional nonimpact cardio cross-training workout.

Base Phase

Training objectives: Build aerobic capacity and endurance, increase injury resistance, and increase muscle activation capacity

WEEK 1   ♦   Proprioceptive Cue: Falling Forward

MONDAY	Off	

TUESDAY	**Base Run + Drills**
	    Run 2 miles @ base pace
	    Running No Arms 20 seconds
	    One-Leg Hop 20 seconds	

WEDNESDAY	**Hill Repetitions**
	    Dynamic stretching warm-up
	    1-mile warm-up @ recovery pace
	    1×30-second hill repetition @ relaxed sprint speed
	    1-mile cool-down @ recovery pace	

THURSDAY	<u>Optional Nonimpact</u>
	<u>Cardio Cross-Training Workout</u>
	20–30 minutes @ recovery pace
	(You may break this workout into a
	10–15-minute warm-up before and a
	10–15-minute cool-down after your
	resistance workout.)
		Resistance Workout
		    1 set each
		    Lying Hip Abduction
		    Cook Hip Lift
		    Kneeling Overhead Draw-In
		    Knee Fall-Out
		    Squat Jump

FRIDAY	**Fartlek Run**
	    Dynamic stretching warm-up
	    Run 2 miles @ base pace w/2×30-second intervals @ 1-mile pace
	        "sprinkled in"	

SATURDAY	**Resistance Workout** *1 set each* Lying Hip Abduction Cook Hip Lift Kneeling Overhead Draw-In Knee Fall-Out Broad Jump
SUNDAY	**Base Run** Run 3 miles @ base pace

WEEK 2 ◆ Proprioceptive Cue: Navel to Spine

MONDAY	Off
TUESDAY	**Base Run + Drills** Run 2.5 miles @ base pace High Knees 2 × 20 seconds Bounding 2 × 20 seconds
WEDNESDAY	**Hill Repetitions** Dynamic stretching warm-up 1-mile warm-up @ recovery pace 4 × 30-second hill repetitions @ relaxed sprint speed w/2-minute active recoveries 1-mile cool-down @ recovery pace

THURSDAY	Optional Nonimpact Cardio Cross-Training Workout 20–30 minutes @ recovery pace	**Resistance Workout** *2 sets each* Lying Hip Abduction Cook Hip Lift Kneeling Overhead Draw-In Knee Fall-Out Split Squat Jump

FRIDAY	**Fartlek Run** Dynamic stretching warm-up Run 2.5 miles @ base pace w/4 × 30-second intervals @ 1-mile pace "sprinkled in"
SATURDAY	**Resistance Workout** *2 sets each* Lying Hip Abduction Cook Hip Lift Kneeling Overhead Draw-In Knee Fall-Out Wall Jump
SUNDAY	**Base Run** Run 4 miles @ base pace

WEEK 3 ◆ Proprioceptive Cue: Running on Water

MONDAY	Off
TUESDAY	**Base Run + Drills** Run 3 miles @ base pace Stiff-Legged Run 2 × 20 seconds Running No Arms 2 × 20 seconds
WEDNESDAY	**Hill Repetitions** Dynamic stretching warm-up 1-mile warm-up @ recovery pace 6 × 30-second hill repetitions @ relaxed sprint speed w/2-minute active recoveries 1-mile cool-down @ recovery pace

THURSDAY	<u>Optional Nonimpact Cardio Cross-Training Workout</u> 20–30 minutes @ recovery pace	**Resistance Workout** *3 sets each* Lying Hip Abduction Cook Hip Lift Kneeling Overhead Draw-In Knee Fall-Out Squat Jump

FRIDAY	**Fartlek Run** Dynamic stretching warm-up Run 3 miles @ base pace w/6 × 30-second intervals @ 1-mile pace "sprinkled in"
SATURDAY	**Resistance Workout** *3 sets each* Lying Hip Abduction Cook Hip Lift Kneeling Overhead Draw-In Knee Fall-Out Broad Jump
SUNDAY	**Base Run** Run 5 miles @ base pace

WEEK 4 (Recovery) ♦ Proprioceptive Cue: Pulling the Road

MONDAY	Off
TUESDAY	**Base Run + Drills** Run 3 miles @ base pace One-Leg Hop 20 seconds High Knees 20 seconds
WEDNESDAY	**Hill Repetitions** Dynamic stretching warm-up 1-mile warm-up @ recovery pace 4 × 30-second hill repetitions @ relaxed sprint speed w/2-minute active recoveries 1-mile cool-down @ recovery pace

THURSDAY	<u>Optional Nonimpact Cardio Cross-Training Workout</u> 20–30 minutes @ recovery pace	**Resistance Workout** *1 set each* Single-Leg Squat Oblique Bridge Lying Draw-In w/Hip Flexion Quadruped *2 sets each* Lying Hip Abduction Cook Hip Lift Kneeling Overhead Draw-In Knee Fall-Out Single-Leg Squat Jump

FRIDAY	**Fartlek Run** Dynamic stretching warm-up Run 3 miles @ base pace w/4 × 30-second intervals @ 1-mile pace "sprinkled in"
SATURDAY	**Resistance Workout** *1 set each* Single-Leg Squat Oblique Bridge Lying Draw-In w/Hip Flexion Quadruped

SATURDAY (continued)	**Resistance Workout** *2 sets each* Lying Hip Abduction Cook Hip Lift Kneeling Overhead Draw-In Knee Fall-Out Wall Jump
SUNDAY	**Base Run** Run 4 miles @ base pace

Build 1 Phase

Training objectives: Continue to increase aerobic capacity and endurance; increase fatigue resistance at 3,000m pace and marathon pace; begin to develop efficiency at 5K pace

WEEK 5 ◆ Proprioceptive Cue: Scooting

MONDAY	Off	
TUESDAY	**Base Run + Drills** Run 3 miles @ base pace High Knees 20 seconds Bounding 20 seconds	
WEDNESDAY	**400m Intervals @ 3,000m Pace** Dynamic stretching warm-up 1-mile warm-up @ recovery pace 3 × 400m intervals @ 3,000m pace w/3-minute active recoveries 1-mile cool-down @ recovery pace	
THURSDAY	Optional Nonimpact Cardio Cross-Training Workout 20–30 minutes @ recovery pace	**Resistance Workout** *2 sets each* Single-Leg Squat Oblique Bridge Lying Draw-In w/Hip Flexion Quadruped *1 set each* Lying Hip Abduction Cook Hip Lift Kneeling Overhead Draw-In Knee Fall-Out Single-Leg Squat Jump
FRIDAY	**30-30 Intervals** Dynamic stretching warm-up 1-mile warm-up @ recovery pace 8 × 30 seconds @ 5 K pace w/30-second active recoveries 1-mile cool-down @ recovery pace	

SATURDAY	**Resistance Workout**
	2 sets each
	Single-Leg Squat
	Oblique Bridge
	Lying Draw-In w/Hip Flexion
	Quadruped
	1 set each
	Lying Hip Abduction
	Cook Hip Lift
	Kneeling Overhead Draw-In
	Knee Fall-Out
	Wall Jump
SUNDAY	**Marathon-Pace Run**
	Run 4 miles @ marathon pace

WEEK 6 ♦ Proprioceptive Cue: Pounding the Ground

MONDAY	Off
TUESDAY	**Base Run + Drills** Run 4 miles @ base pace Stiff-Legged Run 20 seconds Running No Arms 20 seconds
WEDNESDAY	**400m Intervals @ 3,000m Pace** Dynamic stretching warm-up 1-mile warm-up @ recovery pace 5 × 400m intervals @ 3,000m pace w/3-minute active recoveries 1-mile cool-down @ recovery pace
THURSDAY	Optional Nonimpact Cardio Cross-Training Workout 20–30 minutes @ recovery pace <td>**Resistance Workout** *3 sets each* Single-Leg Squat Oblique Bridge Lying Draw-In w/Hip Flexion Quadruped *2 sets* Squat Jump</td>
FRIDAY	**30-30 Intervals** Dynamic stretching warm-up 1-mile warm-up @ recovery pace 10 × 30 seconds @ 5 K pace w/30-second active recoveries 1-mile cool-down @ recovery pace
SATURDAY	**Resistance Workout** *3 sets each* Single-Leg Squat Oblique Bridge Lying Draw-In w/Hip Flexion Quadruped *2 sets* Single-Leg Squat Jump
SUNDAY	**Marathon-Pace Run** Run 5 miles @ marathon pace

WEEK 7 ◆ Proprioceptive Cue: Driving the Thigh

MONDAY	Off	

TUESDAY	**Base Run + Drills**
	   Run 5 miles @ base pace
	   Steep Hill Sprints 20 seconds
	   One-Leg Hop 20 seconds	

WEDNESDAY	**400m Intervals @ 3,000m Pace**
	   Dynamic stretching warm-up
	   1-mile warm-up @ recovery pace
	   7 × 400m intervals @ 3,000m pace w/3-minute active recoveries
	   1-mile cool-down @ recovery pace	

THURSDAY	<u>Optional Nonimpact
	Cardio Cross-Training Workout</u>
	20–30 minutes @ recovery pace
		Resistance Workout
		   2 sets each
		   Single-Leg Squat
		   Oblique Bridge
		   Lying Draw-In w/Hip Flexion
		   Quadruped
		   Split Squat Jump
		
		   1 set each
		   Box Lunge
		   Stability Ball Leg Curl
		   Forearms to Palms Bridge
		   Dead Bug

FRIDAY	**30-30 Intervals**
	   Dynamic stretching warm-up
	   1-mile warm-up @ recovery pace
	   12 × 30 seconds @ 5 K pace w/30-second active recoveries
	   1-mile cool-down @ recovery pace	

SATURDAY	**Resistance Workout**
	   2 sets each
	   Single-Leg Squat
	   Oblique Bridge
	   Lying Draw-In w/Hip Flexion
	   Quadruped
	   Single-Leg Box Jump	

(continued)

WEEK 7 ◆ Proprioceptive Cue: Driving the Thigh
(continued)

SATURDAY (continued)	**Resistance Workout** *1 set each* Box Lunge Stability Ball Leg Curl Forearms to Palms Bridge Dead Bug
SUNDAY	**Marathon-Pace Run** Run 6 miles @ marathon pace

WEEK 8 (Recovery) ◆ Proprioceptive Cue: Floppy Feet

MONDAY	Off
TUESDAY	**Base Run + Drills** Run 4 miles @ base pace High Knees 20 seconds Bounding 20 seconds
WEDNESDAY	**400m Intervals @ 3,000m Pace** Dynamic stretching warm-up 1-mile warm-up @ recovery pace 6 × 400m intervals @ 3,000m pace w/3-minute active recoveries 1-mile cool-down @ recovery pace
THURSDAY	<u>Optional Nonimpact</u> <u>Cardio Cross-Training Workout</u> 20–30 minutes @ recovery pace **Resistance Workout** *1 set each* Single-Leg Squat Oblique Bridge Lying Draw-In w/Hip Flexion Quadruped *2 sets each* Box Lunge Stability Ball Leg Curl Forearms to Palms Bridge Dead Bug Broad Jump
FRIDAY	**30-30 Intervals** Dynamic stretching warm-up 1-mile warm-up @ recovery pace 10 × 30 seconds @ 5 K pace w/30-second active recoveries 1-mile cool-down @ recovery pace
SATURDAY	**Resistance Workout** *1 set each* Single-Leg Squat Oblique Bridge Lying Draw-In w/Hip Flexion Quadruped

(continued)

WEEK 8 (Recovery) ♦ Proprioceptive Cue: Floppy Feet
(continued)

SATURDAY
(continued)
	Resistance Workout
	   2 sets each
	   Box Lunge
	   Stability Ball Leg Curl
	   Forearms to Palms Bridge
	   Dead Bug
	   Wall Jump

SUNDAY	**Marathon-Pace Run** Run 5 miles @ marathon pace

Build 2 Phase

Training objectives: Increase fatigue resistance at 3,000m pace and half-marathon pace; continue to build efficiency at 5K pace

WEEK 9 ◆ Proprioceptive Cue: Butt Squeeze

MONDAY	Off
TUESDAY	**Base Run + Drills** Run 4.5 miles @ base pace Stiff-Legged Run 20 seconds Running No Arms 20 seconds
WEDNESDAY	**600m Intervals @ 3,000m Pace** Dynamic stretching warm-up 1-mile warm-up @ recovery pace 4 × 600m intervals @ 3,000m pace w/3-minute active recoveries 1-mile cool-down @ recovery pace
THURSDAY	<u>Optional Nonimpact</u> <u>Cardio Cross-Training Workout</u> 20–30 minutes @ recovery pace **Resistance Workout** *3 sets each* Box Lunge Stability Ball Leg Curl Forearms to Palms Bridge Dead Bug Wall Jump
FRIDAY	**60-60 Intervals** Dynamic stretching warm-up 1-mile warm-up @ recovery pace 6 × 1 minute @ 5K pace w/1-minute active recoveries 1-mile cool-down @ recovery pace
SATURDAY	**Resistance Workout** *3 sets each* Box Lunge Forearms to Palms Bridge Stability Ball Leg Curl Dead Bug Single-Leg Box Jump
SUNDAY	**Tempo Run** 1-mile warm-up @ recovery pace 3 miles @ half-marathon pace 1-mile cool-down @ recovery pace

WEEK 10 ♦ Proprioceptive Cue: Feeling Symmetry

MONDAY	Off
TUESDAY	**Base Run + Drills** Run 5 miles @ base pace Stiff-Legged Run 20 seconds Running No Arms 20 seconds
WEDNESDAY	**600m Intervals @ 3,000m Pace** Dynamic stretching warm-up 1-mile warm-up @ recovery pace 5 × 600m intervals @ 3,000m pace w/3-minute active recoveries 1-mile cool-down @ recovery pace

THURSDAY	<u>Optional Nonimpact</u>
	<u>Cardio Cross-Training Workout</u>
	20–30 minutes @ recovery pace **Resistance Workout**
	   1 set each
	   Lying Hip Abduction
	   Single-Leg Squat
	   Box Lunge
	   Stability Ball Leg Curl
	   Squat Jump

FRIDAY	**60-60 Intervals** Dynamic stretching warm-up 1-mile warm-up @ recovery pace 7 × 1 minute @ 5K pace w/1-minute active recoveries 1-mile cool-down @ recovery pace
SATURDAY	**Resistance Workout** *1 set each* Cook Hip Lift Oblique Bridge Forearms to Palms Bridge Stability Ball Leg Curl Split Squat Jump
SUNDAY	**Tempo Run** 1-mile warm-up @ recovery pace 3.5 miles @ half-marathon pace 1-mile cool-down @ recovery pace

WEEK 11 ◆ Proprioceptive Cue: Axle Between the Knees

MONDAY	Off
TUESDAY	**Base Run + Drills** Run 5.5 miles @ base pace Steep Hill Sprints 20 seconds One-Leg Hop 20 seconds
WEDNESDAY	**600m Intervals @ 3,000m Pace** Dynamic stretching warm-up 1-mile warm-up @ recovery pace 6 × 600m intervals @ 3,000m pace w/3-minute active recoveries 1-mile cool-down @ recovery pace

THURSDAY	<u>Optional Nonimpact</u> <u>Cardio Cross-Training Workout</u>
	20–30 minutes @ recovery pace **Resistance Workout**
	    1 set each
	    Lying Hip Abduction
	    Single-Leg Squat
	    Box Lunge
	    Stability Ball Leg Curl
	    Single-Leg Squat Jump

FRIDAY	**60-60 Intervals** Dynamic stretching warm-up 1-mile warm-up @ recovery pace 8 × 1 minute @ 5K pace w/1-minute active recoveries 1-mile cool-down @ recovery pace
SATURDAY	**Resistance Workout** *1 set each* Cook Hip Lift Oblique Bridge Forearms to Palms Bridge Stability Ball Leg Curl Broad Jump
SUNDAY	**Tempo Run** 1-mile warm-up @ recovery pace 4 miles @ half-marathon pace 1-mile cool-down @ recovery pace

WEEK 12 (Recovery) ◆ Proprioceptive Cue: Running Against a Wall

MONDAY	Off	
TUESDAY	**Base Run + Drills** Run 4.5 miles @ base pace High Knees 20 seconds Bounding 20 seconds	
WEDNESDAY	**600m Intervals @ 3,000m Pace** Dynamic stretching warm-up 1-mile warm-up @ recovery pace 4 × 600m intervals @ 3,000m pace w/3-minute active recoveries 1-mile cool-down @ recovery pace	
THURSDAY	<u>Optional Nonimpact</u> <u>Cardio Cross-Training Workout</u> 20–30 minutes @ recovery pace	**Resistance Workout** *1 set each* Lying Hip Abduction Single-Leg Squat Box Lunge Stability Ball Leg Curl Wall Jump
FRIDAY	**60-60 Intervals** Dynamic stretching warm-up 1-mile warm-up @ recovery pace 6 × 1 minute @ 5K pace w/1-minute active recoveries 1-mile cool-down @ recovery pace	
SATURDAY	**Resistance Workout** *1 set each* Cook Hip Lift Oblique Bridge Forearms to Palms Bridge Stability Ball Leg Curl	
SUNDAY	**5K Tune-up Race or Time Trial** Dynamic stretching warm-up 1-mile warm-up @ recovery pace 5K tune-up race or time trial 1-mile cool-down @ recovery pace	

Peak Phase

Training objectives: Achieve peak fatigue resistance and efficiency at 5K pace; adapt and recover for peak race day

WEEK 13 ◆ Proprioceptive Cue: Falling Forward

MONDAY	Off	
TUESDAY	**Base Run + Drills** Run 5.5 miles @ base pace High Knees 20 seconds Bounding 20 seconds	
WEDNESDAY	**Mixed Intervals** Dynamic stretching warm-up 1-mile warm-up @ recovery pace 1×1 mile @ 10K pace, 2-minute active recovery 1×1K @ 5K pace, 2-minute active recovery 1×600m @ 3,000m pace, 2-minute active recovery 1×300m @ 1-mile pace 1-mile cool-down @ recovery pace	
THURSDAY	Optional Nonimpact Cardio Cross-Training Workout 20–30 minutes @ recovery pace	**Resistance Workout** *1 set each* Lying Hip Abduction Single-Leg Squat Box Lunge Stability Ball Leg Curl Wall Jump
FRIDAY	**1K Intervals @ 5K Pace** Dynamic stretching warm-up 1-mile warm-up @ recovery pace 3×1K @ 5K pace w/2-minute active recoveries 1-mile cool-down @ recovery pace	

(continued)

WEEK 13 ♦ Proprioceptive Cue: Falling Forward
(continued)

SATURDAY	**Resistance Workout**
	1 set each
	Cook Hip Lift
	Oblique Bridge
	Forearms to Palms Bridge
	Stability Ball Leg Curl
	Single-Leg Box Jump
SUNDAY	**Tempo Run**
	1-mile warm-up @ recovery pace
	3 miles @ 10K pace
	1-mile cool-down @ recovery pace

WEEK 14 ♦ Proprioceptive Cue: Navel to Spine

MONDAY	Off
TUESDAY	**Base Run + Drills** Run 6 miles @ base pace Stiff-Legged Run 20 seconds Running No Arms 20 seconds
WEDNESDAY	**Mixed Intervals** Dynamic stretching warm-up 1-mile warm-up @ recovery pace 1×1 mile @ 10K pace, 90-second active recovery 1×1K @ 5K pace, 90-second active recovery 1×600m @ 3,000m pace, 90-second active recovery 1×300m @ 1-mile pace 1-mile cool-down @ recovery pace

THURSDAY	<u>Optional Nonimpact</u> <u>Cardio Cross-Training Workout</u> 20–30 minutes @ recovery pace	**Resistance Workout** *1 set each* Lying Hip Abduction Single-Leg Squat Box Lunge Stability Ball Leg Curl Squat Jump

FRIDAY	**1K Intervals @ 5K Pace** Dynamic stretching warm-up 1-mile warm-up @ recovery pace 4×1K @ 5K pace w/2-minute active recoveries 1-mile cool-down @ recovery pace
SATURDAY	**Resistance Workout** *1 set each* Cook Hip Lift Oblique Bridge Forearms to Palms Bridge Stability Ball Leg Curl Split Squat Jump
SUNDAY	**Tempo Run** 1-mile warm-up @ recovery pace 3.5 miles @ 10K pace 1-mile cool-down @ recovery pace

WEEK 15 ◆ Proprioceptive Cue: Running on Water

MONDAY	Off
TUESDAY	**Base Run + Drills** Run 5 miles @ base pace Steep Hill Sprints 20 seconds One-Leg Hop 20 seconds
WEDNESDAY	**Mixed Intervals** Dynamic stretching warm-up 1-mile warm-up @ recovery pace 1×1 mile @ 10K pace, 1-minute active recovery 1×1K @ 5K pace, 1-minute active recovery 1×600m @ 3,000m pace, 1-minute active recovery 1×300m @ 1-mile pace 1-mile cool-down @ recovery pace

THURSDAY	<u>Optional Nonimpact</u> <u>Cardio Cross-Training Workout</u> 20–30 minutes @ recovery pace	**Resistance Workout** *1 set each* Lying Hip Abduction Single-Leg Squat Box Lunge Stability Ball Leg Curl Single-Leg Squat Jump

FRIDAY	**1K Intervals @ 5K Pace** Dynamic stretching warm-up 1-mile warm-up @ recovery pace 4×1K @ 5K pace w/90-second active recoveries 1-mile cool-down @ recovery pace
SATURDAY	**Resistance Workout** *1 set each* Cook Hip Lift Oblique Bridge Forearms to Palms Bridge Stability Ball Leg Curl Broad Jump
SUNDAY	**Tempo Run** 1-mile warm-up @ recovery pace 3 miles @ 10K pace 1-mile cool-down @ recovery pace

WEEK 16 (Taper) ◆ Proprioceptive Cue: Your Choice

MONDAY	Off
TUESDAY	**Base Run** Run 4.5 miles @ base pace
WEDNESDAY	**Mixed Intervals** Dynamic stretching warm-up 1-mile warm-up @ recovery pace 1 × 1K @ 5K pace, 1-minute active recovery 1 × 600m @ 3,000m pace, 1-minute active recovery 1 × 300m @ 1-mile pace 1-mile cool-down @ recovery pace
THURSDAY	<u>Optional Nonimpact</u> <u>Cardio Cross-Training Workout</u> 20–30 minutes @ recovery pace **Resistance Workout** *1 set each* Lying Hip Abduction Single-Leg Squat Box Lunge Stability Ball Leg Curl
FRIDAY	**1K Intervals @ 5K Pace** Dynamic stretching warm-up 1-mile warm-up @ recovery pace 2 × 1K @ 5K pace w/2-minute active recovery 1-mile cool-down @ recovery pace
SATURDAY	Off
SUNDAY	**5K Peak Race** Dynamic stretching warm-up 1-mile warm-up @ recovery pace 5K peak race 1-mile cool-down @ recovery pace

LEVEL 2

Use this plan if you are most comfortable with a 5K training plan that features six runs per week and a maximum run distance of ten miles. The plan also includes two resistance workouts and one optional nonimpact endurance workout per week.

Base Phase

Training objectives: Build aerobic capacity and endurance, increase injury resistance, and increase muscle activation capacity

WEEK 1 ◆ Proprioceptive Cue: Falling Forward

MONDAY	Off	
TUESDAY	**Base Run + Drills** Run 5 miles @ base pace Running No Arms 20 seconds One-Leg Hop 20 seconds	
WEDNESDAY	**Hill Repetitions** Dynamic stretching warm-up 2-mile warm-up @ recovery pace 2 × 30-second hill repetitions @ relaxed sprint speed w/2-minute active recovery 2-mile cool-down @ recovery pace	
THURSDAY	**Base Run + Drills** Run 5 miles @ base pace Running No Arms 20 seconds One-Leg Hop 20 seconds or Nonimpact Cardio Cross-Training Workout 20–40 minutes @ recovery pace	**Resistance Workout** *1 set each* Lying Hip Abduction Cook Hip Lift Kneeling Overhead Draw-In Knee Fall-Out Squat Jump
FRIDAY	**Fartlek Run** Dynamic stretching warm-up Run 5 miles @ base pace w/2 × 30-second intervals @ 1-mile pace "sprinkled in"	

SATURDAY	Base Run + Drills	Resistance Workout
	Run 5 miles @ base pace Running No Arms 20 seconds One-Leg Hop 20 seconds	*1 set each* Lying Hip Abduction Cook Hip Lift Kneeling Overhead Draw-In Knee Fall-Out Broad Jump
SUNDAY	Base Run	
	Run 6 miles @ base pace	

WEEK 2 ◆ Proprioceptive Cue: Navel to Spine

MONDAY	Off	
TUESDAY	**Base Run + Drills** Run 5.5 miles @ base pace High Knees 2×20 seconds Bounding 2×20 seconds	
WEDNESDAY	**Hill Repetitions** Dynamic stretching warm-up 2-mile warm-up @ recovery pace 6×30-second hill repetitions @ relaxed sprint speed w/2-minute active recoveries 2-mile cool-down @ recovery pace	
THURSDAY	**Base Run + Drills** Run 5 miles @ base pace High Knees 2×20 seconds Bounding 2×20 seconds *or* Nonimpact Cardio Cross-Training Workout 20–40 minutes @ recovery pace	**Resistance Workout** *2 sets each* Lying Hip Abduction Cook Hip Lift Kneeling Overhead Draw-In Knee Fall-Out Split Squat Jump
FRIDAY	**Fartlek Run** Dynamic stretching warm-up Run 5.5 miles @ base pace w/6×30-second intervals @ 1-mile pace "sprinkled in"	
SATURDAY	**Base Run + Drills** Run 5 miles @ base pace High Knees 2×20 seconds Bounding 2×20 seconds	**Resistance Workout** *2 sets each* Lying Hip Abduction Cook Hip Lift Kneeling Overhead Draw-In Knee Fall-Out Wall Jump
SUNDAY	**Base Run** Run 7 miles @ base pace	

WEEK 3 ◆ Proprioceptive Cue: Running on Water

MONDAY	Off
TUESDAY	**Base Run + Drills** Run 6 miles @ base pace Stiff-Legged Run 2 × 20 seconds Running No Arms 2 × 20 seconds
WEDNESDAY	**Hill Repetitions** Dynamic stretching warm-up 2-mile warm-up @ recovery pace 8 × 30-second hill repetitions @ relaxed sprint speed 2-mile cool-down @ recovery pace
THURSDAY	**Base Run + Drills** Run 6 miles @ base pace Stiff-Legged Run 2 × 20 seconds Running No Arms 2 × 20 seconds *or* Nonimpact Cardio Cross-Training Workout 20–40 minutes @ recovery pace	**Resistance Workout** *3 sets each* Lying Hip Abduction Cook Hip Lift Kneeling Overhead Draw-In Knee Fall-Out Squat Jump
FRIDAY	**Fartlek Run** Dynamic stretching warm-up Run 6 miles @ base pace w/8 × 30-second intervals @ 1-mile pace "sprinkled in"
SATURDAY	**Base Run + Drills** Run 5 miles @ base pace Stiff-Legged Run 2 × 20 seconds Running No Arms 2 × 20 seconds	**Resistance Workout** *3 sets each* Lying Hip Abduction Cook Hip Lift Kneeling Overhead Draw-In Knee Fall-Out Broad Jump
SUNDAY	**Base Run** Run 8 miles @ base pace

WEEK 4 (Recovery) ◆ Proprioceptive Cue: Pulling the Road

MONDAY	Off	
TUESDAY	**Base Run + Drills** Run 5 miles @ base pace One-Leg Hop 20 seconds High Knees 20 seconds	
WEDNESDAY	**Hill Repetitions** Dynamic stretching warm-up 2-mile warm-up @ recovery pace 6 × 30-second hill repetitions @ relaxed sprint speed w/2-minute active recoveries 2-mile cool-down @ recovery pace	
THURSDAY	**Recovery Run** 2–5 miles @ recovery pace *or* Nonimpact Cardio Cross-Training Workout 20–40 minutes @ recovery pace	**Resistance Workout** *1 set each* Single-Leg Squat Oblique Bridge Lying Draw-In w/Hip Flexion Quadruped *2 sets each* Lying Hip Abduction Cook Hip Lift Kneeling Overhead Draw-In Knee Fall-Out Single-Leg Squat Jump
FRIDAY	**Fartlek Run** Dynamic stretching warm-up Run 5 miles @ base pace w/4 × 30-second intervals @ 1-mile pace "sprinkled in"	
SATURDAY	**Recovery Run** 2–5 miles @ recovery pace	**Resistance Workout** *1 set each* Single-Leg Squat Oblique Bridge Lying Draw-In w/Hip Flexion Quadruped

SATURDAY (continued)	Recovery Run	Resistance Workout *2 sets each* Lying Hip Abduction Cook Hip Lift Kneeling Overhead Draw-In Knee Fall-Out Wall Jump
SUNDAY	**Base Run** Run 5 miles @ base pace	

Build 1 Phase

Training objectives: Continue to increase aerobic capacity and endurance; increase fatigue resistance at 3,000m pace and marathon pace; begin to develop efficiency at 5K pace

WEEK 5 ◆ Proprioceptive Cue: Scooting

MONDAY	Off	
TUESDAY	**Base Run + Drills** Run 6 miles @ base pace High Knees 2 × 20 seconds Bounding 2 × 20 seconds	
WEDNESDAY	**400m Intervals @ 3,000m Pace** Dynamic stretching warm-up 1.5-mile warm-up @ recovery pace 6 × 400m intervals @ 3,000m pace w/3-minute active recoveries 1.5-mile cool-down @ recovery pace	
THURSDAY	**Recovery Run** 2–6 miles @ recovery pace *or* Nonimpact Cardio Cross-Training Workout 20–45 minutes @ recovery pace	**Resistance Workout** *2 sets each* Single-Leg Squat Oblique Bridge Lying Draw-In w/Hip Flexion Quadruped *1 set each* Lying Hip Abduction Cook Hip Lift Kneeling Overhead Draw-In Knee Fall-Out Single-Leg Squat Jump
FRIDAY	**30-30 Intervals** Dynamic stretching warm-up 2-mile warm-up @ recovery pace 10 × 30 seconds @ 5K pace w/30-second active recoveries 2-mile cool-down @ recovery pace	

SATURDAY	**Recovery Run** 2–6 miles @ recovery pace	**Resistance Workout** *2 sets each* Single-Leg Squat Oblique Bridge Lying Draw-In w/Hip Flexion Quadruped *1 set each* Lying Hip Abduction Cook Hip Lift Kneeling Overhead Draw-In Knee Fall-Out Wall Jump
SUNDAY	**Marathon-Pace Run** 1-mile warm-up @ recovery pace 6 miles @ marathon pace 1-mile recovery-pace cool-down	

WEEK 6 ◆ Proprioceptive Cue: Pounding the Ground

MONDAY	Off	
TUESDAY	**Base Run + Drills** Run 6 miles @ base pace Stiff-Legged Run 2 × 20 seconds Running No Arms 2 × 20 seconds	
WEDNESDAY	**400m Intervals @ 3,000m Pace** Dynamic stretching warm-up 1.5-mile warm-up @ recovery pace 8 × 400m intervals @ 3,000m pace w/3-minute active recoveries 1.5-mile cool-down @ recovery pace	
THURSDAY	**Recovery Run** 2–6 miles @ recovery pace *or* Nonimpact Cardio Cross-Training Workout 20–45 minutes @ recovery pace	**Resistance Workout** *3 sets each* Single-Leg Squat Oblique Bridge Lying Draw-In w/Hip Flexion Quadruped *2 sets* Squat Jump
FRIDAY	**30-30 Intervals** Dynamic stretching warm-up 2-mile warm-up @ recovery pace 12 × 30 seconds @ 5K pace w/30-second active recoveries 2-mile cool-down @ recovery pace	
SATURDAY	**Recovery Run** 2–6 miles @ recovery pace	**Resistance Workout** *3 sets each* Single-Leg Squat Oblique Bridge Lying Draw-In w/Hip Flexion Quadruped *2 sets* Single-Leg Squat Jump
SUNDAY	**Marathon-Pace Run** 1-mile warm-up @ recovery pace 7 miles @ marathon pace 1-mile cool-down @ recovery pace	

WEEK 7 ◆ Proprioceptive Cue: Driving the Thigh

MONDAY	Off
TUESDAY	**Base Run + Drills** Run 6 miles @ base pace Steep Hill Sprints 2 × 20 seconds One-Leg Hop 2 × 20 seconds
WEDNESDAY	**400m Intervals @ 3,000m Pace** Dynamic stretching warm-up 1.5-mile warm-up @ recovery pace 10 × 400m intervals @ 3,000m pace w/3-minute active recoveries 1.5-mile cool-down @ recovery pace

THURSDAY	**Recovery Run** 2–6 miles @ recovery pace *or* Nonimpact Cardio Cross-Training Workout 20–45 minutes @ recovery pace	**Resistance Workout** *2 sets each* Single-Leg Squat Oblique Bridge Lying Draw-In w/Hip Flexion Quadruped Split Squat Jump *1 set each* Box Lunge Stability Ball Leg Curl Forearms to Palms Bridge Dead Bug

FRIDAY	**30-30 Intervals** Dynamic stretching warm-up 2-mile warm-up @ recovery pace 16 × 30 seconds @ 5K pace w/30-second active recoveries 2-mile cool-down @ recovery pace

SATURDAY	**Recovery Run** 2–6 miles @ recovery pace	**Resistance Workout** *2 sets each* Single-Leg Squat Oblique Bridge Lying Draw-In w/Hip Flexion Quadruped Single-Leg Box Jump

(continued)

WEEK 7 ◆ Proprioceptive Cue: Driving the Thigh
(continued)

SATURDAY (continued)	Recovery Run	Resistance Workout
		1 set each Box Lunge Stability Ball Leg Curl Forearms to Palms Bridge Dead Bug
SUNDAY	**Marathon-Pace Run** 1-mile warm-up @ recovery pace 8 miles @ marathon pace 1-mile cool-down @ recovery pace	

WEEK 8 (Recovery) ◆ Proprioceptive Cue: Floppy Feet

MONDAY	Off	
TUESDAY	**Base Run + Drills** Run 5 miles @ base pace High Knees 20 seconds Bounding 20 seconds	
WEDNESDAY	**400m Intervals @ 3,000m Pace** Dynamic stretching warm-up 1.5-mile warm-up @ recovery pace 6 × 400m intervals @ 3,000m pace w/3-minute active recoveries 1.5-mile cool-down @ recovery pace	
THURSDAY	**Recovery Run** 2–6 miles @ recovery pace *or* Nonimpact Cardio Cross-Training Workout 20–45 minutes @ recovery pace	**Resistance Workout** *1 set each* Single-Leg Squat Oblique Bridge Lying Draw-In w/Hip Flexion Quadruped *2 sets each* Box Lunge Stability Ball Leg Curl Forearms to Palms Bridge Dead Bug Broad Jump
FRIDAY	**30-30 Intervals** Dynamic stretching warm-up 2-mile warm-up @ recovery pace 12 × 30-seconds @ 5K pace w/30-second active recoveries 2-mile cool-down @ recovery pace	
SATURDAY	**Recovery Run** 2–6 miles @ recovery pace	**Resistance Workout** *1 set each* Single-Leg Squat Oblique Bridge Lying Draw-In w/Hip Flexion Quadruped

(continued)

WEEK 8 (Recovery) ◆ Proprioceptive Cue: Floppy Feet
(continued)

SATURDAY (continued)	Recovery Run	Resistance Workout *2 sets each* Box Lunge Stability Ball Leg Curl Forearms to Palms Bridge Dead Bug Wall Jump
SUNDAY	**Marathon-Pace Run** 1-mile warm-up @ recovery pace 6 miles @ marathon pace 1-mile cool-down @ recovery pace	

Build 2 Phase

Training objectives: Increase fatigue resistance at 3,000m pace and half-marathon pace; continue to build efficiency at 5K pace

WEEK 9 ◆ Proprioceptive Cue: Butt Squeeze

MONDAY	Off	
TUESDAY	**Base Run + Drills** Run 6 miles @ base pace Stiff-Legged Run 2 × 20 seconds Running No Arms 2 × 20 seconds	
WEDNESDAY	**600m Intervals @ 3,000m Pace** Dynamic stretching warm-up 2-mile warm-up @ recovery pace 4 × 600m intervals @ 3,000m pace w/3-minute active recoveries 2-mile cool-down @ recovery pace	
THURSDAY	**Recovery Run** 2–6 miles @ recovery pace *or* <u>Nonimpact Cardio Cross-Training Workout</u> 20–45 minutes @ recovery pace	**Resistance Workout** *3 sets each* Box Lunge Stability Ball Leg Curl Forearms to Palms Bridge Dead Bug Wall Jump
FRIDAY	**60-60 Intervals** Dynamic stretching warm-up 1.5-mile warm-up @ recovery pace 8 × 1 minute @ 5K pace w/1 minute active recoveries 1.5-mile cool-down @ recovery pace	
SATURDAY	**Recovery Run** 2–6 miles @ recovery pace	**Resistance Workout** *3 sets each* Box Lunge Stability Ball Leg Curl Forearms to Palms Bridge Dead Bug Single-Leg Box Jump
SUNDAY	**Tempo Run** 2-mile warm-up @ recovery pace 4 miles @ half-marathon pace 2-mile cool-down @ recovery pace	

WEEK 10 ♦ Proprioceptive Cue: Feeling Symmetry

MONDAY	Off	
TUESDAY	**Base Run + Drills** Run 6.5 miles @ base pace Stiff-Legged Run 2×20 seconds Running No Arms 2×20 seconds	
WEDNESDAY	**600m Intervals @ 3,000m Pace** Dynamic stretching warm-up 2-mile warm-up @ recovery pace 5×600m intervals @ 3,000m pace w/3-minute active recoveries 2-mile cool-down @ recovery pace	
THURSDAY	**Recovery Run** 2–6 miles @ recovery pace or Nonimpact Cardio Cross-Training Workout 20–45 minutes @ recovery pace	**Resistance Workout** *2 sets each* Lying Hip Abduction Single-Leg Squat Box Lunge Stability Ball Leg Curl Squat Jump
FRIDAY	**60-60 Intervals** Dynamic stretching warm-up 1.5-mile warm-up @ recovery pace 9×1 minute @ 5K pace w/1-minute active recoveries 1.5-mile cool-down @ recovery pace	
SATURDAY	**Recovery Run** 2–6 miles @ recovery pace	**Resistance Workout** *2 sets each* Cook Hip Lift Oblique Bridge Forearms to Palms Bridge Stability Ball Leg Curl Split Squat Jump
SUNDAY	**Tempo Run** 2-mile warm-up @ recovery pace 4.5 miles @ half-marathon pace 2-mile cool-down @ recovery pace	

WEEK 11 ♦ Proprioceptive Cue: Axle Between the Knees

MONDAY	Off
TUESDAY	**Base Run + Drills** Run 7 miles @ base pace Steep Hill Sprints 2 × 20 seconds One-Leg Hop 2 × 20 seconds
WEDNESDAY	**600m Intervals @ 3,000m Pace** Dynamic stretching warm-up 2-mile warm-up @ recovery pace 6 × 600m intervals @ 3,000m pace w/3-minute active recoveries 2-mile cool-down @ recovery pace

THURSDAY	**Recovery Run** 2–6 miles @ recovery pace *or* Nonimpact Cardio Cross-Training Workout 20–45 minutes @ recovery pace	**Resistance Workout** *2 sets each* Lying Hip Abduction Single-Leg Squat Box Lunge Stability Ball Leg Curl Single-Leg Squat Jump

FRIDAY	**60-60 Intervals** Dynamic stretching warm-up 1.5-mile warm-up @ recovery pace 10 × 1 minute @ 5K pace w/1-minute active recoveries 1.5-mile cool-down @ recovery pace

SATURDAY	**Recovery Run** 2–6 miles @ recovery pace	**Resistance Workout** *2 sets each* Cook Hip Lift Oblique Bridge Forearms to Palms Bridge Stability Ball Leg Curl Broad Jump

SUNDAY	**Tempo Run** 2-mile warm-up @ recovery pace 5 miles @ half-marathon pace 2-mile cool-down @ recovery pace

WEEK 12 (Recovery) ◆ Proprioceptive Cue: Running Against a Wall

MONDAY	Off	
TUESDAY	**Base Run + Drills** Run 5 miles @ base pace High Knees 20 seconds Bounding 20 seconds	
WEDNESDAY	**600m Intervals @ 3,000m Pace** Dynamic stretching warm-up 2-mile warm-up @ recovery pace 4 × 600m intervals @ 3,000m pace w/3-minute active recoveries 2-mile cool-down @ recovery pace	
THURSDAY	**Recovery Run** 2–6 miles @ recovery pace *or* Nonimpact Cardio Cross-Training Workout 20–45 minutes @ recovery pace	**Resistance Workout** *2 sets each* Lying Hip Abduction Single-Leg Squat Box Lunge Stability Ball Leg Curl Wall Jump
FRIDAY	**60-60 Intervals** Dynamic stretching warm-up 1.5-mile warm-up @ recovery pace 7 × 1 minute @ 5K pace w/1-minute active recoveries 1.5-mile cool-down @ recovery pace	
SATURDAY	**Recovery Run** 2 miles @ recovery pace	**Resistance Workout** *1 set each* Cook Hip Lift Oblique Bridge Forearms to Palms Bridge Stability Ball Leg Curl
SUNDAY	**5K Tune-up Race or Time Trial** Dynamic stretching warm-up 1-mile warm-up @ recovery pace 5K tune-up race or time trial 1-mile cool-down @ recovery pace	

Peak Phase

Training objectives: Achieve peak fatigue resistance and efficiency at 5K pace; adapt and recover for peak race day

WEEK 13 ◆ Proprioceptive Cue: Falling Forward

MONDAY	Off
TUESDAY	**Base Run + Drills** Run 7 miles @ base pace High Knees 2 × 20 seconds Bounding 2 × 20 seconds
WEDNESDAY	**Mixed Intervals** Dynamic stretching warm-up 1-mile warm-up @ recovery pace 1 × 1 mile @ 10K pace, 2-minute active recovery 2 × 1K @ 5K pace, 2-minute active recoveries 2 × 600m @ 3,000m pace, 2-minute active recoveries 1 × 300m @ 1-mile pace 1-mile cool-down @ recovery pace

THURSDAY	**Recovery Run** 2–6 miles @ recovery pace *or* <u>Nonimpact Cardio Cross-Training Workout</u> 20–45 minutes @ recovery pace	**Resistance Workout** *2 sets each* Lying Hip Abduction Single-Leg Squat Box Lunge Stability Ball Leg Curl Wall Jump

FRIDAY	**1K Intervals @ 5K Pace** Dynamic stretching warm-up 2-mile warm-up @ recovery pace 4 × 1K @ 5K pace w/2-minute active recoveries 2-mile cool-down @ recovery pace

(continued)

WEEK 13 ◆ Proprioceptive Cue: Falling Forward
(continued)

SATURDAY	Recovery Run	Resistance Workout
	2–6 miles @ recovery pace	*2 sets each* Cook Hip Lift Oblique Bridge Forearms to Palms Bridge Stability Ball Leg Curl Single-Leg Box Jump
SUNDAY	**Tempo Run** 2-mile warm-up @ recovery pace 3.5 miles @ 10K pace 2-mile cool-down @ recovery pace	

WEEK 14 ◆ Proprioceptive Cue: Navel to Spine

MONDAY	Off
TUESDAY	**Base Run + Drills** Run 6.5 miles @ base pace Stiff-Legged Run 2 × 20 seconds Running No Arms 2 × 20 seconds
WEDNESDAY	**Mixed Intervals** Dynamic stretching warm-up 1-mile warm-up @ recovery pace 1 × 1 mile @ 10K pace, 90-second active recovery 2 × 1K @ 5K pace, 90-second active recoveries 2 × 600m @ 3,000m pace, 90-second active recoveries 1 × 300m @ 1-mile pace 1-mile cool-down @ recovery pace

THURSDAY	**Recovery Run** 2–6 miles @ recovery pace *or* Nonimpact Cardio Cross-Training Workout 20–45 minutes @ recovery pace	**Resistance Workout** *2 sets each* Lying Hip Abduction Single-Leg Squat Box Lunge Stability Ball Leg Curl Squat Jump

FRIDAY	**1K Intervals @ 5K Pace** Dynamic stretching warm-up 2-mile warm-up @ recovery pace 5 × 1K @ 5K pace w/2-minute active recoveries 2-mile cool-down @ recovery pace

SATURDAY	**Recovery Run** 2–6 miles @ recovery pace	**Resistance Workout** *2 sets each* Cook Hip Lift Oblique Bridge Forearms to Palms Bridge Stability Ball Leg Curl Split Squat Jump

SUNDAY	**Tempo Run** 1-mile warm-up @ recovery pace 3.5 miles @ 10K pace 1-mile cool-down @ recovery pace

WEEK 15   ◆   Proprioceptive Cue: Running on Water

MONDAY	Off
TUESDAY	**Base Run + Drills** Run 6 miles @ base pace Steep Hill Sprints 2 × 20 seconds One-Leg Hop 2 × 20 seconds
WEDNESDAY	**Mixed Intervals** Dynamic stretching warm-up 1-mile warm-up @ recovery pace 1 × 1 mile @ 10K pace, 1-minute active recovery 2 × 1K @ 5K pace, 1-minute active recoveries 2 × 600m @ 3,000m pace, 1-minute active recoveries 1 × 300m @ 1-mile pace 1-mile cool-down @ recovery pace

THURSDAY	**Recovery Run** 2–6 miles @ recovery pace *or* Nonimpact Cardio Cross-Training Workout 20–45 minutes @ recovery pace	**Resistance Workout** *2 sets each* Lying Hip Abduction Single-Leg Squat Box Lunge Stability Ball Leg Curl Single-Leg Squat Jump

FRIDAY	**1K Intervals @ 5K Pace** Dynamic stretching warm-up 2-mile warm-up @ recovery pace 5 × 1K @ 5K pace w/90-second active recoveries 2-mile cool-down @ recovery pace

SATURDAY	**Recovery Run** 2–6 miles @ recovery pace	**Resistance Workout** *2 sets each* Cook Hip Lift Oblique Bridge Forearms to Palms Bridge Stability Ball Leg Curl Broad Jump

SUNDAY	**Tempo Run** 2-mile warm-up @ recovery pace 4 miles @ 10K pace 2-mile cool-down @ recovery pace

WEEK 16 (Taper) ♦ Proprioceptive Cue: Your Choice

MONDAY	Off
TUESDAY	**Base Run** Run 5 miles @ base pace
WEDNESDAY	**Mixed Intervals** Dynamic stretching warm-up 1-mile warm-up @ recovery pace 1×1 mile @ 10K pace, 1-minute active recovery 1×1K @ 5K pace, 1-minute active recovery 1×600m @ 3,000m pace, 1-minute active recovery 1×300m @ 1-mile pace 1-mile cool-down @ recovery pace

THURSDAY	**Recovery Run** 2 miles @ recovery pace or Nonimpact Cardio Cross-Training Workout 15–20 minutes @ recovery pace	**Resistance Workout** *1 set each* Lying Hip Abduction Single-Leg Squat Box Lunge Stability Ball Leg Curl

FRIDAY	**1K Intervals @ 5K Pace** Dynamic stretching warm-up 1-mile warm-up @ recovery pace 2×1K @ 5K pace w/2-minute active recovery 1-mile cool-down @ recovery pace
SATURDAY	Off
SUNDAY	**5K Peak Race** Dynamic stretching warm-up 1-mile warm-up @ recovery pace 5K peak race 1-mile cool-down @ recovery pace

LEVEL 3

Use this plan if you are most comfortable with a 5K training plan that features six scheduled runs per week plus up to four additional, optional runs or nonimpact cardio cross-training workouts and a maximum run distance of twelve miles. The plan also includes two resistance workouts per week.

Base Phase

Training objectives: Build aerobic capacity and endurance, increase injury resistance, and increase muscle activation capacity

WEEK 1 ♦ Proprioceptive Cue: Falling Forward

MONDAY	Off	
TUESDAY	**Base Run + Drills** Run 6 miles @ base pace Running No Arms 20 seconds One-Leg Hop 20 seconds	Optional Recovery Run or Cardio Cross-Training Workout 20–60 minutes @ recovery pace
WEDNESDAY	**Hill Repetitions** Dynamic stretching warm-up 2-mile warm-up @ recovery pace 2 × 30-second hill repetitions @ relaxed sprint speed w/ 2-minute active recoveries 2-mile cool-down @ recovery pace	Optional Recovery Run or Cardio Cross-Training Workout 20–60 minutes @ recovery pace
THURSDAY	**Base Run + Drills** Run 6 miles @ base pace Running No Arms 20 seconds One-Leg Hop 20 seconds	**Resistance Workout** *1 set each* Lying Hip Abduction Cook Hip Lift Kneeling Overhead Draw-In Knee Fall-Out Squat Jump
FRIDAY	**Fartlek Run** Dynamic stretching warm-up Run 6 miles @ base pace w/4 × 30-second intervals @ 1-mile pace "sprinkled in"	Optional Recovery Run or Cardio Cross-Training Workout 20–60 minutes @ recovery pace

SATURDAY	**Base Run + Drills** Run 6 miles @ base pace Running No Arms 20 seconds One-Leg Hop 20 seconds	**Resistance Workout** *1 set each* Lying Hip Abduction Cook Hip Lift Kneeling Overhead Draw-In Knee Fall-Out Broad Jump Wall Jump
SUNDAY	**Base Run** Run 7 miles @ base pace	Optional Recovery Run or Cardio Cross-Training Workout 20–60 minutes @ recovery pace

WEEK 2 ◆ Proprioceptive Cue: Navel to Spine

MONDAY	Off	
TUESDAY	**Base Run + Drills** Run 6.5 miles @ base pace High Knees 2×20 seconds Bounding 2×20 seconds	Optional Recovery Run or Cardio Cross-Training Workout 20–60 minutes @ recovery pace

WEDNESDAY	**Hill Repetitions**
	Dynamic stretching warm-up
	2-mile warm-up @ recovery pace
	8×30-second hill repetitions
	  @ relaxed sprint speed
	  w/2-minute active recoveries
	2-mile cool-down @ recovery pace
		Optional Recovery Run or Cardio
		Cross-Training Workout
		20–60 minutes @ recovery pace

THURSDAY	**Base Run + Drills** Run 6.5 miles @ base pace High Knees 2×20 seconds Bounding 2×20 seconds	**Resistance Workout** *2 sets each* Lying Hip Abduction Cook Hip Lift Kneeling Overhead Draw-In Knee Fall-Out Split Squat Jump Single-Leg Squat Jump

FRIDAY	**Fartlek Run**
	Dynamic stretching warm-up
	Run 6 miles @ base pace w/8×
	  30-second intervals @ 1-mile
	  pace "sprinkled in"
		Optional Recovery Run or Cardio
		Cross-Training Workout
		20–60 minutes @ recovery pace

SATURDAY	**Base Run + Drills** Run 6 miles @ base pace High Knees 2×20 seconds Bounding 2×20 seconds	**Resistance Workout** *2 sets each* Lying Hip Abduction Cook Hip Lift Kneeling Overhead Draw-In Knee Fall-Out Wall Jump Single-Leg Box Jump
SUNDAY	**Base Run** Run 8 miles @ base pace	Optional Recovery Run or Cardio Cross-Training Workout 20–60 minutes @ recovery pace

WEEK 3 ♦ Proprioceptive Cue: Running on Water

MONDAY	Off	
TUESDAY	**Base Run + Drills** Run 6.5 miles @ base pace Stiff-Legged Run 2 × 20 seconds Running No Arms 2 × 20 seconds	<u>Optional Recovery Run or Cardio</u> <u>Cross-Training Workout</u> 20–60 minutes @ recovery pace
WEDNESDAY	**Hill Repetitions** Dynamic stretching warm-up 2-mile warm-up @ recovery pace 12 × 30-second hill repetitions @ relaxed sprint speed 2-mile cool-down @ recovery pace	<u>Optional Recovery Run or Cardio</u> <u>Cross-Training Workout</u> 20–60 minutes @ recovery pace
THURSDAY	**Base Run + Drills** Run 6.5 miles @ base pace Stiff-Legged Run 2 × 20 seconds Running No Arms 2 × 20 seconds	**Resistance Workout** *3 sets each* Lying Hip Abduction Cook Hip Lift Kneeling Overhead Draw-In Knee Fall-Out Squat Jump Split Squat Jump
FRIDAY	**Fartlek Run** Dynamic stretching warm-up Run 7 miles @ base pace w/12 × 30-second intervals @ 1-mile pace "sprinkled in"	<u>Optional Recovery Run or Cardio</u> <u>Cross-Training Workout</u> 20–60 minutes @ recovery pace
SATURDAY	**Base Run + Drills** Run 6 miles @ base pace Stiff-Legged Run 2 × 20 seconds Running No Arms 2 × 20 seconds	**Resistance Workout** *3 sets each* Lying Hip Abduction Cook Hip Lift Kneeling Overhead Draw-In Knee Fall-Out Broad Jump Wall Jump
SUNDAY	**Base Run** Run 9 miles @ base pace	<u>Optional Recovery Run or Cardio</u> <u>Cross-Training Workout</u> 20–60 minutes @ recovery pace

WEEK 4 (Recovery) ◆ Proprioceptive Cue: Pulling the Road

MONDAY	Off	
TUESDAY	**Base Run + Drills** Run 6 miles @ base pace One-Leg Hop 20 seconds High Knees 20 seconds	Optional Recovery Run or Cardio Cross-Training Workout 20–60 minutes @ recovery pace

WEDNESDAY	**Hill Repetitions**
	Dynamic stretching warm-up
	2-mile warm-up @ recovery pace
	8 × 30-second hill repetitions
	  @ relaxed sprint speed
	  w/2-minute active recoveries
	2-mile cool-down @ recovery pace
		Optional Recovery Run or Cardio Cross-Training Workout
		20–60 minutes @ recovery pace

THURSDAY	**Recovery Run** 2–5 miles @ recovery pace	**Resistance Workout** *1 set each* Single-Leg Squat Oblique Bridge Lying Draw-In w/Hip Flexion Quadruped *2 sets each* Lying Hip Abduction Cook Hip Lift Kneeling Overhead Draw-In Knee Fall-Out Single-Leg Squat Jump Broad Jump

FRIDAY	**Fartlek Run**
	Dynamic stretching warm-up
	Run 6 miles @ base pace
	  w/8 × 30-second intervals
	  @ 1-mile pace "sprinkled in"
		Optional Recovery Run or Cardio Cross-Training Workout
		20–60 minutes @ recovery pace

SATURDAY	**Recovery Run** 2–5 miles @ recovery pace	**Resistance Workout** *1 set each* Single-Leg Squat Oblique Bridge Lying Draw-In w/Hip Flexion Quadruped *2 sets each* Lying Hip Abduction Cook Hip Lift Kneeling Overhead Draw-In Knee Fall-Out Wall Jump Single-Leg Box Jump
SUNDAY	**Base Run** Run 7 miles @ base pace	

Build 1 Phase

Training objectives: Continue to increase aerobic capacity and endurance; increase fatigue resistance at 3,000m pace and marathon pace; begin to develop efficiency at 5K pace

WEEK 5 ◆ Proprioceptive Cue: Scooting

MONDAY	Off	
TUESDAY	**Base Run + Drills** Run 7 miles @ base pace High Knees 2 × 20 seconds Bounding 2 × 20 seconds	Optional Recovery Run or Cardio Cross-Training Workout 20–60 minutes @ recovery pace

WEDNESDAY	**400m Intervals @ 3,000m Pace**
	Dynamic stretching warm-up
	1.5-mile warm-up @ recovery pace
	10 × 400m intervals @ 3,000m pace
	   w/3-minute active recoveries
	1.5-mile cool-down @ recovery
	   pace
		Optional Recovery Run or Cardio Cross-Training Workout
		20–60 minutes @ recovery pace

THURSDAY	**Recovery/Base Run** 2–6 miles @ recovery/base pace (Do this workout as a recovery run if you did *not* do an afternoon recovery workout following yesterday's interval workout. Otherwise, do this workout as a base workout.)	**Resistance Workout** *2 sets each* Single-Leg Squat Oblique Bridge Lying Draw-In w/Hip Flexion Quadruped Single-Leg Squat Jump Broad Jump *1 set each* Lying Hip Abduction Cook Hip Lift Kneeling Overhead Draw-In Knee Fall-Out
FRIDAY	**30-30 Intervals** Dynamic stretching warm-up 2-mile warm-up @ recovery pace 14 × 30 seconds @ 5K pace w/30- second active recoveries 2-mile cool-down @ recovery pace	Optional Recovery Run or Cardio Cross-Training Workout 20–60 minutes @ recovery pace

SATURDAY	**Recovery/Base Run** 2–6 miles @ recovery/base pace	**Resistance Workout** *2 sets each* Single-Leg Squat Oblique Bridge Lying Draw-In w/Hip Flexion Quadruped Wall Jump Single-Leg Box Jump *1 set each* Lying Hip Abduction Cook Hip Lift Kneeling Overhead Draw-In Knee Fall-Out
SUNDAY	**Marathon-Pace Run** 2-mile warm-up @ recovery pace 6 miles @ marathon pace 2-mile cool-down @ recovery pace	Optional Recovery Run or Cardio Cross-Training Workout 20–60 minutes @ recovery pace

WEEK 6 ♦ Proprioceptive Cue: Pounding the Ground

MONDAY	Off	
TUESDAY	**Base Run + Drills** Run 8 miles @ base pace Stiff-Legged Run 2 × 20 seconds Running No Arms 2 × 20 seconds	Optional Recovery Run or Cardio Cross-Training Workout 20–60 minutes @ recovery pace
WEDNESDAY	**400m Intervals @ 3,000m Pace** Dynamic stretching warm-up 1.5-mile warm-up @ recovery pace 12 × 400m intervals @ 3,000m pace w/3-minute active recoveries 1.5-mile cool-down @ recovery pace	Optional Recovery Run or Cardio Cross-Training Workout 20–60 minutes @ recovery pace
THURSDAY	**Recovery/Base Run** 2–6 miles @ recovery/base pace	**Resistance Workout** *3 sets each* Single-Leg Squat Oblique Bridge Lying Draw-In w/Hip Flexion Quadruped *2 sets each* Squat Jump Split Squat Jump
FRIDAY	**30-30 Intervals** Dynamic stretching warm-up 2-mile warm-up @ recovery pace 16 × 30 seconds @ 5K pace w/ 30-second active recoveries 2-mile cool-down @ recovery pace	Optional Recovery Run or Cardio Cross-Training Workout 20–60 minutes @ recovery pace
SATURDAY	**Recovery/Base Run** 2–6 miles @ recovery/base pace	**Resistance Workout** *3 sets each* Single-Leg Squat Oblique Bridge Lying Draw-In w/Hip Flexion Quadruped *2 sets* Single-Leg Squat Jump

SUNDAY	**Marathon-Pace Run** 2-mile warm-up @ recovery pace 7 miles @ marathon pace 2-mile cool-down @ recovery pace	Optional Recovery Run or Cardio Cross-Training Workout 20–60 minutes @ recovery pace

WEEK 7 ◆ Proprioceptive Cue: Driving the Thigh

MONDAY	Off	
TUESDAY	**Base Run + Drills** Run 9 miles @ base pace Steep Hill Sprints 2 × 20 seconds One-Leg Hop 2 × 20 seconds	<u>Optional Recovery Run or Cardio</u> <u>Cross-Training Workout</u> 20–60 minutes @ recovery pace

WEDNESDAY	**400m Intervals @ 3,000m Pace**
	Dynamic stretching warm-up
	1.5-mile warm-up @ recovery pace
	14 × 400m intervals @ 3,000m
	  pace w/3-minute active
	  recoveries
	1.5-mile cool-down
	  @ recovery pace
		<u>Optional Recovery Run or Cardio</u>
		<u>Cross-Training Workout</u>
		20–60 minutes @ recovery pace

THURSDAY	**Recovery/Base Run** 2–6 miles @ recovery/base pace	**Resistance Workout** *2 sets each* Single-Leg Squat Oblique Bridge Lying Draw-In w/Hip Flexion Quadruped Split Squat Jump Single-Leg Squat Jump *1 set each* Box Lunge Stability Ball Leg Curl Forearms to Palms Bridge Dead Bug

FRIDAY	**30-30 Intervals**
	Dynamic stretching warm-up
	2-mile warm-up @ recovery pace
	22 × 30 seconds @ 5K pace w/
	  30-second active recoveries
	2-mile cool-down @ recovery
	  pace
		<u>Optional Recovery Run or Cardio</u>
		<u>Cross-Training Workout</u>
		20–60 minutes @ recovery pace

SATURDAY	**Recovery/Base Run** 2–6 miles @ recovery/base pace	**Resistance Workout** *2 sets each* Single-Leg Squat Oblique Bridge Lying Draw-In w/Hip Flexion Quadruped Single-Leg Box Jump Squat Jump *1 set each* Box Lunge Stability Ball Leg Curl Forearms to Palms Bridge Dead Bug
SUNDAY	**Marathon-Pace Run** 2-mile warm-up @ recovery pace 8 miles @ marathon pace 2-mile cool-down @ recovery pace	Optional Recovery Run or Cardio Cross-Training Workout 20–60 minutes @ recovery pace

WEEK 8 (Recovery) ◆ Proprioceptive Cue: Floppy Feet

MONDAY	Off	
TUESDAY	**Base Run + Drills** Run 6 miles @ base pace High Knees 20 seconds Bounding 20 seconds	Optional Recovery Run or Cardio Cross-Training Workout 20–60 minutes @ recovery pace
WEDNESDAY	**400m Intervals @ 3,000m Pace** Dynamic stretching warm-up 1.5-mile warm-up @ recovery pace 10 × 400m intervals @ 3,000m pace w/3-minute active recoveries 1.5-mile cool-down @ recovery pace	Optional Recovery Run or Cardio Cross-Training Workout 20–60 minutes @ recovery pace
THURSDAY	**Recovery/Base Run** 2–6 miles @ recovery/base pace	**Resistance Workout** *1 set each* Single-Leg Squat Oblique Bridge Lying Draw-In w/Hip Flexion Quadruped *2 sets each* Box Lunge Stability Ball Leg Curl Forearms to Palms Bridge Dead Bug Broad Jump Wall Jump
FRIDAY	**30-30 Intervals** Dynamic stretching warm-up 2-mile warm-up @ recovery pace 14 × 30 seconds @ 5K pace w/30-second active recoveries 2-mile cool-down @ recovery pace	Optional Recovery Run or Cardio Cross-Training Workout 20–60 minutes @ recovery pace

SATURDAY	**Recovery/Base Run** 2–6 miles @ recovery/base pace	**Resistance Workout** *1 set each* Single-Leg Squat Oblique Bridge Lying Draw-In w/Hip Flexion Quadruped *2 sets each* Box Lunge Stability Ball Leg Curl Forearms to Palms Bridge Dead Bug Wall Jump Single-Leg Box Jump
SUNDAY	**Marathon-Pace Run** 2-mile warm-up @ recovery pace 6 miles @ marathon pace 2-mile cool-down @ recovery pace	

Build 2 Phase

Training objectives: Increase fatigue resistance at 3,000m pace and half-marathon pace; continue to build efficiency at 5K pace

WEEK 9 ◆ Proprioceptive Cue: Butt Squeeze

MONDAY	Off	
TUESDAY	**Base Run + Drills** Run 8 miles @ base pace Stiff-Legged Run 2 × 20 seconds Running No Arms 2 × 20 seconds	Optional Recovery Run or Cardio Cross-Training Workout 20–60 minutes @ recovery pace
WEDNESDAY	**600m Intervals @ 3,000m Pace** Dynamic stretching warm-up 2-mile warm-up @ recovery pace 6 × 600m intervals @ 3,000m pace w/3-minute active recoveries 2-mile cool-down @ recovery pace	Optional Recovery Run or Cardio Cross-Training Workout 20–60 minutes @ recovery pace
THURSDAY	**Recovery/Base Run** 2–6 miles @ recovery/base pace	**Resistance Workout** *3 sets each* Box Lunge Stability Ball Leg Curl Forearms to Palms Bridge Dead Bug Wall Jump Single-Leg Box Jump
FRIDAY	**60-60 Intervals** Dynamic stretching warm-up 1.5-mile warm-up @ recovery pace 10 × 1-minute @ 5K pace w/1-minute active recoveries 1.5-mile cool-down @ recovery pace	Optional Recovery Run or Cardio Cross-Training Workout 20–60 minutes @ recovery pace
SATURDAY	**Recovery/Base Run** 2–6 miles @ recovery/base pace	**Resistance Workout** *3 sets each* Box Lunge Stability Ball Leg Curl Forearms to Palms Bridge

SATURDAY (continued)	**Recovery/Base Run**	**Resistance Workout** *3 sets each (cont.)* Dead Bug Single-Leg Box Jump Squat Jump
SUNDAY	**Tempo Run** 2-mile warm-up @ recovery pace 5 miles @ half-marathon pace 2-mile cool-down @ recovery pace	Optional Recovery Run or Cardio Cross-Training Workout 20–60 minutes @ recovery pace

WEEK 10   ◆   Proprioceptive Cue: Feeling Symmetry

MONDAY	Off	
TUESDAY	**Base Run + Drills** Run 9 miles @ base pace Stiff-Legged Run 2 × 20 seconds Running No Arms 2 × 20 seconds	<u>Optional Recovery Run or Cardio Cross-Training Workout</u> 20–60 minutes @ recovery pace
WEDNESDAY	**600m Intervals @ 3,000m Pace** Dynamic stretching warm-up 2-mile warm-up @ recovery pace 7 × 600m intervals @ 3,000m pace 　w/3-minute active recoveries 2-mile cool-down @ recovery pace	<u>Optional Recovery Run or Cardio Cross-Training Workout</u> 20–60 minutes @ recovery pace
THURSDAY	**Recovery/Base Run** 2–6 miles @ recovery/base pace	**Resistance Workout** *2 sets each* Lying Hip Abduction Single-Leg Squat Box Lunge Stability Ball Leg Curl Squat Jump Split Squat Jump
FRIDAY	**60-60 Intervals** Dynamic stretching warm-up 1.5-mile warm-up @ recovery pace 12 × 1 minute @ 5K pace 　w/1-minute active recoveries 1.5-mile cool-down @ recovery 　pace	<u>Optional Recovery Run or Cardio Cross-Training Workout</u> 20–60 minutes @ recovery pace
SATURDAY	**Recovery/Base Run** 2–6 miles @ recovery/base pace	**Resistance Workout** *2 sets each* Cook Hip Lift Oblique Bridge Forearms to Palms Bridge Stability Ball Leg Curl Split Squat Jump Single-Leg Squat Jump

| SUNDAY | **Tempo Run**
2-mile warm-up @ recovery pace
6 miles @ half-marathon pace
2-mile cool-down @ recovery pace | <u>Optional Recovery Run or Cardio</u>
<u>Cross-Training Workout</u>
20–60 minutes @ recovery pace |

WEEK 11 ♦ Proprioceptive Cue: Axle Between the Knees

MONDAY	Off	
TUESDAY	**Base Run + Drills** Run 10 miles @ base pace Steep Hill Sprints 2 × 20 seconds One-Leg Hop 2 × 20 seconds	<u>Optional Recovery Run or Cardio Cross-Training Workout</u> 20–60 minutes @ recovery pace
WEDNESDAY	**600m Intervals @ 3,000m Pace** Dynamic stretching warm-up 2-mile warm-up @ recovery pace 8 × 600m intervals @ 3,000m pace w/3-minute active recoveries 2-mile cool-down @ recovery pace	<u>Optional Recovery Run or Cardio Cross-Training Workout</u> 20–60 minutes @ recovery pace
THURSDAY	**Recovery/Base Run** 2–6 miles @ recovery/base pace	**Resistance Workout** *2 sets each* Lying Hip Abduction Single-Leg Squat Box Lunge Stability Ball Leg Curl Single-Leg Squat Jump Broad Jump
FRIDAY	**60-60 Intervals** Dynamic stretching warm-up 1.5-mile warm-up @ recovery pace 12 × 1 minute @ 5K pace w/1-minute active recoveries 1.5-mile cool-down @ recovery pace	<u>Optional Recovery Run or Cardio Cross-Training Workout</u> 20–60 minutes @ recovery pace
SATURDAY	**Recovery/Base Run** 2–6 miles @ recovery/base pace	**Resistance Workout** *2 sets each* Cook Hip Lift Oblique Bridge Forearms to Palms Bridge Stability Ball Leg Curl Broad Jump Wall Jump

| SUNDAY | **Tempo Run**
2-mile warm-up @ recovery pace
7 miles @ half-marathon pace
2-mile cool-down @ recovery pace | Optional Recovery Run or Cardio
Cross-Training Workout
20–60 minutes @ recovery pace |

WEEK 12 (Recovery) ◆ Proprioceptive Cue: Running Against a Wall

MONDAY	Off	
TUESDAY	**Base Run + Drills** Run 6 miles @ base pace High Knees 20 seconds Bounding 20 seconds	Optional Recovery Run or Cardio Cross-Training Workout 20–60 minutes @ recovery pace
WEDNESDAY	**600m Intervals @ 3,000m Pace** Dynamic stretching warm-up 2-mile warm-up @ recovery pace 6 × 600m intervals @ 3,000m pace w/3-minute active recoveries 2-mile cool-down @ recovery pace	Optional Recovery Run or Cardio Cross-Training Workout 20–60 minutes @ recovery pace
THURSDAY	**Recovery/Base Run** 2–6 miles @ recovery/base pace	**Resistance Workout** *2 sets each* Lying Hip Abduction Single-Leg Squat Box Lunge Stability Ball Leg Curl Wall Jump Single-Leg Box Jump
FRIDAY	**60-60 Intervals** Dynamic stretching warm-up 1.5-mile warm-up @ recovery pace 8 × 1 minute @ 5K pace w/1 minute active recoveries 1.5-mile cool-down @ recovery pace	Optional Recovery Run or Cardio Cross-Training Workout 20–60 minutes @ recovery pace
SATURDAY	**Recovery Run** 2 miles @ recovery pace	**Resistance Workout** *1 set each* Cook Hip Lift Oblique Bridge Forearms to Palms Bridge Stability Ball Leg Curl
SUNDAY	**5K Tune-up Race or Time Trial** Dynamic stretching warm-up 2-mile warm-up @ recovery pace 5K tune-up race or time trial 2-mile cool-down @ recovery pace	

Peak Phase

Training objectives: Achieve peak fatigue resistance and efficiency at 5K pace; adapt and recover for peak race day

WEEK 13 ◆ Proprioceptive Cue: Falling Forward

MONDAY	Off	
TUESDAY	**Base Run + Drills** Run 9 miles @ base pace High Knees 2 × 20 seconds Bounding 2 × 20 seconds	<u>Optional Recovery Run or Cardio</u> <u>Cross-Training Workout</u> 20–60 minutes @ recovery pace

WEDNESDAY	**Mixed Intervals**
	Dynamic stretching warm-up
	1-mile warm-up @ recovery pace
	2 × 1 mile @ 10K pace, 2-minute
	    active recoveries
	2 × 1K @ 5K pace, 2-minute active
	    recoveries
	2 × 600m @ 3,000m pace,
	    2-minute active recoveries
	2 × 300m @ 1-mile pace
	1-mile cool-down @ recovery pace
		<u>Optional Recovery Run or Cardio</u>
		<u>Cross-Training Workout</u>
		20–60 minutes @ recovery pace

THURSDAY	**Recovery/Base Run** 2–6 miles @ recovery/base pace	**Resistance Workout** *2 sets each* Lying Hip Abduction Single-Leg Squat Box Lunge Stability Ball Leg Curl Wall Jump Single-Leg Box Jump
FRIDAY	**1K Intervals @ 5K Pace** Dynamic stretching warm-up 2-mile warm-up @ recovery pace 5 × 1K @ 5K pace w/2-minute active recoveries 2-mile cool-down @ recovery pace	<u>Optional Recovery Run or Cardio</u> <u>Cross-Training Workout</u> 20–60 minutes @ recovery pace

(continued)

WEEK 13 ◆ Proprioceptive Cue: Falling Forward
(continued)

SATURDAY	**Recovery/Base Run** 2–6 miles @ recovery/base pace	**Resistance Workout** *2 sets each* Cook Hip Lift Oblique Bridge Forearms to Palms Bridge Stability Ball Leg Curl Single-Leg Box Jump Squat Jump
SUNDAY	**Tempo Run** 2-mile warm-up @ recovery pace 4 miles @ 10K pace 2-mile cool-down @ recovery pace	Optional Recovery Run or Cardio Cross-Training Workout 20–60 minutes @ recovery pace

WEEK 14 ◆ Proprioceptive Cue: Navel to Spine

MONDAY	Off	
TUESDAY	**Base Run + Drills** Run 8 miles @ base pace Stiff-Legged Run 2 × 20 seconds Running No Arms 2 × 20 seconds	Optional Recovery Run or Cardio Cross-Training Workout 20–60 minutes @ recovery pace
WEDNESDAY	**Mixed Intervals** Dynamic stretching warm-up 1-mile warm-up @ recovery pace 2 × 1 mile @ 10K pace, 90-second active recoveries 2 × 1K @ 5K pace, 90-second active recoveries 2 × 600m @ 3,000m pace, 90-second active recoveries 2 × 300m @ 1-mile pace 1-mile cool-down @ recovery pace	Optional Recovery Run or Cardio Cross-Training Workout 20–60 minutes @ recovery pace
THURSDAY	**Recovery/Base Run** 2–6 miles @ recovery/base pace	**Resistance Workout** *2 sets each* Lying Hip Abduction Single-Leg Squat Box Lunge Stability Ball Leg Curl Squat Jump Split Squat Jump
FRIDAY	**1K Intervals @ 5K Pace** Dynamic stretching warm-up 2-mile warm-up @ recovery pace 6 × 1K @ 5K pace w/2-minute active recoveries 2-mile cool-down @ recovery pace	Optional Recovery Run or Cardio Cross-Training Workout 20–60 minutes @ recovery pace

(continued)

WEEK 14 ◆ Proprioceptive Cue: Navel to Spine
(continued)

SATURDAY	**Recovery/Base Run** 2–6 miles @ recovery/base pace	**Resistance Workout** *2 sets each* Cook Hip Lift Oblique Bridge Forearms to Palms Bridge Stability Ball Leg Curl Split Squat Jump Single-Leg Squat Jump
SUNDAY	**Tempo Run** 1-mile warm-up @ recovery pace 4.5 miles @ 10K pace 1-mile cool-down @ recovery pace	Optional Recovery Run or Cardio Cross-Training Workout 20–60 minutes @ recovery pace

WEEK 15 ◆ Proprioceptive Cue: Running on Water

MONDAY	Off	
TUESDAY	**Base Run + Drills** Run 7 miles @ base pace Steep Hill Sprints 2 × 20 seconds One-Leg Hop 2 × 20 seconds	<u>Optional Recovery Run or Cardio Cross-Training Workout</u> 20–60 minutes @ recovery pace
WEDNESDAY	**Mixed Intervals** Dynamic stretching warm-up 1-mile warm-up @ recovery pace 2 × 1 mile @ 10K pace, 1-minute active recoveries 2 × 1K @ 5K pace, 1-minute active recoveries 2 × 600m @ 3,000m pace, 1-minute active recoveries 2 × 300m @ 1-mile pace 1-mile cool-down @ recovery pace	<u>Optional Recovery Run or Cardio Cross-Training Workout</u> 20–60 minutes @ recovery pace
THURSDAY	**Recovery/Base Run** 2–6 miles @ recovery/base pace	**Resistance Workout** *2 sets each* Lying Hip Abduction Single-Leg Squat Box Lunge Stability Ball Leg Curl Single-Leg Squat Jump
FRIDAY	**1K Intervals @ 5K Pace** Dynamic stretching warm-up 2-mile warm-up @ recovery pace 6 × 1K @ 5K pace w/90-second active recoveries 2-mile cool-down @ recovery pace	<u>Optional Recovery Run or Cardio Cross-Training Workout</u> 20–60 minutes @ recovery pace

(continued)

WEEK 15 ◆ Proprioceptive Cue: Running on Water
(continued)

SATURDAY	Recovery/Base Run 2–6 miles @ recovery/base pace	Resistance Workout *2 sets each* Cook Hip Lift Oblique Bridge Forearms to Palms Bridge Stability Ball Leg Curl Broad Jump Wall Jump
SUNDAY	Tempo Run 2-mile warm-up @ recovery pace 5 miles @ 10K pace 2-mile cool-down @ recovery pace	Optional Recovery Run or Cardio Cross-Training Workout 20–60 minutes @ recovery pace

WEEK 16 (Taper) ◆ Proprioceptive Cue: Your Choice

MONDAY	Off	
TUESDAY	**Base Run** Run 6 miles @ base pace	Optional Recovery Run or Cardio Cross-Training Workout 20–60 minutes @ recovery pace
WEDNESDAY	**Mixed Intervals** Dynamic stretching warm-up 1-mile warm-up @ recovery pace 1×1 mile @ 10K pace, 1-minute active recovery 1×1K @ 5K pace, 1-minute active recovery 1×600m @ 3,000m pace, 1-minute active recovery 1×300m @ 1-mile pace 1-mile cool-down @ recovery pace	
THURSDAY	**Recovery Run** 4 miles @ recovery pace	**Resistance Workout** *1 set each* Lying Hip Abduction Single-Leg Squat Box Lunge Stability Ball Leg Curl
FRIDAY	**1K Intervals @ 5K Pace** Dynamic stretching warm-up 1-mile warm-up @ recovery pace 2×1K @ 5K pace w/2-minute active recovery 1-mile cool-down @ recovery pace	
SATURDAY	Off	
SUNDAY	**5K Peak Race** Dynamic stretching warm-up 2-mile warm-up @ recovery pace 5K peak race 2-mile cool-down @ recovery pace	

CHAPTER ◆ 12

BRAIN TRAINING PLANS: 10K

For competitive runners, 10 kilometers (or 6.2 miles) is considered a critical distance, because in most cases the faster you can run this distance, the faster you can run *any* distance, from one mile to a marathon. Your 10K time is like a barometer of your overall running fitness, and training to improve your 10K time is one of the best ways to take your running to the next level generally.

The same distance has similar significance for beginning runners. For this group, training to complete a 10K race is one of the best and most efficient ways to improve general health and fitness. You can slog through a 5K without being particularly fit. On the other hand, once you begin to train for races beyond 10K, you quickly enter the zone of diminishing returns: more and more training for smaller and smaller gains. Ten kilometers is the sweet spot.

There are three 10K training plans in this chapter: Level 1, Level 2, and Level 3. Each plan is eighteen weeks long and includes a 5K tune-up race/breakthrough workout at the end of Week 12 and a 10K tune-up race/breakthrough workout at the end of Week 15, in addition to the 10K peak race at the end of Week 18. The eighteen weeks are divided into Base, Build 1, Build 2, and Peak phases. Each of the first three phases is four weeks in duration; the Peak phase lasts six weeks. Weeks 4, 8, 12, and 15 are reduced-volume recovery weeks, and Week 18 is a reduced-volume taper week. Monday is a rest day in all three plans.

There are three key workouts per week in each plan: a speed workout on Wednesdays, an intensive endurance workout on Fridays, and an extensive endurance workout on Sundays. Key workouts are indicated by shaded boxes.

LEVEL 1

Use this plan if you are most comfortable with a 10K training plan that features four runs per week and a maximum run distance of 8 miles. The plan also includes two resistance workouts per week and one optional nonimpact cardio cross-training workout.

Base Phase

Training objectives: Build aerobic capacity and endurance, increase injury resistance, and increase muscle activation capacity

WEEK 1 ♦ Proprioceptive Cue: Falling Forward

MONDAY	Off	
TUESDAY	**Base Run + Drills** Run 2 miles @ base pace Running No Arms 20 seconds One-Leg Hop 20 seconds	
WEDNESDAY	**Hill Repetitions** Dynamic stretching warm-up 1-mile warm-up @ recovery pace 1×30-second hill repetition @ relaxed sprint speed 1-mile cool-down @ recovery pace	
THURSDAY	<u>Optional Nonimpact Cardio</u> <u>Cross-Training Workout</u> 20–30 minutes @ recovery pace (You may break this workout into a 10–15-minute warm-up before and a 10–15-minute cool-down after your resistance workout.)	**Resistance Workout** *1 set each* Lying Hip Abduction Cook Hip Lift Kneeling Overhead Draw-In Knee Fall-Out Squat Jump
FRIDAY	**Fartlek Run** Dynamic stretching warm-up Run 2 miles @ base pace w/2×30-second intervals @ 1-mile pace "sprinkled in"	

SATURDAY	**Resistance Workout** *1 set each* Lying Hip Abduction Cook Hip Lift Kneeling Overhead Draw-In Knee Fall-Out Broad Jump
SUNDAY	**Base Run** Run 3 miles @ base pace

WEEK 2 ◆ Proprioceptive Cue: Navel to Spine

MONDAY	Off
TUESDAY	**Base Run + Drills** Run 2.5 miles @ base pace High Knees 2 × 20 seconds Bounding 2 × 20 seconds
WEDNESDAY	**Hill Repetitions** Dynamic stretching warm-up 1-mile warm-up @ recovery pace 4 × 30-second hill repetitions @ relaxed sprint speed w/2-minute active recoveries 1-mile cool-down @ recovery pace

THURSDAY	Optional Nonimpact Cardio Cross-Training Workout 20–30 minutes @ recovery pace	**Resistance Workout** *2 sets each* Lying Hip Abduction Cook Hip Lift Kneeling Overhead Draw-In Knee Fall-Out Split Squat Jump

FRIDAY	**Fartlek Run** Dynamic stretching warm-up Run 2.5 miles @ base pace w/4 × 30-second intervals @ 1-mile pace "sprinkled in"
SATURDAY	**Resistance Workout** *2 sets each* Lying Hip Abduction Cook Hip Lift Kneeling Overhead Draw-In Knee Fall-Out Wall Jump
SUNDAY	**Base Run** Run 4 miles @ base pace

WEEK 3 ◆ Proprioceptive Cue: Running on Water

MONDAY	Off
TUESDAY	**Base Run + Drills** Run 3 miles @ base pace Stiff-Legged Run 2 × 20 seconds Running No Arms 2 × 20 seconds
WEDNESDAY	**Hill Repetitions** Dynamic stretching warm-up 1-mile warm-up @ recovery pace 5 × 45-second hill repetitions @ 1-mile pace w/2-minute active recoveries 1-mile cool-down @ recovery pace

THURSDAY	<u>Optional Nonimpact Cardio</u>
	<u>Cross-Training Workout</u>
	20–30 minutes @ recovery pace **Resistance Workout**
	    3 sets each
	    Lying Hip Abduction
	    Cook Hip Lift
	    Kneeling Overhead Draw-In
	    Knee Fall-Out
	    Squat Jump

FRIDAY	**Fartlek Run** Dynamic stretching warm-up Run 3 miles @ base pace w/5 × 45-second intervals @ 1-mile pace "sprinkled in"
SATURDAY	**Resistance Workout** *3 sets each* Lying Hip Abduction Cook Hip Lift Kneeling Overhead Draw-In Knee Fall-Out Broad Jump
SUNDAY	**Base Run** Run 5 miles @ base pace

WEEK 4 (Recovery) ◆ Proprioceptive Cue: Pulling the Road

MONDAY	Off
TUESDAY	**Base Run + Drills** Run 3 miles @ base pace One-Leg Hop 20 seconds High Knees 20 seconds
WEDNESDAY	**Hill Repetitions** Dynamic stretching warm-up 1-mile warm-up @ recovery pace 3 × 1-minute hill repetitions @ 1-mile pace w/2-minute active recoveries 1-mile cool-down @ recovery pace

THURSDAY	Optional Nonimpact Cardio Cross-Training Workout 20–30 minutes @ recovery pace	**Resistance Workout** *1 set each* Single-Leg Squat Oblique Bridge Lying Draw-In w/Hip Flexion Quadruped *2 sets each* Lying Hip Abduction Cook Hip Lift Kneeling Overhead Draw-In Knee Fall-Out Single-Leg Squat Jump

FRIDAY	**Fartlek Run** Dynamic stretching warm-up Run 3 miles @ base pace w/3 × 1-minute intervals @ 1-mile pace "sprinkled in"
SATURDAY	**Resistance Workout** *1 set each* Single-Leg Squat Oblique Bridge Lying Draw-In w/Hip Flexion Quadruped *2 sets each* Lying Hip Abduction Cook Hip Lift

SATURDAY (continued)	**Resistance Workout** *2 sets each (cont.)* Kneeling Overhead Draw-In Knee Fall-Out Wall Jump
SUNDAY	**Base Run** Run 4 miles @ base pace

Build 1 Phase

Training objectives: Continue to increase aerobic capacity and endurance; increase fatigue resistance at 3,000m pace and marathon pace; begin to develop efficiency at 10K pace

WEEK 5 ◆ Proprioceptive Cue: Scooting

MONDAY	Off	
TUESDAY	**Base Run + Drills** Run 3 miles @ base pace High Knees 2 × 20 seconds Bounding 2 × 20 seconds	
WEDNESDAY	**400m Intervals @ 3,000m Pace** Dynamic stretching warm-up 1-mile warm-up @ recovery pace 4 × 400m intervals @ 3,000m pace w/3-minute active recoveries 1-mile cool-down @ recovery pace	
THURSDAY	Optional Nonimpact Cardio Cross-Training Workout 20–30 minutes @ recovery pace	**Resistance Workout** *2 sets each* Single-Leg Squat Oblique Bridge Lying Draw-In w/Hip Flexion Quadruped *1 set each* Lying Hip Abduction Cook Hip Lift Kneeling Overhead Draw-In Knee Fall-Out Single-Leg Squat Jump
FRIDAY	**1K Intervals @ 10K Pace** Dynamic stretching warm-up 1-mile warm-up @ recovery pace 2 × 1K @ 10K pace w/2-minute active recoveries 1-mile recovery-pace cool-down	

SATURDAY	**Resistance Workout**
	2 sets each
	Single-Leg Squat
	Oblique Bridge
	Lying Draw-In w/Hip Flexion
	Quadruped
	1 set each
	Lying Hip Abduction
	Cook Hip Lift
	Kneeling Overhead Draw-In
	Knee Fall-Out
	Wall Jump
SUNDAY	**Base Run**
	Run 6 miles @ base pace

WEEK 6 ◆ Proprioceptive Cue: Pounding the Ground

MONDAY	Off	
TUESDAY	**Base Run + Drills** Run 4 miles @ base pace Stiff-Legged Run 2×20 seconds Running No Arms 2×20 seconds	
WEDNESDAY	**400m Intervals @ 3,000m Pace** Dynamic stretching warm-up 1-mile warm-up @ recovery pace 6×400m intervals @ 3,000m pace w/3-minute active recoveries 1-mile cool-down @ recovery pace	
THURSDAY	<u>Optional Nonimpact Cardio</u> <u>Cross-Training Workout</u> 20–30 minutes @ recovery pace	**Resistance Workout** *3 sets each* Single-Leg Squat Oblique Bridge Lying Draw-In w/Hip Flexion Quadruped *2 sets* Squat Jump
FRIDAY	**1K Intervals @ 10K Pace** Dynamic stretching warm-up 1-mile warm-up @ recovery pace 3×1K @ 10K pace w/2-minute active recoveries 1-mile recovery-pace cool-down	
SATURDAY	**Resistance Workout** *3 sets each* Single-Leg Squat Oblique Bridge Lying Draw-In w/Hip Flexion Quadruped *2 sets* Single-Leg Squat Jump	
SUNDAY	**Base Run** Run 7 miles @ base pace	

WEEK 7 ◆ Proprioceptive Cue: Driving the Thigh

MONDAY	Off	
TUESDAY	**Base Run + Drills** Run 5 miles @ base pace Steep Hill Sprints 2 × 20 seconds One-Leg Hop 2 × 20 seconds	
WEDNESDAY	**400m Intervals @ 3,000m Pace** Dynamic stretching warm-up 1-mile warm-up @ recovery pace 8 × 400m intervals @ 3,000m pace w/3-minute active recoveries 1-mile cool-down @ recovery pace	
THURSDAY	Optional Nonimpact Cardio Cross-Training Workout 20–30 minutes @ recovery pace	**Resistance Workout** *2 sets each* Single-Leg Squat Oblique Bridge Lying Draw-In w/Hip Flexion Quadruped Split Squat Jump *1 set each* Box Lunge Stability Ball Leg Curl Forearms to Palms Bridge Dead Bug
FRIDAY	**1K Intervals @ 10K Pace** Dynamic stretching warm-up 1-mile warm-up @ recovery pace 4 × 1K @ 10K pace w/2-minute active recoveries 1-mile recovery-pace cool-down	

(continued)

WEEK 7 ♦ Proprioceptive Cue: Driving the Thigh
(continued)

SATURDAY	Resistance Workout
	2 sets each
	Single-Leg Squat
	Oblique Bridge
	Lying Draw-In w/Hip Flexion
	Quadruped
	Single-Leg Box Jump
	1 set each
	Box Lunge
	Stability Ball Leg Curl
	Forearms to Palms Bridge
	Dead Bug
SUNDAY	**Base Run**
	Run 8 miles @ base pace

WEEK 8 (Recovery) ◆ Proprioceptive Cue: Floppy Feet

MONDAY	Off	
TUESDAY	**Base Run + Drills** Run 4 miles @ base pace High Knees 20 seconds Bounding 20 seconds	
WEDNESDAY	**400m Intervals @ 3,000m Pace** Dynamic stretching warm-up 1-mile warm-up @ recovery pace 6 × 400m intervals @ 3,000m pace w/3-minute active recoveries 1-mile cool-down @ recovery pace	
THURSDAY	Optional Nonimpact Cardio Cross-Training Workout 20–30 minutes @ recovery pace	**Resistance Workout** *1 set each* Single-Leg Squat Oblique Bridge Lying Draw-In w/Hip Flexion Quadruped *2 sets each* Box Lunge Stability Ball Leg Curl Forearms to Palms Bridge Dead Bug Broad Jump
FRIDAY	**1K Intervals @ 10K Pace** Dynamic stretching warm-up 1-mile warm-up @ recovery pace 3 × 1K @ 10K pace w/2-minute active recoveries 1-mile recovery-pace cool-down	

(continued)

WEEK 8 (Recovery) ♦ Proprioceptive Cue: Floppy Feet
(continued)

SATURDAY	**Resistance Workout**
	1 set each
	Single-Leg Squat
	Oblique Bridge
	Lying Draw-In w/Hip Flexion
	Quadruped
	2 sets each
	Box Lunge
	Stability Ball Leg Curl
	Forearms to Palms Bridge
	Dead Bug
	Wall Jump
SUNDAY	**Base Run**
	Run 6 miles @ base pace

Build 2

Training objectives: Increase fatigue resistance at 5K pace and half-marathon pace; continue to build efficiency at 10K pace

WEEK 9 ◆ Proprioceptive Cue: Butt Squeeze

MONDAY	Off
TUESDAY	**Base Run + Drills** Run 5 miles @ base pace Stiff-Legged Run 2×20 seconds Running No Arms 2×20 seconds
WEDNESDAY	**1K Intervals @ 5K Pace** Dynamic stretching warm-up 1-mile warm-up @ recovery pace 3×1K intervals @ 5K pace w/3-minute active recoveries 1-mile cool-down @ recovery pace
THURSDAY	<u>Optional Nonimpact Cardio</u> <u>Cross-Training Workout</u> 20–30 minutes @ recovery pace **Resistance Workout** _3 sets each_ Box Lunge Stability Ball Leg Curl Forearms to Palms Bridge Dead Bug Wall Jump
FRIDAY	**2K Intervals @ 10K Pace** Dynamic stretching warm-up 1-mile warm-up @ recovery pace 2×2K @ 10K pace w/2-minute active recoveries 1-mile recovery-pace cool-down
SATURDAY	**Resistance Workout** _3 sets each_ Box Lunge Stability Ball Leg Curl Forearms to Palms Bridge Dead Bug Single-Leg Box Jump
SUNDAY	**Progression Base Run** Run 6 miles Start @ recovery pace; gradually increase pace every mile Run last mile @ half-marathon pace

WEEK 10 ◆ Proprioceptive Cue: Feeling Symmetry

MONDAY	Off
TUESDAY	**Base Run + Drills** Run 5.5 miles @ base pace Stiff-Legged Run 2 × 20 seconds Running No Arms 2 × 20 seconds
WEDNESDAY	**1K Intervals @ 5K Pace** Dynamic stretching warm-up 1-mile warm-up @ recovery pace 4 × 1K intervals @ 5K pace w/3-minute active recoveries 1-mile cool-down @ recovery pace
THURSDAY	<u>Optional Nonimpact Cardio</u> <u>Cross-Training Workout</u> 20–30 minutes @ recovery pace **Resistance Workout** *1 set each* Lying Hip Abduction Single-Leg Squat Box Lunge Stability Ball Leg Curl Squat Jump
FRIDAY	**2K Intervals @ 10K Pace** Dynamic stretching warm-up 1-mile warm-up @ recovery pace 3 × 2K @ 10K pace w/2-minute active recoveries 1-mile recovery-pace cool-down
SATURDAY	**Resistance Workout** *1 set each* Cook Hip Lift Oblique Bridge Forearms to Palms Bridge Stability Ball Leg Curl Split Squat Jump
SUNDAY	**Progression Base Run** Run 7 miles Start @ recovery pace; gradually increase pace every mile Run last mile @ half-marathon pace

WEEK 11 ♦ Proprioceptive Cue: Axle Between the Knees

MONDAY	Off
TUESDAY	**Base Run + Drills** Run 6 miles @ base pace Steep Hill Sprints 2×20 seconds One-Leg Hop 2×20 seconds
WEDNESDAY	**1K Intervals @ 5K Pace** Dynamic stretching warm-up 1-mile warm-up @ recovery pace 4×1K intervals @ 5K pace w/2-minute active recoveries 1-mile cool-down @ recovery pace

THURSDAY	<u>Optional Nonimpact Cardio</u> <u>Cross-Training Workout</u> 20–30 minutes @ recovery pace	**Resistance Workout** *1 set each* Lying Hip Abduction Single-Leg Squat Box Lunge Stability Ball Leg Curl Single-Leg Squat Jump

FRIDAY	**2K Intervals @ 10K Pace** Dynamic stretching warm-up 1-mile warm-up @ recovery pace 3×2K @ 10K pace w/90-second active recoveries 1-mile recovery-pace cool-down
SATURDAY	**Resistance Workout** *1 set each* Cook Hip Lift Oblique Bridge Forearms to Palms Bridge Stability Ball Leg Curl Broad Jump
SUNDAY	**Progression Base Run** Run 8 miles Start @ recovery pace; gradually increase pace every mile Run last mile @ half-marathon pace

WEEK 12 (Recovery) ◆ Proprioceptive Cue: Running Against a Wall

MONDAY	Off
TUESDAY	**Base Run + Drills** Run 4.5 miles @ base pace High Knees 20 seconds Bounding 20 seconds
WEDNESDAY	**1K Intervals @ 5K Pace** Dynamic stretching warm-up 1-mile warm-up @ recovery pace 3 × 1K intervals @ 5K pace w/3-minute active recoveries 1-mile cool-down @ recovery pace

THURSDAY	<u>Optional Nonimpact Cardio</u> <u>Cross-Training Workout</u> 20–30 minutes @ recovery pace	**Resistance Workout** *1 set each* Lying Hip Abduction Single-Leg Squat Box Lunge Stability Ball Leg Curl Wall Jump

FRIDAY	**2K Intervals @ 10K Pace** Dynamic stretching warm-up 1-mile warm-up @ recovery pace 2 × 2K @ 10K pace w/2-minute active recovery 1-mile recovery-pace cool-down
SATURDAY	**Resistance Workout** *1 set each* Cook Hip Lift Oblique Bridge Forearms to Palms Bridge Stability Ball Leg Curl
SUNDAY	**5K Tune-up Race or Time Trial** Dynamic stretching warm-up 1-mile warm-up @ recovery pace 5K tune-up race or time trial 1-mile recovery-pace cool-down

Peak Phase

Training objectives: Achieve peak fatigue resistance and efficiency at 10K pace; adapt and recover for peak race day

WEEK 13 ◆ Proprioceptive Cue: Falling Forward

MONDAY	Off	
TUESDAY	**Base Run + Drills** Run 6 miles @ base pace High Knees 2 × 20 seconds Bounding 2 × 20 seconds	
WEDNESDAY	**Mixed Intervals** Dynamic stretching warm-up 1-mile warm-up @ recovery pace 1 × 2K @ half-marathon pace, 2-minute active recovery 1 × 1 mile @ 10K pace, 2-minute active recovery 1 × 1K @ 5K pace, 2-minute active recovery 1 × 800m @ 3,000m pace 1-mile cool-down @ recovery pace	
THURSDAY	Optional Nonimpact Cardio Cross-Training Workout 20–30 minutes @ recovery pace	**Resistance Workout** *1 set each* Lying Hip Abduction Single-Leg Squat Box Lunge Stability Ball Leg Curl Wall Jump
FRIDAY	**3K Intervals @ 10K Pace** Dynamic stretching warm-up 1-mile warm-up @ recovery pace 2 × 3K @ 10K pace w/3-minute active recovery 1-mile recovery-pace cool-down	

(continued)

WEEK 13 ♦ Proprioceptive Cue: Falling Forward
(continued)

SATURDAY	**Resistance Workout** *1 set each* Cook Hip Lift Oblique Bridge Forearms to Palms Bridge Stability Ball Leg Curl Single-Leg Box Jump
SUNDAY	**Half-Marathon-Pace Tempo Run** 1-mile warm-up @ recovery pace 4 miles @ half-marathon pace 1-mile recovery-pace cool-down

WEEK 14 ◆ Proprioceptive Cue: Navel to Spine

MONDAY	Off
TUESDAY	**Base Run + Drills** Run 6 miles @ base pace Stiff-Legged Run 2 × 20 seconds Running No Arms 2 × 20 seconds
WEDNESDAY	**Mixed Intervals** Dynamic stretching warm-up 1-mile warm-up @ recovery pace 1 × 2K @ half-marathon pace, 2-minute active recovery 1 × 1 mile @ 10K pace, 2-minute active recovery 1 × 1K @ 5K pace, 2-minute active recovery 1 × 800m @ 3,000m pace 1-mile cool-down @ recovery pace

THURSDAY	<u>Optional Nonimpact Cardio</u> <u>Cross-Training Workout</u> 20–30 minutes @ recovery pace	**Resistance Workout** *1 set each* Lying Hip Abduction Single-Leg Squat Box Lunge Stability Ball Leg Curl Squat Jump

FRIDAY	**3K Intervals @ 10K Pace** Dynamic stretching warm-up 1-mile warm-up @ recovery pace 2 × 3K @ 10K pace w/2-minute active recovery 1-mile recovery-pace cool-down
SATURDAY	**Resistance Workout** *1 set each* Cook Hip Lift Oblique Bridge Forearms to Palms Bridge Stability Ball Leg Curl Split Squat Jump
SUNDAY	**Half-Marathon-Pace Tempo Run** 1-mile warm-up @ recovery pace 4 miles @ half-marathon pace 1-mile recovery-pace cool-down

WEEK 15 (Recovery) ◆ Proprioceptive Cue: Running on Water

MONDAY	Off	
TUESDAY	**Base Run + Drills** Run 5 miles @ base pace Steep Hill Sprints 20 seconds One-Leg Hop 20 seconds	
WEDNESDAY	**Mixed Intervals** Dynamic stretching warm-up 1-mile warm-up @ recovery pace 1×2K @ half-marathon pace, 2-minute active recovery 1×1 mile @ 10K pace, 2-minute active recovery 1×1K @ 5K pace, 2-minute active recovery 1-mile cool-down @ recovery pace	
THURSDAY	Optional Nonimpact Cardio Cross-Training Workout 20–30 minutes @ recovery pace	**Resistance Workout** *1 set each* Lying Hip Abduction Single-Leg Squat Box Lunge Stability Ball Leg Curl Single-Leg Squat Jump
FRIDAY	**3K Intervals @ 10K Pace** Dynamic stretching warm-up 1-mile warm-up @ recovery pace 2×3K @ 10K pace w/3-minute active recovery 1-mile recovery-pace cool-down	
SATURDAY	**Resistance Workout** *1 set each* Cook Hip Lift Oblique Bridge Forearms to Palms Bridge Stability Ball Leg Curl Broad Jump	
SUNDAY	**10K Tune-up Race or Time Trial** Dynamic stretching warm-up 1-mile warm-up @ recovery pace 10K tune-up race or time trial 1-mile recovery-pace cool-down	

WEEK 16 ◆ Proprioceptive Cue: Pulling the Road

MONDAY	Off
TUESDAY	**Base Run + Drills** Run 6 miles @ base pace Stiff-Legged Run 2 × 20 seconds Running No Arms 2 × 20 seconds
WEDNESDAY	**Mixed Intervals** Dynamic stretching warm-up 1-mile warm-up @ recovery pace 1 × 2K @ half-marathon pace, 90-second active recovery 1 × 1 mile @ 10K pace, 90-second active recovery 1 × 1K @ 5K pace, 90-second active recovery 1 × 800m @ 3,000m pace 1-mile cool-down @ recovery pace

THURSDAY	Optional Nonimpact Cardio Cross-Training Workout 20–30 minutes @ recovery pace	**Resistance Workout** *1 set each* Lying Hip Abduction Single-Leg Squat Box Lunge Stability Ball Leg Curl Squat Jump

FRIDAY	**3K Intervals @ 10K Pace** Dynamic stretching warm-up 1-mile warm-up @ recovery pace 2 × 3K @ 10K pace w/90-second active recovery 1-mile recovery-pace cool-down
SATURDAY	**Resistance Workout** *1 set each* Cook Hip Lift Oblique Bridge Forearms to Palms Bridge Stability Ball Leg Curl Split Squat Jump
SUNDAY	**Half-Marathon-Pace Tempo Run** 1-mile warm-up @ recovery pace 5 miles @ half-marathon pace 1-mile recovery-pace cool-down

WEEK 17 ✦ Proprioceptive Cue: Driving the Thigh

MONDAY	Off	
TUESDAY	**Base Run + Drills** Run 6 miles @ base pace Stiff-Legged Run 2×20 seconds Running No Arms 2×20 seconds	
WEDNESDAY	**Mixed Intervals** Dynamic stretching warm-up 1-mile warm-up @ recovery pace 1×2K @ half-marathon pace, 1-minute active recovery 1×1 mile @ 10K pace, 1-minute active recovery 1×1K @ 5K pace, 1-minute active recovery 1×800m @ 3,000m pace 1-mile cool-down @ recovery pace	
THURSDAY	Optional Nonimpact Cardio Cross-Training Workout 20–30 minutes @ recovery pace	**Resistance Workout** *1 set each* Lying Hip Abduction Single-Leg Squat Box Lunge Stability Ball Leg Curl Squat Jump
FRIDAY	**3K Intervals @ 10K Pace** Dynamic stretching warm-up 1-mile warm-up @ recovery pace 2×3K @ 10K pace w/1-minute active recovery 1-mile recovery-pace cool-down	
SATURDAY	**Resistance Workout** *1 set each* Cook Hip Lift Oblique Bridge Forearms to Palms Bridge Stability Ball Leg Curl Split Squat Jump	
SUNDAY	**Half-Marathon-Pace Tempo Run** 1-mile warm-up @ recovery pace 6 miles @ half-marathon pace 1-mile recovery-pace cool-down	

WEEK 18 (Taper) ◆ Proprioceptive Cue: Your Choice

MONDAY	Off	
TUESDAY	**Base Run + Drills** Run 5 miles @ base pace Stiff-Legged Run 20 seconds Running No Arms 20 seconds	
WEDNESDAY	**Mixed Intervals** Dynamic stretching warm-up 1-mile warm-up @ recovery pace 1×2K @ half-marathon pace, 1-minute active recovery 1×1 mile @ 10K pace, 1-minute active recovery 1×1K @ 5K pace 1-mile cool-down @ recovery pace	
THURSDAY	Optional Nonimpact Cardio Cross-Training Workout 20–30 minutes @ recovery pace	**Resistance Workout** *1 set each* Lying Hip Abduction Single-Leg Squat Box Lunge Stability Ball Leg Curl Squat Jump
FRIDAY	**3K Interval @ 10K Pace** Dynamic stretching warm-up 1-mile warm-up @ recovery pace 1×3K @ 10K pace 1-mile recovery-pace cool-down	
SATURDAY	Off	
SUNDAY	**10K Peak Race** Dynamic stretching warm-up 1-mile warm-up @ recovery pace 10K race or time trial 1-mile recovery-pace cool-down	

LEVEL 2

Use this plan if you are most comfortable with a 10K training plan that features six runs per week and a maximum run distance of 11 miles. The plan also includes two resistance workouts per week and one optional nonimpact cardio cross-training workout.

Base Phase

Training objectives: Build aerobic capacity and endurance, increase injury resistance, and increase muscle activation capacity

WEEK 1 ♦ Proprioceptive Cue: Falling Forward

MONDAY	Off	
TUESDAY	**Base Run + Drills** Run 4 miles @ base pace Running No Arms 20 seconds One-Leg Hop 20 seconds	
WEDNESDAY	**Hill Repetitions** Dynamic stretching warm-up 2-mile warm-up @ recovery pace 1 × 30-second hill repetition @ relaxed sprint speed 2-mile cool-down @ recovery pace	
THURSDAY	**Base Run** Run 4 miles @ base pace or Nonimpact Cardio Cross-Training Workout 20–30 minutes @ recovery pace	**Resistance Workout** *1 set each* Lying Hip Abduction Cook Hip Lift Kneeling Overhead Draw-In Knee Fall-Out Squat Jump
FRIDAY	**Fartlek Run** Dynamic stretching warm-up Run 4 miles @ base pace w/ 2 × 30-second intervals @ 1-mile pace "sprinkled in"	

SATURDAY	**Base Run** Run 4 miles @ base pace	**Resistance Workout** *1 set each* Lying Hip Abduction Cook Hip Lift Kneeling Overhead Draw-In Knee Fall-Out Broad Jump
SUNDAY	**Base Run** Run 5 miles @ base pace	

WEEK 2 ◆ Proprioceptive Cue: Navel to Spine

MONDAY	Off	
TUESDAY	**Base Run + Drills** Run 4.5 miles @ base pace High Knees 2 × 20 seconds Bounding 2 × 20 seconds	
WEDNESDAY	**Hill Repetitions** Dynamic stretching warm-up 2-mile warm-up @ recovery pace 6 × 30-second hill repetitions @ relaxed sprint speed w/2-minute active recoveries 2-mile cool-down @ recovery pace	
THURSDAY	**Base Run** Run 4.5 miles @ base pace *or* Nonimpact Cardio Cross-Training Workout 25–35 minutes @ recovery pace	**Resistance Workout** *2 sets each* Lying Hip Abduction Cook Hip Lift Kneeling Overhead Draw-In Knee Fall-Out Split Squat Jump
FRIDAY	**Fartlek Run** Dynamic stretching warm-up Run 4.5 miles @ base pace w/6 × 30-second intervals @ 1-mile pace "sprinkled in"	
SATURDAY	**Base Run** Run 4.5 miles @ base pace	**Resistance Workout** *2 sets each* Lying Hip Abduction Cook Hip Lift Kneeling Overhead Draw-In Knee Fall-Out Wall Jump
SUNDAY	**Base Run** Run 6 miles @ base pace	

WEEK 3 ♦ Proprioceptive Cue: Running on Water

MONDAY	Off
TUESDAY	**Base Run + Drills** Run 5 miles @ base pace Stiff-Legged Run 2 × 20 seconds Running No Arms 2 × 20 seconds
WEDNESDAY	**Hill Repetitions** Dynamic stretching warm-up 2-mile warm-up @ recovery pace 7 × 45-second hill repetitions @ 1-mile pace w/2-minute active recoveries 2-mile cool-down @ recovery pace
THURSDAY	**Base Run** Run 5 miles @ base pace *or* Nonimpact Cardio Cross-Training Workout 30–40 minutes @ recovery pace **Resistance Workout** *3 sets each* Lying Hip Abduction Cook Hip Lift Kneeling Overhead Draw-In Knee Fall-Out Squat Jump
FRIDAY	**Fartlek Run** Dynamic stretching warm-up Run 5 miles @ base pace w/7 × 45-second intervals @ 1-mile pace "sprinkled in"
SATURDAY	**Base Run** Run 5 miles @ base pace **Resistance Workout** *3 sets each* Lying Hip Abduction Cook Hip Lift Kneeling Overhead Draw-In Knee Fall-Out Broad Jump
SUNDAY	**Base Run** Run 7 miles @ base pace

WEEK 4 (Recovery) ◆ Proprioceptive Cue: Pulling the Road

MONDAY	Off		
TUESDAY	**Base Run + Drills** Run 4 miles @ base pace One-Leg Hop 20 seconds High Knees 20 seconds		
WEDNESDAY	**Hill Repetitions** Dynamic stretching warm-up 2-mile warm-up @ recovery pace 3×1-minute hill repetitions @ 1-mile pace w/2-minute active recoveries 2-mile cool-down @ recovery pace		
THURSDAY	**Base Run** Run 4 miles @ base pace *or* <u>Nonimpact Cardio Cross-Training Workout</u> 20–30 minutes @ recovery pace	**Resistance Workout** *1 set each* Single-Leg Squat Oblique Bridge Lying Draw-In w/Hip Flexion Quadruped *2 sets each* Lying Hip Abduction Cook Hip Lift Kneeling Overhead Draw-In Knee Fall-Out Single-Leg Squat Jump	
FRIDAY	**Fartlek Run** Dynamic stretching warm-up Run 4 miles @ base pace w/3×1-minute intervals @ 1-mile pace "sprinkled in"		
SATURDAY	**Base Run** Run 4 miles @ base pace	**Resistance Workout** *1 set each* Single-Leg Squat Oblique Bridge Lying Draw-In w/Hip Flexion Quadruped	

SATURDAY (continued)	Base Run	Resistance Workout *2 sets each* Lying Hip Abduction Cook Hip Lift Kneeling Overhead Draw-In Knee Fall-Out Wall Jump
SUNDAY	**Base Run** Run 5 miles @ base pace	

Build 1 Phase

Training objectives: Continue to increase aerobic capacity and endurance; increase fatigue resistance at 3,000m pace and marathon pace; begin to develop efficiency at 10K pace

WEEK 5 ◆ Proprioceptive Cue: Scooting

MONDAY	Off	
TUESDAY	**Base Run + Drills** Run 5.5 miles @ base pace High Knees 2×20 seconds Bounding 2×20 seconds	
WEDNESDAY	**400m Intervals @ 3,000m Pace** Dynamic stretching warm-up 1.5-mile warm-up @ recovery pace 6×400m intervals @ 3,000m pace w/3-minute active recoveries 1.5-mile cool-down @ recovery pace	
THURSDAY	**Recovery Run** 2–6 miles @ recovery pace *or* Nonimpact Cardio Cross-Training Workout 20–45 minutes @ recovery pace	**Resistance Workout** *2 sets each* Single-Leg Squat Oblique Bridge Lying Draw-In w/Hip Flexion Quadruped *1 set each* Lying Hip Abduction Cook Hip Lift Kneeling Overhead Draw-In Knee Fall-Out Single-Leg Squat Jump
FRIDAY	**1K Intervals @ 10K Pace** Dynamic stretching warm-up 1.5-mile warm-up @ recovery pace 3×1K @ 10K pace w/2-minute active recoveries 1.5-mile recovery-pace cool-down	

| SATURDAY | **Recovery Run**
2–6 miles @ recovery pace | **Resistance Workout**
2 sets each
Single-Leg Squat
Oblique Bridge
Lying Draw-In w/Hip Flexion
Quadruped

1 set each
Lying Hip Abduction
Cook Hip Lift
Kneeling Overhead Draw-In
Knee Fall-Out
Wall Jump |
| SUNDAY | **Base Run**
Run 8 miles @ base pace | |

WEEK 6 ◆ Proprioceptive Cue: Pounding the Ground

MONDAY	Off	
TUESDAY	**Base Run + Drills** Run 6 miles @ base pace Stiff-Legged Run 2×20 seconds Running No Arms 2×20 seconds	
WEDNESDAY	**400m Intervals @ 3,000m Pace** Dynamic stretching warm-up 1.5-mile warm-up @ recovery pace 8×400m intervals @ 3,000m pace w/3-minute active recoveries 1.5-mile cool-down @ recovery pace	
THURSDAY	**Recovery Run** 2–6 miles @ recovery pace *or* <u>Nonimpact Cardio Cross-Training Workout</u> 20–45 minutes @ recovery pace	**Resistance Workout** *3 sets each* Single-Leg Squat Oblique Bridge Lying Draw-In w/Hip Flexion Quadruped *2 sets* Squat Jump
FRIDAY	**1K Intervals @ 10K Pace** Dynamic stretching warm-up 1.5-mile warm-up @ recovery pace 4×1K @ 10K pace w/2-minute active recoveries 1.5-mile recovery-pace cool-down	
SATURDAY	**Recovery Run** 2–6 miles @ recovery pace	**Resistance Workout** *3 sets each* Single-Leg Squat Oblique Bridge Lying Draw-In w/Hip Flexion Quadruped *2 sets* Single-Leg Squat Jump
SUNDAY	**Base Run** Run 9 miles @ base pace	

WEEK 7 ◆ Proprioceptive Cue: Driving the Thigh

MONDAY	Off
TUESDAY	**Base Run + Drills** Run 6.5 miles @ base pace Steep Hill Sprints 2 × 20 seconds One-Leg Hop 2 × 20 seconds
WEDNESDAY	**400m Intervals @ 3,000m Pace** Dynamic stretching warm-up 1.5-mile warm-up @ recovery pace 10 × 400m intervals @ 3,000m pace w/3-minute active recoveries 1.5-mile cool-down @ recovery pace

THURSDAY	**Recovery Run** 2–6 miles @ recovery pace *or* Nonimpact Cardio Cross-Training Workout 20–45 minutes @ recovery pace	**Resistance Workout** *2 sets each* Single-Leg Squat Oblique Bridge Lying Draw-In w/Hip Flexion Quadruped Split Squat Jump *1 set each* Box Lunge Stability Ball Leg Curl Forearms to Palms Bridge Dead Bug

FRIDAY	**1K Intervals @ 10K Pace** Dynamic stretching warm-up 1.5-mile warm-up @ recovery pace 5 × 1K @ 10K pace w/2-minute active recoveries 1.5-mile recovery-pace cool-down

SATURDAY	**Recovery Run** 2–6 miles @ recovery pace	**Resistance Workout** *2 sets each* Single-Leg Squat Oblique Bridge Lying Draw-In w/Hip Flexion Quadruped Single-Leg Box Jump

(continued)

WEEK 7 ◆ Proprioceptive Cue: Driving the Thigh
(continued)

SATURDAY (continued)	Recovery Run	Resistance Workout *1 set each* Box Lunge Stability Ball Leg Curl Forearms to Palms Bridge Dead Bug
SUNDAY	**Endurance Run** Run 10 miles @ base pace	

WEEK 8 (Recovery) ◆ Proprioceptive Cue: Floppy Feet

MONDAY	Off	
TUESDAY	**Base Run + Drills** Run 5 miles @ base pace High Knees 20 seconds Bounding 20 seconds	
WEDNESDAY	**400m Intervals @ 3,000m Pace** Dynamic stretching warm-up 1-mile warm-up @ recovery pace 6 × 400m intervals @ 3,000m pace w/3-minute active recoveries 1-mile cool-down @ recovery pace	
THURSDAY	**Recovery Run** 2–6 miles @ recovery pace *or* <u>Nonimpact Cardio Cross-Training Workout</u> 20–45 minutes @ recovery pace	**Resistance Workout** *1 set each* Single-Leg Squat Oblique Bridge Lying Draw-In w/Hip Flexion Quadruped *2 sets each* Box Lunge Stability Ball Leg Curl Forearms to Palms Bridge Dead Bug Broad Jump
FRIDAY	**1K Intervals @ 10K Pace** Dynamic stretching warm-up 1.5-mile warm-up @ recovery pace 4 × 1K @ 10K pace w/2-minute active recoveries 1.5-mile recovery-pace cool-down	
SATURDAY	**Recovery Run** 2–6 miles @ recovery pace	**Resistance Workout** *1 set each* Single-Leg Squat Oblique Bridge Lying Draw-In w/Hip Flexion Quadruped

(continued)

WEEK 8 (Recovery) ◆ Proprioceptive Cue: Floppy Feet
(continued)

SATURDAY (continued)	Recovery Run	Resistance Workout *2 sets each* Box Lunge Stability Ball Leg Curl Forearms to Palms Bridge Dead Bug Wall Jump
SUNDAY	Base Run Run 7 miles @ base pace	

Build 2 Phase

Training objectives: Increase fatigue resistance at 5K pace and half-marathon pace; continue to build efficiency at 10K pace

WEEK 9 ◆ Proprioceptive Cue: Butt Squeeze

MONDAY	Off	
TUESDAY	**Base Run + Drills** Run 6.5 miles @ base pace Stiff-Legged Run 2 × 20 seconds Running No Arms 2 × 20 seconds	
WEDNESDAY	**1K Intervals @ 5K Pace** Dynamic stretching warm-up 1.5-mile warm-up @ recovery pace 3 × 1K intervals @ 5K pace w/3-minute active recoveries 1.5-mile cool-down @ recovery pace	
THURSDAY	**Recovery Run** 2–6 miles @ recovery pace *or* Nonimpact Cardio Cross-Training Workout 20–45 minutes @ recovery pace	**Resistance Workout** *3 sets each* Box Lunge Stability Ball Leg Curl Forearms to Palms Bridge Dead Bug Wall Jump
FRIDAY	**2K Intervals @ 10K Pace** Dynamic stretching warm-up 1.5-mile warm-up @ recovery pace 3 × 2K @ 10K pace w/2-minute active recoveries 1.5-mile recovery-pace cool-down	
SATURDAY	**Recovery Run** 2–6 miles @ recovery pace	**Resistance Workout** *3 sets each* Box Lunge Stability Ball Leg Curl Forearms to Palms Bridge Dead Bug Single-Leg Box Jump
SUNDAY	**Progression Base Run** Run 9 miles Start @ recovery pace; gradually increase pace every other mile Run last mile @ half-marathon pace	

WEEK 10 ◆ Proprioceptive Cue: Feeling Symmetry

MONDAY	Off
TUESDAY	**Base Run + Drills** Run 7 miles @ base pace Stiff-Legged Run 2×20 seconds Running No Arms 2×20 seconds
WEDNESDAY	**1K Intervals @ 5K Pace** Dynamic stretching warm-up 1.5-mile warm-up @ recovery pace 4×1K intervals @ 5K pace w/3-minute active recoveries 1.5-mile cool-down @ recovery pace

THURSDAY	**Recovery Run** 2–6 miles @ recovery pace *or* <u>Nonimpact Cardio Cross-Training Workout</u> 20–45 minutes @ recovery pace	**Resistance Workout** *2 sets each* Lying Hip Abduction Single-Leg Squat Box Lunge Stability Ball Leg Curl Squat Jump

FRIDAY	**2K Intervals @ 10K Pace** Dynamic stretching warm-up 1.5-mile warm-up @ recovery pace 3×2K @ 10K pace w/2-minute active recoveries 1.5-mile recovery-pace cool-down

SATURDAY	**Recovery Run** 2–6 miles @ recovery pace	**Resistance Workout** *2 sets each* Cook Hip Lift Oblique Bridge Forearms to Palms Bridge Stability Ball Leg Curl Split Squat Jump

SUNDAY	**Progression Run** Run 10 miles Start @ recovery pace; gradually increase pace every other mile Run last 2 miles @ half-marathon pace

WEEK 11 ◆ Proprioceptive Cue: Axle Between the Knees

MONDAY	Off
TUESDAY	**Base Run + Drills** Run 7.5 miles @ base pace Steep Hill Sprints 2 × 20 seconds One-Leg Hop 2 × 20 seconds
WEDNESDAY	**1K Intervals @ 5K Pace** Dynamic stretching warm-up 1.5-mile warm-up @ recovery pace 5 × 1K intervals @ 5K pace w/2-minute active recoveries 1.5-mile cool-down @ recovery pace

THURSDAY	**Recovery Run** 2–6 miles @ recovery pace *or* Nonimpact Cardio Cross-Training Workout 20–45 minutes @ recovery pace	**Resistance Workout** *2 sets each* Lying Hip Abduction Single-Leg Squat Box Lunge Stability Ball Leg Curl Single-Leg Squat Jump

FRIDAY	**2K Intervals @ 10K Pace** Dynamic stretching warm-up 1.5-mile warm-up @ recovery pace 4 × 2K @ 10K pace w/90-second active recoveries 1.5-mile recovery-pace cool-down

SATURDAY	**Recovery Run** 2–6 miles @ recovery pace	**Resistance Workout** *2 sets each* Cook Hip Lift Oblique Bridge Forearms to Palms Bridge Stability Ball Leg Curl Broad Jump

SUNDAY	**Progression Run** Run 11 miles Start @ recovery pace; gradually increase pace every other mile Run last 2 miles @ half-marathon pace

WEEK 12 (Recovery) ◆ Proprioceptive Cue: Running Against a Wall

MONDAY	Off	
TUESDAY	**Base Run + Drills** Run 6 miles @ base pace High Knees 20 seconds Bounding 20 seconds	
WEDNESDAY	**1K Intervals @ 5K Pace** Dynamic stretching warm-up 1.5-mile warm-up @ recovery pace 3 × 1K intervals @ 5K pace w/3-minute active recoveries 1.5-mile cool-down @ recovery pace	
THURSDAY	**Recovery Run** 2–6 miles @ recovery pace *or* <u>Nonimpact Cardio Cross-Training Workout</u> 20–45 minutes @ recovery pace	**Resistance Workout** *2 sets each* Lying Hip Abduction Single-Leg Squat Box Lunge Stability Ball Leg Curl Wall Jump
FRIDAY	**2K Intervals @ 10K Pace** Dynamic stretching warm-up 1.5-mile warm-up @ recovery pace 3 × 2K @ 10K pace w/2-minute active recoveries 1.5-mile recovery-pace cool-down	
SATURDAY	**Recovery Run** 2 miles @ recovery pace	**Resistance Workout** *1 set each* Cook Hip Lift Oblique Bridge Forearms to Palms Bridge Stability Ball Leg Curl
SUNDAY	**5K Tune-up Race or Time Trial** Dynamic stretching warm-up 1.5-mile warm-up @ recovery pace 5K tune-up race or time trial 1.5-mile recovery-pace cool-down	

Peak Phase

Training objectives: Achieve peak fatigue resistance and efficiency at 10K pace; adapt and recover for peak race day

WEEK 13 ◆ Proprioceptive Cue: Falling Forward

MONDAY	Off	
TUESDAY	**Base Run + Drills** Run 7 miles @ base pace High Knees 2 × 20 seconds Bounding 2 × 20 seconds	
WEDNESDAY	**Mixed Intervals** Dynamic stretching warm-up 1-mile warm-up @ recovery pace 1 × 2K @ half-marathon pace, 2-minute active recovery 1 × 1 mile @ 10K pace, 2-minute active recovery 1 × 1K @ 5K pace, 2-minute active recovery 2 × 800m @ 3,000m pace, 2-minute active recoveries 1-mile cool-down @ recovery pace	
THURSDAY	**Recovery Run** 2–6 miles @ recovery pace *or* Nonimpact Cardio Cross-Training Workout 20–45 minutes @ recovery pace	**Resistance Workout** *2 sets each* Lying Hip Abduction Single-Leg Squat Box Lunge Stability Ball Leg Curl Wall Jump
FRIDAY	**3K Intervals @ 10K Pace** Dynamic stretching warm-up 1.5-mile warm-up @ recovery pace 3 × 3K @ 10K pace w/3-minute active recoveries 1.5-mile recovery-pace cool-down	

(continued)

WEEK 13 ◆ Proprioceptive Cue: Falling Forward
(continued)

SATURDAY	Recovery Run
	  2–6 miles @ recovery pace
		Resistance Workout
		  2 sets each
		  Cook Hip Lift
		  Oblique Bridge
		  Forearms to Palms Bridge
		  Stability Ball Leg Curl
		  Single-Leg Box Jump

SUNDAY	**Half-Marathon-Pace Tempo Run**
	  2-mile warm-up @ recovery pace
	  4 miles @ half-marathon pace
	  2-mile recovery-pace cool-down	

WEEK 14 ◆ Proprioceptive Cue: Navel to Spine

MONDAY	Off
TUESDAY	**Base Run + Drills** Run 7.5 miles @ base pace Stiff-Legged Run 2 × 20 seconds Running No Arms 2 × 20 seconds
WEDNESDAY	**Mixed Intervals** Dynamic stretching warm-up 1-mile warm-up @ recovery pace 1 × 2K @ half-marathon pace, 2-minute active recovery 1 × 1 mile @ 10K pace, 2-minute active recovery 2 × 1K @ 5K pace, 2-minute active recoveries 2 × 800m @ 3,000m pace, 2-minute active recoveries 1-mile cool-down @ recovery pace

THURSDAY	**Recovery Run** 2–6 miles @ recovery pace *or* <u>Nonimpact Cardio Cross-Training Workout</u> 20–45 minutes @ recovery pace	**Resistance Workout** *2 sets each* Lying Hip Abduction Single-Leg Squat Box Lunge Stability Ball Leg Curl Squat Jump

FRIDAY	**3K Intervals @ 10K Pace** Dynamic stretching warm-up 1.5-mile warm-up @ recovery pace 3 × 3K @ 10K pace w/2-minute active recoveries 1.5-mile recovery-pace cool-down

SATURDAY	**Recovery Run** 2–6 miles @ recovery pace	**Resistance Workout** *2 sets each* Cook Hip Lift Oblique Bridge Forearms to Palms Bridge Stability Ball Leg Curl Split Squat Jump

SUNDAY	**Half-Marathon-Pace Tempo Run** 2-mile warm-up @ recovery pace 5-miles @ half-marathon pace 2-mile recovery-pace cool-down

WEEK 15 (Recovery) ◆ Proprioceptive Cue: Running on Water

MONDAY	Off	
TUESDAY	**Base Run + Drills** Run 6 miles @ base pace Steep Hill Sprints 20 seconds One-Leg Hop 20 seconds	
WEDNESDAY	**Mixed Intervals** Dynamic stretching warm-up 1-mile warm-up @ recovery pace 1×2K @ half-marathon pace, 2-minute active recovery 1×1 mile @ 10K pace, 2-minute active recovery 1×1K @ 5K pace, 2-minute active recovery 2×800m @ 3,000m pace 1-mile cool-down @ recovery pace	
THURSDAY	**Recovery Run** 2–6 miles @ recovery pace *or* Nonimpact Cardio Cross-Training Workout 20–45 minutes @ recovery pace	**Resistance Workout** *2 sets each* Lying Hip Abduction Single-Leg Squat Box Lunge Stability Ball Leg Curl Single-Leg Squat Jump
FRIDAY	**3K Intervals @ 10K Pace** Dynamic stretching warm-up 1.5-mile warm-up @ recovery pace 2×3K @ 10K pace w/3-minute active recoveries 1.5-mile recovery-pace cool-down	
SATURDAY	**Recovery Run** 2 miles @ recovery pace	**Resistance Workout** *2 sets each* Cook Hip Lift Oblique Bridge Forearms to Palms Bridge Stability Ball Leg Curl Broad Jump
SUNDAY	**10K Tune-up Race or Time Trial** Dynamic stretching warm-up 1.5-mile warm-up @ recovery pace 10K tune-up race or time trial 1.5-mile recovery-pace cool-down	

WEEK 16 ◆ Proprioceptive Cue: Pulling the Road

MONDAY	Off
TUESDAY	**Base Run + Drills** Run 8 miles @ base pace Stiff-Legged Run 2 × 20 seconds Running No Arms 2 × 20 seconds
WEDNESDAY	**Mixed Intervals** Dynamic stretching warm-up 1-mile warm-up @ recovery pace 1 × 2K @ half-marathon pace, 90-second active recovery 1 × 1 mile @ 10K pace, 90-second active recovery 2 × 1K @ 5K pace, 90-second active recoveries 2 × 800m @ 3,000m pace, 90-second active recoveries 1-mile cool-down @ recovery pace

THURSDAY	**Recovery Run** 2–6 miles @ recovery pace *or* <u>Nonimpact Cardio Cross-Training Workout</u> 20–45 minutes @ recovery pace	**Resistance Workout** *2 sets each* Lying Hip Abduction Single-Leg Squat Box Lunge Stability Ball Leg Curl Squat Jump

FRIDAY	**3K Intervals @ 10K Pace** Dynamic stretching warm-up 1.5-mile warm-up @ recovery pace 3 × 3K @ 10K pace w/90-second active recoveries 1.5-mile recovery-pace cool-down

SATURDAY	**Recovery Run** 2–6 miles @ recovery pace	**Resistance Workout** *2 sets each* Cook Hip Lift Oblique Bridge Forearms to Palms Bridge Stability Ball Leg Curl Split Squat Jump

SUNDAY	**Half-Marathon-Pace Tempo Run** 2-mile warm-up @ recovery pace 6 miles @ half-marathon pace 2-mile recovery-pace cool-down

WEEK 17 ◆ Proprioceptive Cue: Scooting

MONDAY	Off	
TUESDAY	**Base Run + Drills** Run 7 miles @ base pace Stiff-Legged Run 2×20 seconds Running No Arms 2×20 seconds	
WEDNESDAY	**Mixed Intervals** Dynamic stretching warm-up 1-mile warm-up @ recovery pace 1×2K @ half-marathon pace, 1-minute active recovery 1×1 mile @ 10K pace, 1-minute active recovery 2×1K @ 5K pace, 1-minute active recoveries 2×800m @ 3,000m pace, 1-minute active recoveries 1-mile cool-down @ recovery pace	
THURSDAY	**Recovery Run** 2–6 miles @ recovery pace *or* <u>Nonimpact Cardio Cross-Training Workout</u> 20–45 minutes @ recovery pace	**Resistance Workout** *2 sets each* Lying Hip Abduction Single-Leg Squat Box Lunge Stability Ball Leg Curl Squat Jump
FRIDAY	**3K Intervals @ 10K Pace** Dynamic stretching warm-up 1.5-mile warm-up @ recovery pace 3×3K @ 10K pace w/1-minute active recoveries 1.5-mile recovery-pace cool-down	
SATURDAY	**Recovery Run** 2–6 miles @ recovery pace	**Resistance Workout** *2 sets each* Cook Hip Lift Oblique Bridge Forearms to Palms Bridge Stability Ball Leg Curl Split Squat Jump
SUNDAY	**Half-Marathon-Pace Tempo Run** 2-mile warm-up @ recovery pace 6 miles @ half-marathon pace 2-mile recovery-pace cool-down	

WEEK 18 (Taper) ◆ Proprioceptive Cue: Your Choice

MONDAY	Off	
TUESDAY	**Base Run + Drills** Run 6 miles @ base pace Stiff-Legged Run 20 seconds Running No Arms 20 seconds	
WEDNESDAY	**Mixed Intervals** Dynamic stretching warm-up 1-mile warm-up @ recovery pace 1×2K @ half-marathon pace, 1-minute active recovery 1×1 mile @ 10K pace, 1-minute active recovery 1×1K @ 5K pace, 1-minute active recovery 1×800m @ 3,000m pace 1-mile cool-down @ recovery pace	
THURSDAY	**Recovery Run** 2–6 miles @ recovery pace *or* Nonimpact Cardio Cross-Training Workout 20–45 minutes @ recovery pace	**Resistance Workout** *1 set each* Lying Hip Abduction Single-Leg Squat Box Lunge Stability Ball Leg Curl Squat Jump
FRIDAY	**3K Interval @ 10K Pace** Dynamic stretching warm-up 1.5-mile warm-up @ recovery pace 1×3K @ 10K pace 1.5-mile recovery-pace cool-down	
SATURDAY	Off	
SUNDAY	**10K Peak Race** Dynamic stretching warm-up 1.5-mile warm-up @ recovery pace 10K peak race 1.5-mile recovery-pace cool-down	

LEVEL 3

Use this plan if you are most comfortable with a 10K training plan that features six scheduled runs per week plus up to four additional, optional recovery runs or nonimpact cardio cross-training workouts and a maximum run distance of 12 miles. There are also two scheduled resistance workouts each week.

Base Phase

Training objectives: Build aerobic capacity and endurance, increase injury resistance, and increase muscle activation capacity

WEEK 1 ◆ Proprioceptive Cue: Falling Forward

MONDAY	Off	
TUESDAY	**Base Run + Drills** Run 6 miles @ base pace Running No Arms 20 seconds One-Leg Hop 20 seconds	Optional Recovery Run or Cardio Cross-Training Workout 20–60 minutes @ recovery pace
WEDNESDAY	**Hill Repetitions** Dynamic stretching warm-up 2-mile warm-up @ recovery pace 2 × 30-second hill repetitions @ relaxed sprint speed, 2-minute active recoveries 2-mile cool-down @ recovery pace	Optional Recovery Run or Cardio Cross-Training Workout 20–60 minutes @ recovery pace
THURSDAY	**Base Run** Run 6 miles @ base pace	**Resistance Workout** *1 set each* Lying Hip Abduction Cook Hip Lift Kneeling Overhead Draw-In Knee Fall-Out Squat Jump
FRIDAY	**Fartlek Run** Dynamic stretching warm-up Run 6 miles @ base pace w/2 × 30-second intervals @ 1-mile pace "sprinkled in"	Optional Recovery Run or Cardio Cross-Training Workout 20–60 minutes @ recovery pace

SATURDAY	**Base Run** Run 6 miles @ base pace	**Resistance Workout** *1 set each* Lying Hip Abduction Cook Hip Lift Kneeling Overhead Draw-In Knee Fall-Out Broad Jump
SUNDAY	**Base Run** Run 7 miles @ base pace	Optional Recovery Run or Cardio Cross-Training Workout 20–60 minutes @ recovery pace

WEEK 2 ◆ Proprioceptive Cue: Navel to Spine

MONDAY	Off	
TUESDAY	**Base Run + Drills** Run 6.5 miles @ base pace High Knees 2 × 20 seconds Bounding 2 × 20 seconds	Optional Recovery Run or Cardio Cross-Training Workout 20–60 minutes @ recovery pace
WEDNESDAY	**Hill Repetitions** Dynamic stretching warm-up 2-mile warm-up @ recovery pace 8 × 30-second hill repetitions @ relaxed sprint speed w/2-minute active recoveries 2-mile cool-down @ recovery pace	Optional Recovery Run or Cardio Cross-Training Workout 20–60 minutes @ recovery pace
THURSDAY	**Base Run** Run 6.5 miles @ base pace	**Resistance Workout** *2 sets each* Lying Hip Abduction Cook Hip Lift Kneeling Overhead Draw-In Knee Fall-Out Split Squat Jump
FRIDAY	**Fartlek Run** Dynamic stretching warm-up Run 6.5 miles @ base pace w/8 × 30-second intervals @ 1-mile pace "sprinkled in"	Optional Recovery Run or Cardio Cross-Training Workout 20–60 minutes @ recovery pace
SATURDAY	**Base Run** Run 6.5 miles @ base pace	**Resistance Workout** *2 sets each* Lying Hip Abduction Cook Hip Lift Kneeling Overhead Draw-In Knee Fall-Out Wall Jump
SUNDAY	**Base Run** Run 8 miles @ base pace	Optional Recovery Run or Cardio Cross-Training Workout 20–60 minutes @ recovery pace

WEEK 3 ♦ Proprioceptive Cue: Running on Water

MONDAY	Off	
TUESDAY	**Base Run + Drills** Run 7 miles @ base pace Stiff-Legged Run 2 × 20 seconds Running No Arms 2 × 20 seconds	Optional Recovery Run or Cardio Cross-Training Workout 20–60 minutes @ recovery pace
WEDNESDAY	**Hill Repetitions** Dynamic stretching warm-up 2-mile warm-up @ recovery pace 12 × 45-second hill repetitions @ 1-mile pace w/2-minute active recoveries 2-mile cool-down @ recovery pace	Optional Recovery Run or Cardio Cross-Training Workout 20–60 minutes @ recovery pace
THURSDAY	**Base Run** Run 7 miles @ base pace	**Resistance Workout** *3 sets each* Lying Hip Abduction Cook Hip Lift Kneeling Overhead Draw-In Knee Fall-Out Squat Jump
FRIDAY	**Fartlek Run** Dynamic stretching warm-up Run 7 miles @ base pace w/12 × 45-second intervals @ 1-mile pace "sprinkled in"	Optional Recovery Run or Cardio Cross-Training Workout 20–60 minutes @ recovery pace
SATURDAY	**Base Run** Run 7 miles @ base pace	**Resistance Workout** *3 sets each* Lying Hip Abduction Cook Hip Lift Kneeling Overhead Draw-In Knee Fall-Out Broad Jump
SUNDAY	**Base Run** Run 8 miles @ base pace	Optional Recovery Run or Cardio Cross-Training Workout 20–60 minutes @ recovery pace

WEEK 4 (Recovery) ◆ Proprioceptive Cue: Pulling the Road

MONDAY	Off	
TUESDAY	**Base Run + Drills** Run 5 miles @ base pace One-Leg Hop 20 seconds High Knees 20 seconds	<u>Optional Recovery Run or Cardio</u> <u>Cross-Training Workout</u> 20–60 minutes @ recovery pace

WEDNESDAY	**Hill Repetitions**
	Dynamic stretching warm-up
	2-mile warm-up @ recovery pace
	6×1-minute hill repetitions
	    @ 1-mile pace w/2-minute
	    active recoveries
	2-mile cool-down @ recovery
	    pace
		<u>Optional Recovery Run or Cardio</u>
		<u>Cross-Training Workout</u>
		20–60 minutes @ recovery pace

THURSDAY	**Base Run** Run 5 miles @ base pace	**Resistance Workout** *1 set each* Single-Leg Squat Oblique Bridge Lying Draw-In w/Hip Flexion Quadruped *2 sets each* Lying Hip Abduction Cook Hip Lift Kneeling Overhead Draw-In Knee Fall-Out Single-Leg Squat Jump Broad Jump

FRIDAY	**Fartlek Run**
	Dynamic stretching warm-up
	Run 5 miles @ base pace
	    w/6×1-minute intervals @
	    1-mile pace "sprinkled in"
		<u>Optional Recovery Run or Cardio</u>
		<u>Cross-Training Workout</u>
		20–60 minutes @ recovery pace

SATURDAY	**Base Run** Run 5 miles @ base pace	**Resistance Workout** *1 set each* Single-Leg Squat Oblique Bridge Lying Draw-In w/Hip Flexion Quadruped *2 sets each* Lying Hip Abduction Cook Hip Lift Kneeling Overhead Draw-In Knee Fall-Out Wall Jump Single-Leg Box Jump
SUNDAY	**Base Run** Run 6 miles @ base pace	Optional Recovery Run or Cardio Cross-Training Workout 20–60 minutes @ recovery pace

Build 1 Phase

Training objectives: Continue to increase aerobic capacity and endurance; increase fatigue resistance at 3,000m pace and marathon pace; begin to develop efficiency at 10K pace

WEEK 5 ♦ Proprioceptive Cue: Scooting

MONDAY	Off	
TUESDAY	**Base Run + Drills** Run 7 miles @ base pace High Knees 2 × 20 seconds Bounding 2 × 20 seconds	Optional Recovery Run or Cardio Cross-Training Workout 20–60 minutes @ recovery pace

WEDNESDAY	**400m Intervals @ 3,000m Pace**
	Dynamic stretching warm-up
	1.5-mile warm-up @ recovery pace
	10 × 400m intervals @ 3,000m
	    pace w/3-minute active
	    recoveries
	1.5-mile cool-down
	    @ recovery pace
		Optional Recovery Run or Cardio Cross-Training Workout
		20–60 minutes @ recovery pace

THURSDAY	**Recovery/Base Run** 4–8 miles @ recovery/base pace (Do this workout as a recovery run if you did *not* do an afternoon recovery workout following yesterday's interval workout. Otherwise, do this workout as a base workout.)	**Resistance Workout** *2 sets each* Single-Leg Squat Oblique Bridge Lying Draw-In w/Hip Flexion Quadruped *1 set each* Lying Hip Abduction Cook Hip Lift Kneeling Overhead Draw-In Knee Fall-Out Single-Leg Squat Jump Broad Jump

FRIDAY	**1K Intervals @ 10K Pace** Dynamic stretching warm-up 1.5-mile warm-up @ recovery pace 6 × 1K @ 10K pace w/2-minute active recoveries 1.5-mile recovery-pace cool-down	Optional Recovery Run or Cardio Cross-Training Workout 20–60 minutes @ recovery pace
SATURDAY	**Recovery/Base Run** 4–8 miles @ recovery pace	**Resistance Workout** *2 sets each* Single-Leg Squat Oblique Bridge Lying Draw-In w/Hip Flexion Quadruped *1 set each* Lying Hip Abduction Cook Hip Lift Kneeling Overhead Draw-In Knee Fall-Out Wall Jump Single-Leg Box Jump
SUNDAY	**Endurance Run** Run 10 miles @ base pace	Optional Recovery Run or Cardio Cross-Training Workout 20–60 minutes @ recovery pace

WEEK 6 ◆ Proprioceptive Cue: Pounding the Ground

MONDAY	Off	
TUESDAY	**Base Run+ Drills** Run 7.5 miles @ base pace Stiff-Legged Run 2 × 20 seconds Running No Arms 2 × 20 seconds	<u>Optional Recovery Run or Cardio</u> <u>Cross-Training Workout</u> 20–60 minutes @ recovery pace

WEDNESDAY	**400m Intervals @ 3,000m Pace**
	Dynamic stretching warm-up
	1.5-mile warm-up @ recovery pace
	12 × 400m intervals @ 3,000m
	  pace w/3-minute active
	  recoveries
	1.5-mile cool-down @ recovery
	  pace
		<u>Optional Recovery Run or Cardio</u>
		<u>Cross-Training Workout</u>
		20–60 minutes @ recovery pace

THURSDAY	**Recovery/Base Run** 4–8 miles @ recovery pace	**Resistance Workout** *3 sets each* Single-Leg Squat Oblique Bridge Lying Draw-In w/Hip Flexion Quadruped *2 sets each* Squat Jump Split Squat Jump
FRIDAY	**1K Intervals @ 10K Pace** Dynamic stretching warm-up 1.5-mile warm-up @ recovery pace 7 × 1K @ 10K pace w/2-minute active recoveries 1.5-mile recovery-pace cool-down	<u>Optional Recovery Run or Cardio</u> <u>Cross-Training Workout</u> 20–60 minutes @ recovery pace
SATURDAY	**Recovery/Base Run** 4–8 miles @ recovery pace	**Resistance Workout** *3 sets each* Single-Leg Squat Oblique Bridge Lying Draw-In w/Hip Flexion Quadruped *2 sets* Single-Leg Squat Jump
SUNDAY	**Endurance Run** Run 11 miles @ base pace	

WEEK 7 ◆ Proprioceptive Cue: Driving the Thigh

MONDAY	Off	
TUESDAY	**Base Run + Drills** Run 8 miles @ base pace Steep Hill Sprints 2 × 20 seconds One-Leg Hop 2 × 20 seconds	<u>Optional Recovery Run or Cardio</u> <u>Cross-Training Workout</u> 20–60 minutes @ recovery pace

WEDNESDAY	**400m Intervals @ 3,000m Pace**
	Dynamic stretching warm-up
	1.5-mile warm-up @ recovery pace
	14 × 400m intervals @ 3,000m
	   pace w/3-minute active
	   recoveries
	1.5-mile cool-down @ recovery
	   pace
		<u>Optional Recovery Run or Cardio</u>
		<u>Cross-Training Workout</u>
		20–60 minutes @ recovery pace

THURSDAY	**Recovery/Base Run** 4–8 miles @ recovery pace	**Resistance Workout** *2 sets each* Single-Leg Squat Oblique Bridge Lying Draw-In w/Hip Flexion Quadruped Split Squat Jump Single-Leg Squat Jump *1 set each* Box Lunge Stability Ball Leg Curl Forearms to Palms Bridge Dead Bug
FRIDAY	**1K Intervals @ 10K Pace** Dynamic stretching warm-up 1.5-mile warm-up @ recovery pace 8 × 1K @ 10K pace w/2-minute active recoveries 1.5-mile recovery-pace cool-down	<u>Optional Recovery Run or Cardio</u> <u>Cross-Training Workout</u> 20–60 minutes @ recovery pace

(continued)

WEEK 7 ◆ Proprioceptive Cue: Driving the Thigh

(continued)

SATURDAY	Recovery/Base Run	Resistance Workout
	4–8 miles @ recovery pace	*2 sets each* Single-Leg Squat Oblique Bridge Lying Draw-In w/Hip Flexion Quadruped Single-Leg Box Jump *1 set each* Box Lunge Stability Ball Leg Curl Forearms to Palms Bridge Dead Bug
SUNDAY	**Endurance Run** Run 12 miles @ base pace	

WEEK 8 (Recovery) ◆ Proprioceptive Cue: Floppy Feet

MONDAY	Off	
TUESDAY	**Base Run + Drills** Run 6 miles @ base pace High Knees 20 seconds Bounding 20 seconds	<u>Optional Recovery Run or Cardio</u> <u>Cross-Training Workout</u> 20–60 minutes @ recovery pace

WEDNESDAY	**400m Intervals @ 3,000m Pace**
	Dynamic stretching warm-up
	1-mile warm-up @ recovery pace
	8 × 400m intervals @ 3,000m
	    pace w/3-minute active
	    recoveries
	1-mile cool-down @ recovery pace
		<u>Optional Recovery Run or Cardio</u>
		<u>Cross-Training Workout</u>
		20–60 minutes @ recovery pace

THURSDAY	**Recovery/Base Run** 4–8 miles @ recovery pace	**Resistance Workout** *1 set each* Single-Leg Squat Oblique Bridge Lying Draw-In w/Hip Flexion Quadruped *2 sets each* Box Lunge Stability Ball Leg Curl Forearms to Palms Bridge Dead Bug Broad Jump Wall Jump
FRIDAY	**1K Intervals @ 10K Pace** Dynamic stretching warm-up 1.5-mile warm-up @ recovery pace 4 × 1K @ 10K pace w/2-minute active recoveries 1.5-mile recovery-pace cool-down	<u>Optional Recovery Run or Cardio</u> <u>Cross-Training Workout</u> 20–60 minutes @ recovery pace

(continued)

WEEK 8 (Recovery) ◆ Proprioceptive Cue: Floppy Feet
(continued)

SATURDAY	Recovery/Base Run 4–8 miles @ recovery pace	Resistance Workout *1 set each* Single-Leg Squat Oblique Bridge Lying Draw-In w/Hip Flexion Quadruped *2 sets each* Box Lunge Stability Ball Leg Curl Forearms to Palms Bridge Dead Bug Wall Jump Single-Leg Box Jump
SUNDAY	**Base Run** Run 8 miles @ base pace	Optional Recovery Run or Cardio Cross-Training Workout 20–60 minutes @ recovery pace

Build 2

Training objectives: Increase fatigue resistance at 5K pace and half-marathon pace; continue to build efficiency at 10K pace

WEEK 9 ◆ Proprioceptive Cue: Butt Squeeze

MONDAY	Off	
TUESDAY	**Base Run + Drills** Run 7.5 miles @ base pace Stiff-Legged Run 2 × 20 seconds Running No Arms 2 × 20 seconds	Optional Recovery Run or Cardio Cross-Training Workout 20–60 minutes @ recovery pace

WEDNESDAY	**1K Intervals @ 5K Pace**
	Dynamic stretching warm-up
	1.5-mile warm-up @ recovery pace
	4 × 1K intervals @ 5K pace
	  w/3-minute active recoveries
	1.5-mile cool-down @ recovery
	  pace
		Optional Recovery Run or Cardio Cross-Training Workout
		20–60 minutes @ recovery pace

THURSDAY	**Recovery/Base Run** 4–8 miles @ recovery pace	**Resistance Workout** *3 sets each* Box Lunge Stability Ball Leg Curl Forearms to Palms Bridge Dead Bug Wall Jump Single-Leg Box Jump
FRIDAY	**2K Intervals @ 10K Pace** Dynamic stretching warm-up 1.5-mile warm-up @ recovery pace 4 × 2K @ 10K pace w/2-minute active recoveries 1.5-mile recovery-pace cool-down	Optional Recovery Run or Cardio Cross-Training Workout 20–60 minutes @ recovery pace

(continued)

WEEK 9 ◆ Proprioceptive Cue: Butt Squeeze
(continued)

SATURDAY	**Recovery/Base Run** 4–8 miles @ recovery pace	**Resistance Workout** *3 sets each* Box Lunge Stability Ball Leg Curl Forearms to Palms Bridge Dead Bug Single-Leg Box Jump Squat Jump
SUNDAY	**Progression Run** Run 10 miles Start @ recovery pace; gradually increase pace every other mile Run last mile @ half-marathon pace	Optional Recovery Run or Cardio Cross-Training Workout 20–60 minutes @ recovery pace

WEEK 10 ◆ Proprioceptive Cue: Feeling Symmetry

MONDAY	Off	
TUESDAY	**Base Run + Drills** Run 8 miles @ base pace Stiff-Legged Run 2 × 20 seconds Running No Arms 2 × 20 seconds	<u>Optional Recovery Run or Cardio Cross-Training Workout</u> 20–60 minutes @ recovery pace

WEDNESDAY	**1K Intervals @ 5K Pace**
	Dynamic stretching warm-up
	1.5-mile warm-up @ recovery pace
	6 × 1K intervals @ 5K pace
	   w/3-minute active recoveries
	1.5-mile cool-down @ recovery
	   pace
		<u>Optional Recovery Run or Cardio
		Cross-Training Workout</u>
		20–60 minutes @ recovery pace

THURSDAY	**Recovery/Base Run** 4–8 miles @ recovery pace	**Resistance Workout** *2 sets each* Lying Hip Abduction Single-Leg Squat Box Lunge Stability Ball Leg Curl Squat Jump Split Squat Jump
FRIDAY	**2K Intervals @ 10K Pace** Dynamic stretching warm-up 1.5-mile warm-up @ recovery pace 5 × 2K @ 10K pace w/2-minute active recoveries 1.5-mile recovery-pace cool-down	<u>Optional Recovery Run or Cardio Cross-Training Workout</u> 20–60 minutes @ recovery pace
SATURDAY	**Recovery/Base Run** 4–8 miles @ recovery pace	**Resistance Workout** *2 sets each* Cook Hip Lift Oblique Bridge Forearms to Palms Bridge Stability Ball Leg Curl Split Squat Jump Single-Leg Squat Jump

(continued)

WEEK 10 ◆ Proprioceptive Cue: Feeling Symmetry
(continued)

| SUNDAY | **Progression Run**
Run 11 miles
Start @ recovery pace; gradually
    increase pace every other mile
Run last 2 miles @ half-marathon
    pace | Optional Recovery Run or Cardio
Cross-Training Workout
20–60 minutes @ recovery pace |

WEEK 11 ◆ Proprioceptive Cue: Axle Between the Knees

MONDAY	Off	
TUESDAY	**Base Run + Drills** Run 8.5 miles @ base pace Steep Hill Sprints 2 × 20 seconds One-Leg Hop 2 × 20 seconds	<u>Optional Recovery Run or Cardio Cross-Training Workout</u> 20–60 minutes @ recovery pace

WEDNESDAY	**1K Intervals @ 5K Pace**
	Dynamic stretching warm-up
	1.5-mile warm-up @ recovery pace
	6 × 1K intervals @ 5K pace
	  w/2-minute active recoveries
	1.5-mile cool-down @ recovery
	  pace
		<u>Optional Recovery Run or Cardio Cross-Training Workout</u>
		20–60 minutes @ recovery pace

THURSDAY	**Recovery/Base Run** 4–8 miles @ recovery pace	**Resistance Workout** *2 sets each* Lying Hip Abduction Single-Leg Squat Box Lunge Stability Ball Leg Curl Single-Leg Squat Jump Broad Jump
FRIDAY	**2K Intervals @ 10K Pace** Dynamic stretching warm-up 1.5-mile warm-up @ recovery pace 5 × 2K @ 10K pace w/90-second active recoveries 1.5-mile recovery-pace cool-down	<u>Optional Recovery Run or Cardio Cross-Training Workout</u> 20–60 minutes @ recovery pace
SATURDAY	**Recovery/Base Run** 4–8 miles @ recovery pace	**Resistance Workout** *2 sets each* Cook Hip Lift Oblique Bridge Forearms to Palms Bridge Stability Ball Leg Curl Broad Jump Wall Jump

(continued)

WEEK 11 ◆ **Proprioceptive Cue: Axle Between the Knees**
(continued)

| SUNDAY | **Progression Run**
Run 12 miles
Start @ recovery pace; gradually
   increase pace every other mile
Run last 2 miles @ half-marathon
   pace | Optional Recovery Run or Cardio
Cross-Training Workout
20–60 minutes @ recovery pace |

WEEK 12 (Recovery) ◆ Proprioceptive Cue: Running Against a Wall

MONDAY	Off	
TUESDAY	**Base Run + Drills** Run 6 miles @ base pace High Knees 20 seconds Bounding 20 seconds	<u>Optional Recovery Run or Cardio Cross-Training Workout</u> 20–60 minutes @ recovery pace

WEDNESDAY	**1K Intervals @ 5K Pace**
	Dynamic stretching warm-up
	1.5-mile warm-up @ recovery pace
	4 × 1K intervals @ 5K pace
	   w/3-minute active recoveries
	1.5-mile cool-down @ recovery
	   pace
		<u>Optional Recovery Run or Cardio Cross-Training Workout</u>
		20–60 minutes @ recovery pace

THURSDAY	**Recovery/Base Run** 4–8 miles @ recovery pace	**Resistance Workout** *2 sets each* Lying Hip Abduction Single-Leg Squat Box Lunge Stability Ball Leg Curl Wall Jump Single-Leg Box Jump
FRIDAY	**2K Intervals @ 10K Pace** Dynamic stretching warm-up 1.5-mile warm-up @ recovery pace 3 × 2K @ 10K pace w/2-minute active recoveries 1.5-mile recovery-pace cool-down	
SATURDAY	**Recovery Run** 2 miles @ recovery pace	**Resistance Workout** *1 set each* Cook Hip Lift Oblique Bridge Forearms to Palms Bridge Stability Ball Leg Curl

(continued)

WEEK 12 (Recovery) ◆ Proprioceptive Cue: Running Against a Wall

(continued)

SUNDAY	5K Tune-up Race or Time Trial
	Dynamic stretching warm-up
	2-mile warm-up @ recovery pace
	5K tune-up race or time trial
	2-mile recovery-pace cool-down

Peak Phase

Training objectives: Achieve peak fatigue resistance and efficiency at 10K pace; adapt and recover for peak race day

WEEK 13 ◆ Proprioceptive Cue: Falling Forward

MONDAY	Off	
TUESDAY	**Base Run + Drills** Run 8.5 miles @ base pace High Knees 2 × 20 seconds Bounding 2 × 20 seconds	Optional Recovery Run or Cardio Cross-Training Workout 20–60 minutes @ recovery pace

WEDNESDAY	**Mixed Intervals**
	Dynamic stretching warm-up
	1-mile warm-up @ recovery pace
	1 × 2K @ half-marathon pace,
	  2-minute active recovery
	1 × 1 mile @ 10K pace, 2-minute
	  active recovery
	2 × 1K @ 5K pace, 2-minute active
	  recoveries
	2 × 800m @ 3,000m pace,
	  2-minute active recoveries
	1-mile cool-down @ recovery pace
		Optional Recovery Run or Cardio Cross-Training Workout
		20–60 minutes @ recovery pace

THURSDAY	**Recovery/Base Run** 4–8 miles @ recovery pace	**Resistance Workout** *2 sets each* Lying Hip Abduction Single-Leg Squat Box Lunge Stability Ball Leg Curl Wall Jump Single-Leg Box Jump
FRIDAY	**3K Intervals @ 10K Pace** Dynamic stretching warm-up 1.5-mile warm-up @ recovery pace 3 × 3K @ 10K pace w/3-minute active recoveries 1.5-mile recovery-pace cool-down	Optional Recovery Run or Cardio Cross-Training Workout 20–60 minutes @ recovery pace

(continued)

WEEK 13 ◆ Proprioceptive Cue: Falling Forward
(continued)

SATURDAY	**Recovery/Base Run** 4–8 miles @ recovery pace	**Resistance Workout** *2 sets each* Cook Hip Lift Oblique Bridge Forearms to Palms Bridge Stability Ball Leg Curl Single-Leg Box Jump Squat Jump
SUNDAY	**Half-Marathon-Pace Tempo Run** 2-mile warm-up @ recovery pace 5 miles @ half-Marathon pace 2-mile recovery-pace cool-down	<u>Optional Recovery Run or Cardio</u> <u>Cross-Training Workout</u> 20–60 minutes @ recovery pace

WEEK 14 ◆ Proprioceptive Cue: Navel to Spine

MONDAY	Off	
TUESDAY	**Base Run + Drills** Run 9 miles @ base pace Stiff-Legged Run 2 × 20 seconds Running No Arms 2 × 20 seconds	Optional Recovery Run or Cardio Cross-Training Workout 20–60 minutes @ recovery pace

WEDNESDAY	**Mixed Intervals**
	Dynamic stretching warm-up
	1-mile warm-up @ recovery pace
	1 × 2K @ half-marathon pace,
	    2-minute active recovery
	2 × 1 mile @ 10K pace, 2-minute
	    active recoveries
	2 × 1K @ 5K pace, 2-minute active
	    recoveries
	2 × 800m @ 3,000m pace,
	    2-minute active recoveries
	1-mile cool-down @ recovery pace
		Optional Recovery Run or Cardio
		Cross-Training Workout
		20–60 minutes @ recovery pace

THURSDAY	**Recovery/Base Run** 4–8 miles @ recovery pace	**Resistance Workout** *2 sets each* Lying Hip Abduction Single-Leg Squat Box Lunge Stability Ball Leg Curl Squat Jump
FRIDAY	**3K Intervals @ 10K Pace** Dynamic stretching warm-up 1.5-mile warm-up @ recovery pace 4 × 3K @ 10K pace w/ 2-minute active recoveries 1.5-mile recovery-pace cool-down	Optional Recovery Run or Cardio Cross-Training Workout 20–60 minutes @ recovery pace

(continued)

WEEK 14 ◆ Proprioceptive Cue: Navel to Spine
(continued)

SATURDAY	Recovery/Base Run	Resistance Workout
	4–8 miles @ recovery pace	*2 sets each* Cook Hip Lift Oblique Bridge Forearms to Palms Bridge Stability Ball Leg Curl Split Squat Jump Single-Leg Squat Jump
SUNDAY	**Half-Marathon-Pace Tempo Run** 2-mile warm-up @ recovery pace 6 miles @ half-marathon pace 2-mile recovery-pace cool-down	Optional Recovery Run or Cardio Cross-Training Workout 20–60 minutes @ recovery pace

WEEK 15 (Recovery) ◆ Proprioceptive Cue: Running on Water

MONDAY	Off	
TUESDAY	**Base Run + Drills** Run 6 miles @ base pace Steep Hill Sprints 20 seconds One-Leg Hop 20 seconds	<u>Optional Recovery Run or Cardio Cross-Training Workout</u> 20–60 minutes @ recovery pace
WEDNESDAY	**Mixed Intervals** Dynamic stretching warm-up 1-mile warm-up @ recovery pace 1×2K @ half-marathon pace, 2-minute active recovery 1×1 mile @ 10K pace, 2-minute active recovery 1×1K @ 5K pace, 2-minute active recovery 2×800m @ 3,000m pace, 2-minute active recoveries 1-mile cool-down @ recovery pace	<u>Optional Recovery Run or Cardio Cross-Training Workout</u> 20–60 minutes @ recovery pace
THURSDAY	**Recovery Run** 2–6 miles @ recovery pace	**Resistance Workout** *2 sets each* Lying Hip Abduction Single-Leg Squat Box Lunge Stability Ball Leg Curl Single-Leg Squat Jump
FRIDAY	**3K Intervals @ 10K Pace** Dynamic stretching warm-up 1.5-mile warm-up @ recovery pace 2×3K @ 10K pace w/3-minute active recoveries 1.5-mile recovery-pace cool-down	
SATURDAY	**Recovery Run** 2 miles @ recovery pace	**Resistance Workout** *2 sets each* Cook Hip Lift Oblique Bridge Forearms to Palms Bridge Stability Ball Leg Curl Broad Jump

(continued)

WEEK 15 (Recovery) ◆ Proprioceptive Cue: Running on Water
(continued)

SUNDAY	**10K Tune-up Race or Time Trial**
	Dynamic stretching warm-up
	2-mile warm-up @ recovery pace
	10K tune-up race or time trial
	2-mile recovery-pace cool-down

WEEK 16 ♦ Proprioceptive Cue: Pulling the Road

MONDAY	Off	
TUESDAY	**Base Run + Drills** Run 10 miles @ base pace Stiff-Legged Run 2 × 20 seconds Running No Arms 2 × 20 seconds	Optional Recovery Run or Cardio Cross-Training Workout 20–60 minutes @ recovery pace

WEDNESDAY	**Mixed Intervals**
	Dynamic stretching warm-up
	1-mile warm-up @ recovery pace
	1 × 2K @ half-marathon pace,
	    90-second active recovery
	2 × 1 mile @ 10K pace, 90-second
	    active recoveries
	2 × 1K @ 5K pace, 90-second
	    active recoveries
	2 × 800m @ 3,000m pace,
	    90-second active recoveries
	1-mile cool-down @ recovery pace
		Optional Recovery Run or Cardio Cross-Training Workout
		20–60 minutes @ recovery pace

THURSDAY	**Recovery/Base Run** 4–8 miles @ recovery pace	**Resistance Workout** *2 sets each* Lying Hip Abduction Single-Leg Squat Box Lunge Stability Ball Leg Curl Squat Jump Split Squat Jump
FRIDAY	**3K Intervals @ 10K Pace** Dynamic stretching warm-up 1.5-mile warm-up @ recovery pace 4 × 3K @ 10K pace w/90-second active recoveries 1.5-mile recovery-pace cool-down	Optional Recovery Run or Cardio Cross-Training Workout 20–60 minutes @ recovery pace

(continued)

WEEK 16 ◆ Proprioceptive Cue: Pulling the Road
(continued)

SATURDAY	**Recovery/Base Run** 4–8 miles @ recovery pace	**Resistance Workout** *2 sets each* Cook Hip Lift Oblique Bridge Forearms to Palms Bridge Stability Ball Leg Curl Split Squat Jump Single-Leg Squat Jump
SUNDAY	**Half-Marathon-Pace Tempo Run** 2-mile warm-up @ recovery pace 7 miles @ half-marathon pace 2-mile recovery-pace cool-down	Optional Recovery Run or Cardio Cross-Training Workout 20–60 minutes @ recovery pace

WEEK 17 ◆ Proprioceptive Cue: Scooting

MONDAY	Off	
TUESDAY	**Base Run + Drills** Run 9 miles @ base pace Stiff-Legged Run 2 × 20 seconds Running No Arms 2 × 20 seconds	Optional Recovery Run or Cardio Cross-Training Workout 20–60 minutes @ recovery pace

WEDNESDAY	**Mixed Intervals**
	Dynamic stretching warm-up
	1-mile warm-up @ recovery pace
	1 × 2K @ half-marathon pace,
	   1-minute active recovery
	2 × 1 mile @ 10K pace, 1-minute
	   active recoveries
	2 × 1K @ 5K pace, 1-minute active
	   recoveries
	2 × 800m @ 3,000m pace,
	   1-minute active recovery
	1-mile cool-down @ recovery pace
		Optional Recovery Run or Cardio
		Cross-Training Workout
		20–60 minutes @ recovery pace

THURSDAY	**Recovery/Base Run** 4–8 miles @ recovery pace	**Resistance Workout** *2 sets each* Lying Hip Abduction Single-Leg Squat Box Lunge Stability Ball Leg Curl Squat Jump Split Squat Jump
FRIDAY	**3K Intervals @ 10K Pace** Dynamic stretching warm-up 1.5-mile warm-up @ recovery pace 3 × 3K @ 10K pace w/1-minute active recoveries 1.5-mile recovery-pace cool-down	Optional Recovery Run or Cardio Cross-Training Workout 20–60 minutes @ recovery pace

(continued)

WEEK 17 ◆ Proprioceptive Cue: Scooting
(continued)

SATURDAY	Recovery/Base Run	Resistance Workout
	4–8 miles @ recovery pace	*2 sets each* Cook Hip Lift Oblique Bridge Forearms to Palms Bridge Stability Ball Leg Curl Split Squat Jump Single-Leg Squat Jump
SUNDAY	**Half-Marathon-Pace Tempo Run** 2-mile warm-up @ recovery pace 7 miles @ half-marathon pace 2-mile recovery-pace cool-down	Optional Recovery Run or Cardio Cross-Training Workout 20–60 minutes @ recovery pace

WEEK 18 (Taper) ◆ Proprioceptive Cue: Your Choice

MONDAY	Off	
TUESDAY	**Base Run + Drills** Run 7 miles @ base pace Stiff-Legged Run 20 seconds Running No Arms 20 seconds	<u>Optional Recovery Run or Cardio</u> <u>Cross-Training Workout</u> 20–60 minutes @ recovery pace
WEDNESDAY	**Mixed Intervals** Dynamic stretching warm-up 1-mile warm-up @ recovery pace 1×2K @ half-marathon pace, 1-minute active recovery 1×1 mile @ 10K pace, 1-minute active recovery 1×1K @ 5K pace, 1-minute active recovery 1×800m @ 3,000m pace 1-mile cool-down @ recovery pace	
THURSDAY	**Recovery Run** 2–6 miles @ recovery pace	**Resistance Workout** *1 set each* Lying Hip Abduction Single-Leg Squat Box Lunge Stability Ball Leg Curl Squat Jump
FRIDAY	**3K Interval @ 10K Pace** Dynamic stretching warm-up 1.5-mile warm-up @ recovery pace 1×3K @ 10K pace 1.5-mile recovery-pace cool-down	
SATURDAY	Off	
SUNDAY	**10K Peak Race** Dynamic stretching warm-up 2-mile warm-up @ recovery pace 10K peak race 2-mile recovery-pace cool-down	

CHAPTER 13

BRAIN TRAINING PLANS: HALF MARATHON

The half marathon has made a huge surge in popularity within the past decade. It's easy to understand why. The half marathon is a long enough distance to present a solid challenge for runners who are looking for a challenge. When you finish or set a PR in a half marathon, you feel you've really done something. On the other hand, the half marathon is a lot more manageable than the traditional big running challenge—the marathon. You don't have to devote nearly as many weekend hours to long endurance runs when preparing for a half marathon, and the body recovers from a half marathon much faster. I often tell other runners, "Don't be fooled by the numbers: A marathon is much more than two half marathons!"

There are three half-marathon training plans in this chapter: Level 1, Level 2, and Level 3. Each plan is twenty weeks long and includes a 5K tune-up race/breakthrough workout at the end of Week 12 and a 10K tune-up race/breakthrough workout at the end of Week 16, in addition to the half-marathon peak race at the end of Week 20. The plans are divided into Base, Build 1, Build 2, and Peak phases. The Base phase is six weeks long, the Build 1 and 2 phases last four weeks apiece, and the Peak phase lasts six weeks. Weeks 4, 8, 12, and 16 are reduced-volume recovery weeks, and Week 20 is a reduced-volume taper week.

There are three key workouts per week in each plan: a speed workout on Wednesdays, an intensive endurance workout on Fridays, and an extensive endurance workout on Sundays. Key workouts are indicated by shaded boxes.

LEVEL 1

Use this plan if you are most comfortable with a half-marathon training plan that features four runs per week and a maximum run distance of 12 miles. The plan also contains one optional nonimpact cardio cross-training workout and two resistance workouts per week.

Base Phase

Training objectives: Build aerobic capacity and endurance, increase injury resistance, and increase muscle activation capacity

WEEK 1 ◆ Proprioceptive Cue: Falling Forward

MONDAY	Off
TUESDAY	**Base Run + Drills** Run 3 miles @ base pace Running No Arms 20 seconds One-Leg Hop 20 seconds
WEDNESDAY	**Hill Repetitions** Dynamic stretching warm-up 1.5-mile warm-up @ recovery pace 1 × 30-second hill repetition @ relaxed sprint speed 1.5-mile cool-down @ recovery pace

THURSDAY	Optional Nonimpact Cardio Cross-Training Workout 20–30 minutes @ recovery pace (You may break this workout into a 10–15-minute warm-up before and a 10–15-minute cool-down after your resistance workout.)	**Resistance Workout** *1 set each* Lying Hip Abduction Cook Hip Lift Kneeling Overhead Draw-In Knee Fall-Out Squat Jump

FRIDAY	**Fartlek Run** Dynamic stretching warm-up Run 3 miles @ base pace w/2 × 30-second intervals @ 1-mile pace "sprinkled in"

(continued)

WEEK 1 ♦ Proprioceptive Cue: Falling Forward
(continued)

SATURDAY	**Resistance Workout** *1 set each* Lying Hip Abduction Cook Hip Lift Kneeling Overhead Draw-In Knee Fall-Out Broad Jump
SUNDAY	**Base Run** Run 4 miles @ base pace

WEEK 2 ◆ Proprioceptive Cue: Navel to Spine

MONDAY	Off

TUESDAY	**Base Run + Drills**
	   Run 3.5 miles @ base pace
	   High Knees 2×20 seconds
	   Bounding 2×20 seconds

WEDNESDAY	**Hill Repetitions**
	   Dynamic stretching warm-up
	   1.5-mile warm-up @ recovery pace
	   4×30-second hill repetitions @ relaxed sprint speed w/2-minute
	      active recoveries
	   1.5-mile cool-down @ recovery pace

THURSDAY	<u>Optional Nonimpact Cardio</u> <u>Cross-Training Workout</u> 20–30 minutes @ recovery pace	**Resistance Workout** *2 sets each* Lying Hip Abduction Cook Hip Lift Kneeling Overhead Draw-In Knee Fall-Out Split Squat Jump

FRIDAY	**Fartlek Run**
	   Dynamic stretching warm-up
	   Run 3.5 miles @ base pace w/4×30-second intervals @ 1-mile pace
	      "sprinkled in"

SATURDAY	**Resistance Workout**
	   2 sets each
	   Lying Hip Abduction
	   Cook Hip Lift
	   Kneeling Overhead Draw-In
	   Knee Fall-Out
	   Wall Jump

SUNDAY	**Base Run** Run 5 miles @ base pace

WEEK 3 ◆ Proprioceptive Cue: Running on Water

MONDAY	Off
TUESDAY	**Base Run + Drills** Run 4 miles @ base pace Stiff-Legged Run 2 × 20 seconds Running No Arms 2 × 20 seconds
WEDNESDAY	**Hill Repetitions** Dynamic stretching warm-up 1.5-mile warm-up @ recovery pace 5 × 45-second hill repetitions @ 1-mile pace w/2-minute active recoveries 1.5-mile cool-down @ recovery pace

THURSDAY	Optional Nonimpact Cardio Cross-Training Workout 20–30 minutes @ recovery pace	**Resistance Workout** *3 sets each* Lying Hip Abduction Cook Hip Lift Kneeling Overhead Draw-In Knee Fall-Out Squat Jump

FRIDAY	**Fartlek Run** Dynamic stretching warm-up Run 4 miles @ base pace w/5 × 45-second intervals @ 1-mile pace "sprinkled in"
SATURDAY	**Resistance Workout** *3 sets each* Lying Hip Abduction Cook Hip Lift Kneeling Overhead Draw-In Knee Fall-Out Broad Jump
SUNDAY	**Base Run** Run 6 miles @ base pace

WEEK 4 (Recovery) ♦ Proprioceptive Cue: Pulling the Road

MONDAY	Off	
TUESDAY	**Base Run + Drills** Run 3 miles @ base pace One-Leg Hop 20 seconds High Knees 20 seconds	
WEDNESDAY	**Hill Repetitions** Dynamic stretching warm-up 1.5-mile warm-up @ recovery pace 3 × 1-minute hill repetitions @ 1-mile pace w/2-minute active recoveries 1.5-mile cool-down @ recovery pace	
THURSDAY	<u>Optional Nonimpact Cardio Cross-Training Workout</u> 20–30 minutes @ recovery pace	**Resistance Workout** *1 set each* Single-Leg Squat Oblique Bridge Lying Draw-In w/Hip Flexion Quadruped *2 sets each* Lying Hip Abduction Cook Hip Lift Kneeling Overhead Draw-In Knee Fall-Out Single-Leg Squat Jump
FRIDAY	**Fartlek Run** Dynamic stretching warm-up Run 3 miles @ base pace w/3 × 1-minute intervals @ 1-mile pace "sprinkled in"	
SATURDAY	**Resistance Workout** *1 set each* Single-Leg Squat Oblique Bridge Lying Draw-In w/Hip Flexion Quadruped	

(continued)

WEEK 4 (Recovery) ◆ Proprioceptive Cue: Pulling the Road
(continued)

SATURDAY (continued)	**Resistance Workout** *2 sets each* Lying Hip Abduction Cook Hip Lift Kneeling Overhead Draw-In Knee Fall-Out Wall Jump
SUNDAY	**Base Run** Run 4 miles @ base pace

WEEK 5 ♦ Proprioceptive Cue: Scooting

MONDAY	Off
TUESDAY	**Base Run + Drills** Run 4.5 miles @ base pace High Knees 2 × 20 seconds Bounding 2 × 20 seconds
WEDNESDAY	**Hill Repetitions** Dynamic stretching warm-up 1-mile warm-up @ recovery pace 4 × 90-second hill repetitions @ 1-mile pace w/2-minute active recoveries 1-mile cool-down @ recovery pace

THURSDAY	<u>Optional Nonimpact Cardio</u> <u>Cross-Training Workout</u> 20–30 minutes @ recovery pace	**Resistance Workout** *2 sets each* Single-Leg Squat Oblique Bridge Lying Draw-In w/Hip Flexion Quadruped *1 set each* Lying Hip Abduction Cook Hip Lift Kneeling Overhead Draw-In Knee Fall-Out Single-Leg Squat Jump

FRIDAY	**Fartlek Run** Dynamic stretching warm-up Run 4.5 miles @ base pace w/4 × 90-second intervals @ 3,000m pace "sprinkled in"
SATURDAY	**Resistance Workout** *2 sets each* Single-Leg Squat Oblique Bridge Lying Draw-In w/Hip Flexion Quadruped

(continued)

WEEK 5 ♦ Proprioceptive Cue: Scooting
(continued)

SATURDAY (continued)	**Resistance Workout** *1 set each* Lying Hip Abduction Cook Hip Lift Kneeling Overhead Draw-In Knee Fall-Out Wall Jump
SUNDAY	**Base Run** Run 6 miles @ base pace

WEEK 6 ◆ Proprioceptive Cue: Pounding the Ground

MONDAY	Off

TUESDAY	**Base Run + Drills**
	    Run 5 miles @ base pace
	    Stiff-Legged Run 2 × 20 seconds
	    Running No Arms 2 × 20 seconds

WEDNESDAY	**Hill Repetitions**
	    Dynamic stretching warm-up
	    1-mile warm-up @ recovery pace
	    5 × 90-second hill repetitions @ 1-mile pace w/2-minute active recoveries
	    1-mile cool-down @ recovery pace

THURSDAY	Optional Nonimpact Cardio
	Cross-Training Workout
	20–30 minutes @ recovery pace
		Resistance Workout
		    3 sets each
		    Single-Leg Squat
		    Oblique Bridge
		    Lying Draw-In w/Hip Flexion
		    Quadruped
		
		    2 sets
		    Squat Jump

FRIDAY	**Fartlek Run**
	    Dynamic stretching warm-up
	    Run 4.5 miles @ base pace w/4 × 90-second intervals @ 3,000m pace
	        "sprinkled in"

SATURDAY	**Resistance Workout**
	    3 sets each
	    Single-Leg Squat
	    Oblique Bridge
	    Lying Draw-In w/Hip Flexion
	    Quadruped
	
	    2 sets
	    Single-Leg Squat Jump

SUNDAY	**Base Run** Run 7 miles @ base pace

Build 1 Phase

Training objectives: Continue to increase aerobic capacity and endurance; increase fatigue resistance at 3,000m pace and 10K pace

WEEK 7 ♦ Proprioceptive Cue: Driving the Thigh

MONDAY	Off
TUESDAY	**Base Run + Drills** Run 6 miles @ base pace Steep Hill Sprints 2 × 20 seconds One-Leg Hop 2 × 20 seconds
WEDNESDAY	**400m Intervals @ 3,000m Pace** Dynamic stretching warm-up 1-mile warm-up @ recovery pace 6 × 400m @ 3,000m pace w/3-minute active recoveries 1-mile cool-down @ recovery pace

THURSDAY	<u>Optional Nonimpact Cardio Cross-Training Workout</u>
	20–30 minutes @ recovery pace **Resistance Workout**
	    2 sets each
	    Single-Leg Squat
	    Oblique Bridge
	    Lying Draw-In w/Hip Flexion
	    Quadruped
	    Split Squat Jump
	
	    1 set each
	    Box Lunge
	    Stability Ball Leg Curl
	    Forearms to Palms Bridge
	    Dead Bug

FRIDAY	**1-Mile Intervals @ 10K Pace** Dynamic stretching warm-up 1-mile warm-up @ recovery pace 2 × 1 mile @ 10K pace w/2-minute active recoveries 1-mile cool-down @ recovery pace

SATURDAY	**Resistance Workout**
	2 sets each
	Single-Leg Squat
	Oblique Bridge
	Lying Draw-In w/Hip Flexion
	Quadruped
	Single-Leg Box Jump
	1 set each
	Box Lunge
	Stability Ball Leg Curl
	Forearms to Palms Bridge
	Dead Bug
SUNDAY	**Base Run**
	Run 8 miles @ base pace

WEEK 8 (Recovery) ◆ Proprioceptive Cue: Floppy Feet

MONDAY	Off
TUESDAY	**Base Run + Drills** Run 4 miles @ base pace High Knees 20 seconds Bounding 20 seconds
WEDNESDAY	**400m Intervals @ 3,000m Pace** Dynamic stretching warm-up 1-mile warm-up @ recovery pace 5×400m @ 3,000m pace w/3-minute active recoveries 1-mile cool-down @ recovery pace

THURSDAY	Optional Nonimpact Cardio Cross-Training Workout 20–30 minutes @ recovery pace	**Resistance Workout** *1 set each* Single-Leg Squat Oblique Bridge Lying Draw-In w/Hip Flexion Quadruped *2 sets each* Box Lunge Stability Ball Leg Curl Forearms to Palms Bridge Dead Bug Broad Jump

FRIDAY	**1-Mile Intervals @ 10K Pace** Dynamic stretching warm-up 1-mile warm-up @ recovery pace 2×1 mile @ 10K pace w/2-minute active recoveries 1-mile cool-down @ recovery pace
SATURDAY	**Resistance Workout** *1 set each* Single-Leg Squat Oblique Bridge Lying Draw-In w/Hip Flexion Quadruped

SATURDAY (continued)	**Resistance Workout** *2 sets each* Box Lunge Stability Ball Leg Curl Forearms to Palms Bridge Dead Bug Wall Jump
SUNDAY	**Base Run** Run 6 miles @ base pace

WEEK 9 ♦ Proprioceptive Cue: Butt Squeeze

MONDAY	Off
TUESDAY	**Base Run + Drills** Run 6 miles @ base pace Stiff-Legged Run 2 × 20 seconds Running No Arms 2 × 20 seconds
WEDNESDAY	**400m Intervals @ 3,000m Pace** Dynamic stretching warm-up 1-mile warm-up @ recovery pace 7 × 400m @ 3,000m pace w/3-minute active recoveries 1-mile cool-down @ recovery pace

THURSDAY	Optional Nonimpact Cardio Cross-Training Workout 20–30 minutes @ recovery pace	**Resistance Workout** *3 sets each* Box Lunge Stability Ball Leg Curl Forearms to Palms Bridge Dead Bug Wall Jump

FRIDAY	**1-Mile Intervals @ 10K Pace** Dynamic stretching warm-up 1-mile warm-up @ recovery pace 3 × 1 mile @ 10K pace w/2-minute active recoveries 1-mile cool-down @ recovery pace
SATURDAY	**Resistance Workout** *3 sets each* Box Lunge Stability Ball Leg Curl Forearms to Palms Bridge Dead Bug Single-Leg Box Jump
SUNDAY	**Base Run** Run 9 miles @ base pace

WEEK 10 ◆ Proprioceptive Cue: Feeling Symmetry

MONDAY	Off
TUESDAY	**Base Run + Drills** Run 5.5 miles @ base pace Stiff-Legged Run 2×20 seconds Running No Arms 2×20 seconds
WEDNESDAY	**400m Intervals @ 3,000m Pace** Dynamic stretching warm-up 1-mile warm-up @ recovery pace 8×400m @ 3,000m pace w/3-minute active recoveries 1-mile cool-down @ recovery pace

THURSDAY	<u>Optional Nonimpact Cardio</u>
	<u>Cross-Training Workout</u>
	20–30 minutes @ recovery pace **Resistance Workout**
	      1 set each
	      Lying Hip Abduction
	      Single-Leg Squat
	      Box Lunge
	      Stability Ball Leg Curl
	      Squat Jump

FRIDAY	**1-Mile Intervals @ 10K Pace** Dynamic stretching warm-up 1-mile warm-up @ recovery pace 3×1 mile @ 10K pace w/2-minute active recoveries 1-mile cool-down @ recovery pace
SATURDAY	**Resistance Workout** *1 set each* Cook Hip Lift Oblique Bridge Forearms to Palms Bridge Stability Ball Leg Curl Split Squat Jump
SUNDAY	**Base Run** Run 9 miles @ base pace

Build 2

Training objectives: Increase fatigue resistance at 5K pace and 10K pace; build efficiency at half-marathon pace

WEEK 11 ◆ Proprioceptive Cue: Axle Between the Knees

MONDAY	Off	
TUESDAY	**Base Run + Drills** Run 6 miles @ base pace Steep Hill Sprints 2×20 seconds One-Leg Hop 2×20 seconds	
WEDNESDAY	**1K Intervals @ 5K Pace** Dynamic stretching warm-up 1-mile warm-up @ recovery pace 3×1K @ 5K pace w/3-minute active recoveries 1-mile cool-down @ recovery pace	
THURSDAY	Optional Nonimpact Cardio Cross-Training Workout 20–30 minutes @ recovery pace	**Resistance Workout** *1 set each* Lying Hip Abduction Single-Leg Squat Box Lunge Stability Ball Leg Curl Single-Leg Squat Jump
FRIDAY	**Tempo Run @ 10K Pace** Dynamic stretching warm-up 1-mile warm-up @ recovery pace 2.5 miles @ 10K pace 1-mile cool-down @ recovery pace	
SATURDAY	**Resistance Workout** *1 set each* Cook Hip Lift Oblique Bridge Forearms to Palms Bridge Stability Ball Leg Curl Broad Jump	

SUNDAY	**Progression Run**
	Run 10 miles
	Start @ recovery pace; gradually increase pace every other mile
	Run last mile @ half-marathon pace

WEEK 12 (Recovery) ◆ Proprioceptive Cue: Running Against a Wall

MONDAY	Off	
TUESDAY	**Base Run + Drills** Run 4.5 miles @ base pace High Knees 20 seconds Bounding 20 seconds	
WEDNESDAY	**1K Intervals @ 5K Pace** Dynamic stretching warm-up 1-mile warm-up @ recovery pace 3 × 1K @ 5K pace w/3-minute active recoveries 1-mile cool-down @ recovery pace	
THURSDAY	<u>Optional Nonimpact Cardio</u> <u>Cross-Training Workout</u> 20–30 minutes @ recovery pace	**Resistance Workout** *1 set each* Lying Hip Abduction Single-Leg Squat Box Lunge Stability Ball Leg Curl Wall Jump
FRIDAY	**Tempo Run @ 10K Pace** Dynamic stretching warm-up 1-mile warm-up @ recovery pace 2 miles @ 10K pace 1-mile cool-down @ recovery pace	
SATURDAY	**Resistance Workout** *1 set each* Cook Hip Lift Oblique Bridge Forearms to Palms Bridge Stability Ball Leg Curl	
SUNDAY	**5K Tune-up Race or Time Trial** Dynamic stretching warm-up 1-mile warm-up @ recovery pace 5K tune-up race or time trial 1-mile cool-down @ recovery pace	

WEEK 13 ♦ Proprioceptive Cue: Falling Forward

MONDAY	Off
TUESDAY	**Base Run + Drills** Run 6 miles @ base pace High Knees 2 × 20 seconds Bounding 2 × 20 seconds
WEDNESDAY	**1K Intervals @ 5K Pace** Dynamic stretching warm-up 1-mile warm-up @ recovery pace 4 × 1K intervals @ 5K pace w/3-minute active recoveries 1-mile cool-down @ recovery pace
THURSDAY	<u>Optional Nonimpact Cardio</u> <u>Cross-Training Workout</u> 20–30 minutes @ recovery pace **Resistance Workout** *1 set each* Lying Hip Abduction Single-Leg Squat Box Lunge Stability Ball Leg Curl Wall Jump
FRIDAY	**Tempo Run @ 10K Pace** Dynamic stretching warm-up 1-mile warm-up @ recovery pace 3 miles @ 10K pace 1-mile cool-down @ recovery pace
SATURDAY	**Resistance Workout** *1 set each* Cook Hip Lift Oblique Bridge Forearms to Palms Bridge Stability Ball Leg Curl Single-Leg Box Jump
SUNDAY	**Progression Run** Run 11 miles Start @ recovery pace; gradually increase pace every other mile Run last mile @ half-marathon pace

WEEK 14 ◆ Proprioceptive Cue: Navel to Spine

MONDAY	Off
TUESDAY	**Base Run + Drills** Run 6 miles @ base pace Stiff-Legged Run 2 × 20 seconds Running No Arms 2 × 20 seconds
WEDNESDAY	**1K Intervals @ 5K Pace** Dynamic stretching warm-up 1-mile warm-up @ recovery pace 4 × 1K intervals @ 5K pace w/3-minute active recoveries 1-mile cool-down @ recovery pace

THURSDAY	Optional Nonimpact Cardio Cross-Training Workout 20–30 minutes @ recovery pace	**Resistance Workout** *1 set each* Lying Hip Abduction Single-Leg Squat Box Lunge Stability Ball Leg Curl Squat Jump

FRIDAY	**Tempo Run @ 10K Pace** Dynamic stretching warm-up 1-mile warm-up @ recovery pace 4 miles @ 10K pace 1-mile cool-down @ recovery pace
SATURDAY	**Resistance Workout** *1 set each* Cook Hip Lift Oblique Bridge Forearms to Palms Bridge Stability Ball Leg Curl Split Squat Jump
SUNDAY	**Progression Run** Run 12 miles Start @ recovery pace; gradually increase pace every other mile Run last mile @ half-marathon pace

Peak Phase

Training objectives: Achieve peak fatigue resistance and efficiency at half-marathon pace; adapt and recover for peak race day

WEEK 15 ◆ Proprioceptive Cue: Running on Water

MONDAY	Off	
TUESDAY	**Base Run + Drills** Run 6 miles @ base pace Steep Hill Sprints 20 seconds One-Leg Hop 20 seconds	
WEDNESDAY	**Mixed Intervals** Dynamic stretching warm-up 1-mile warm-up @ recovery pace 1 × 2K @ half-marathon pace, 3-minute active recovery 1 × 1 mile @ 10K pace, 3-minute active recovery 1 × 1K @ 5K pace, 3-minute active recovery 1 × 800m @ 3,000m pace 1-mile cool-down @ recovery pace	
THURSDAY	Optional Nonimpact Cardio Cross-Training Workout 20–30 minutes @ recovery pace	**Resistance Workout** *1 set each* Lying Hip Abduction Single-Leg Squat Box Lunge Stability Ball Leg Curl Single-Leg Squat Jump
FRIDAY	**Tempo Run @ Half-Marathon Pace** 1-mile warm-up @ recovery pace 5 miles @ half-marathon pace 1-mile cool-down @ recovery pace	
SATURDAY	**Resistance Workout** *1 set each* Cook Hip Lift Oblique Bridge	

(continued)

WEEK 15 ◆ Proprioceptive Cue: Running on Water
(continued)

SATURDAY (continued)	**Resistance Workout** *1 set each (cont.)* Forearms to Palms Bridge Stability Ball Leg Curl Broad Jump
SUNDAY	**Marathon-Pace Run** 1-mile warm-up @ recovery pace 8 miles @ marathon pace 1-mile cool-down @ recovery pace

WEEK 16 (Recovery) ♦ Proprioceptive Cue: Pulling the Road

MONDAY	Off
TUESDAY	**Base Run + Drills** Run 5 miles @ base pace Stiff-Legged Run 2 × 20 seconds Running No Arms 2 × 20 seconds
WEDNESDAY	**Mixed Intervals** Dynamic stretching warm-up 1-mile warm-up @ recovery pace 1 × 2K @ half-marathon pace, 3-minute active recovery 1 × 1 mile @ 10K pace, 3-minute active recovery 1 × 1K @ 5K pace 1-mile cool-down @ recovery pace

THURSDAY	Optional Nonimpact Cardio Cross-Training Workout 20–30 minutes @ recovery pace	**Resistance Workout** *1 set each* Lying Hip Abduction Single-Leg Squat Box Lunge Stability Ball Leg Curl Squat Jump

FRIDAY	**Tempo Run @ Half-Marathon Pace** 1-mile warm-up @ recovery pace 4 miles @ half-marathon pace 1-mile cool-down @ recovery pace
SATURDAY	**Resistance Workout** *1 set each* Cook Hip Lift Oblique Bridge Forearms to Palms Bridge Stability Ball Leg Curl Split Squat Jump
SUNDAY	**10K Tune-up Race or Time Trial** Dynamic stretching warm-up 1-mile warm-up @ recovery pace 10K tune-up race or time trial 1-mile cool-down @ recovery pace

WEEK 17 ♦ Proprioceptive Cue: Scooting

MONDAY	Off
TUESDAY	**Base Run + Drills** Run 6 miles @ base pace Stiff-Legged Run 2 × 20 seconds Running No Arms 2 × 20 seconds
WEDNESDAY	**Mixed Intervals** Dynamic stretching warm-up 1-mile warm-up @ recovery pace 1 × 2K @ half-marathon pace, 2-minute active recovery 1 × 1 mile @ 10K pace, 2-minute active recovery 1 × 1K @ 5K pace, 2-minute active recovery 1 × 800m @ 3,000m pace 1-mile cool-down @ recovery pace

THURSDAY	<u>Optional Nonimpact Cardio</u> <u>Cross-Training Workout</u> 20–30 minutes @ recovery pace	**Resistance Workout** *1 set each* Lying Hip Abduction Single-Leg Squat Box Lunge Stability Ball Leg Curl Squat Jump

FRIDAY	**Tempo Run @ Half-Marathon Pace** 1-mile warm-up @ recovery pace 5.5 miles @ half-marathon pace 1-mile cool-down @ recovery pace
SATURDAY	**Resistance Workout** *1 set each* Cook Hip Lift Oblique Bridge Forearms to Palms Bridge Stability Ball Leg Curl Split Squat Jump
SUNDAY	**Marathon-Pace Run** 1-mile warm-up @ recovery pace 8 miles @ marathon pace 1-mile cool-down @ recovery pace

WEEK 18 ◆ Proprioceptive Cue: Pounding the Ground

MONDAY	Off
TUESDAY	**Base Run + Drills** Run 6 miles @ base pace Stiff-Legged Run 2×20 seconds Running No Arms 2×20 seconds
WEDNESDAY	**Mixed Intervals** Dynamic stretching warm-up 1-mile warm-up @ recovery pace 1×2K @ half-marathon pace, 90-second active recovery 1×1 mile @ 10K pace, 90-second active recovery 1×1K @ 5K pace, 90-second active recovery 1×800m @ 3,000m pace 1-mile cool-down @ recovery pace
THURSDAY	<u>Optional Nonimpact Cardio</u> <u>Cross-Training Workout</u> 20–30 minutes @ recovery pace **Resistance Workout** *1 set each* Lying Hip Abduction Single-Leg Squat Box Lunge Stability Ball Leg Curl Squat Jump
FRIDAY	**Tempo Run @ Half-Marathon Pace** 1-mile warm-up @ recovery pace 6 miles @ half-marathon pace 1-mile cool-down @ recovery pace
SATURDAY	**Resistance Workout** *1 set each* Cook Hip Lift Oblique Bridge Quadruped Dead Bug Single-Leg Squat Jump
SUNDAY	**Marathon-Pace Run** 1-mile warm-up @ recovery pace 9 miles @ marathon pace 1-mile cool-down @ recovery pace

WEEK 19 ✦ Proprioceptive Cue: Driving the Thigh

MONDAY	Off
TUESDAY	**Base Run + Drills** Run 6 miles @ base pace Steep Hill Sprints 2 × 20 seconds One-Leg Hop 2 × 20 seconds
WEDNESDAY	**Mixed Intervals** Dynamic stretching warm-up 1-mile warm-up @ recovery pace 1 × 2K @ half-marathon pace, 1-minute active recovery 1 × 1 mile @ 10K pace, 1-minute active recovery 1 × 1K @ 5K pace, 1-minute active recovery 1 × 800m @ 3,000m pace 1-mile cool-down @ recovery pace

THURSDAY	Optional Nonimpact Cardio Cross-Training Workout 20–30 minutes @ recovery pace	**Resistance Workout** *1 set each* Kneeling Overhead Draw-In Lying Draw-In w/Hip Flexion Box Lunge Stability Ball Leg Curl Broad Jump

FRIDAY	**Tempo Run @ Half-Marathon Pace** 1-mile warm-up @ recovery pace 5.5 miles @ half-marathon pace 1-mile cool-down @ recovery pace
SATURDAY	**Resistance Workout** *1 set each* Cook Hip Lift Oblique Bridge Quadruped Dead Bug Single-Leg Squat Jump
SUNDAY	**Marathon-Pace Run** 1-mile warm-up @ recovery pace 8 miles @ marathon pace 1-mile cool-down @ recovery pace

WEEK 20 (Taper) ◆ Proprioceptive Cue: Your Choice

MONDAY	Off
TUESDAY	**Base Run + Drills** Run 5 miles @ base pace High Knees 20 seconds Bounding 20 seconds
WEDNESDAY	**Mixed Intervals** Dynamic stretching warm-up 1-mile warm-up @ recovery pace 1×2K @ half-marathon pace, 2-minute active recovery 1×1 mile @ 10K pace, 2-minute active recovery 1×1K @ 5K pace, 2-minute active recovery 1-mile cool-down @ recovery pace

THURSDAY	Optional Nonimpact Cardio Cross-Training Workout 20–30 minutes @ recovery pace	**Resistance Workout** *1 set each* Kneeling Overhead Draw-In Lying Draw-In w/Hip Flexion Box Lunge Stability Ball Leg Curl

FRIDAY	**Tempo Run @ Half-Marathon Pace** 1-mile warm-up @ recovery pace 2 miles @ half-marathon pace 1-mile cool-down @ recovery pace
SATURDAY	Off
SUNDAY	**Half-Marathon Peak Race** 1-mile warm-up @ recovery pace Half Marathon 1-mile cool-down @ recovery pace

LEVEL 2

Use this plan if you are most comfortable with a half-marathon training plan that features six runs per week and a maximum run distance of fourteen miles. The plan also contains one optional nonimpact cardio cross-training workout and two resistance workouts per week.

Base Phase

Training objectives: Build aerobic capacity and endurance, increase injury resistance, and increase muscle activation capacity

WEEK 1 ◆ Proprioceptive Cue: Falling Forward

MONDAY	Off	
TUESDAY	**Base Run + Drills** Run 4 miles @ base pace Running No Arms 20 seconds One-Leg Hop 20 seconds	
WEDNESDAY	**Hill Repetitions** Dynamic stretching warm-up 2-mile warm-up @ recovery pace 1 × 30-second hill repetition @ relaxed sprint speed 2-mile cool-down @ recovery pace	
THURSDAY	**Base Run** Run 4 miles @ base pace *or* Nonimpact Cardio Cross-Training Workout 20–30 minutes @ recovery pace	**Resistance Workout** *1 set each* Lying Hip Abduction Cook Hip Lift Kneeling Overhead Draw-In Knee Fall-Out Squat Jump
FRIDAY	**Fartlek Run** Dynamic stretching warm-up Run 4 miles @ base pace w/2 × 30-second intervals @ 1-mile pace "sprinkled in"	

SATURDAY	**Base Run** Run 4 miles @ base pace	**Resistance Workout** *1 set each* Lying Hip Abduction Cook Hip Lift Kneeling Overhead Draw-In Knee Fall-Out Broad Jump
SUNDAY	**Base Run** Run 6 miles @ base pace	

WEEK 2 ◆ Proprioceptive Cue: Navel to Spine

MONDAY	Off	
TUESDAY	**Base Run + Drills** Run 4.5 miles @ base pace High Knees 2 × 20 seconds Bounding 2 × 20 seconds	
WEDNESDAY	**Hill Repetitions** Dynamic stretching warm-up 2-mile warm-up @ recovery pace 6 × 30-second hill repetitions @ relaxed sprint speed w/2-minute active recoveries 2-mile cool-down @ recovery pace	
THURSDAY	**Base Run** Run 4.5 miles @ base pace *or* Nonimpact Cardio Cross-Training Workout 25–35 minutes @ recovery pace	**Resistance Workout** *2 sets each* Lying Hip Abduction Cook Hip Lift Kneeling Overhead Draw-In Knee Fall-Out Split Squat Jump
FRIDAY	**Fartlek Run** Dynamic stretching warm-up Run 4.5 miles @ base pace w/6 × 30-second intervals @ 1-mile pace "sprinkled in"	
SATURDAY	**Base Run** Run 4.5 miles @ base pace	**Resistance Workout** *2 sets each* Lying Hip Abduction Cook Hip Lift Kneeling Overhead Draw-In Knee Fall-Out Wall Jump
SUNDAY	**Base Run** Run 7 miles @ base pace	

WEEK 3 ♦ Proprioceptive Cue: Running on Water

MONDAY	Off
TUESDAY	**Base Run + Drills** Run 5 miles @ base pace Stiff-Legged Run 2 × 20 seconds Running No Arms 2 × 20 seconds
WEDNESDAY	**Hill Repetitions** Dynamic stretching warm-up 2-mile warm-up @ recovery pace 6 × 45-second hill repetitions @ 1-mile pace w/2-minute active recoveries 2-mile cool-down @ recovery pace

THURSDAY	**Base Run** Run 5 miles @ base pace *or* <u>Nonimpact Cardio Cross-Training Workout</u> 30–40 minutes @ recovery pace	**Resistance Workout** *3 sets each* Lying Hip Abduction Cook Hip Lift Kneeling Overhead Draw-In Knee Fall-Out Squat Jump

FRIDAY	**Fartlek Run** Dynamic stretching warm-up Run 4 miles @ base pace w/6 × 45-second intervals @ 1-mile pace "sprinkled in"

SATURDAY	**Base Run** Run 5 miles @ base pace	**Resistance Workout** *3 sets each* Lying Hip Abduction Cook Hip Lift Kneeling Overhead Draw-In Knee Fall-Out Broad Jump

SUNDAY	**Base Run** Run 8 miles @ base pace

WEEK 4 (Recovery) ◆ Proprioceptive Cue: Pulling the Road

MONDAY	Off
TUESDAY	**Base Run + Drills** Run 4 miles @ base pace One-Leg Hop 20 seconds High Knees 20 seconds
WEDNESDAY	**Hill Repetitions** Dynamic stretching warm-up 2-mile warm-up @ recovery pace 4 × 1-minute hill repetitions @ 1-mile pace w/2-minute active recoveries 2-mile cool-down @ recovery pace

THURSDAY	**Base Run** Run 4 miles @ base pace *or* Nonimpact Cardio Cross-Training Workout 25–35 minutes @ recovery pace	**Resistance Workout** *1 set each* Single-Leg Squat Oblique Bridge Lying Draw-In w/Hip Flexion Quadruped *2 sets each* Lying Hip Abduction Cook Hip Lift Kneeling Overhead Draw-In Knee Fall-Out Single-Leg Squat Jump

FRIDAY	**Fartlek Run** Dynamic stretching warm-up Run 4 miles @ base pace w/4 × 1-minute intervals @ 1-mile pace "sprinkled in"

SATURDAY	**Base Run** Run 4 miles @ base pace	**Resistance Workout** *1 set each* Single-Leg Squat Oblique Bridge Lying Draw-In w/Hip Flexion Quadruped

SATURDAY (continued)	**Base Run**	**Resistance Workout** *2 sets each* Lying Hip Abduction Cook Hip Lift Kneeling Overhead Draw-In Knee Fall-Out Wall Jump
SUNDAY	**Base Run** Run 6 miles @ base pace	

WEEK 5 ◆ Proprioceptive Cue: Scooting

MONDAY	Off
TUESDAY	**Base Run + Drills** Run 5.5 miles @ base pace High Knees 2 × 20 seconds Bounding 2 × 20 seconds

WEDNESDAY	**Hill Repetitions** Dynamic stretching warm-up 1.5-mile warm-up @ recovery pace 6 × 90-second hill repetitions @ 1-mile pace w/2-minute active recoveries 1.5-mile cool-down @ recovery pace

THURSDAY	**Base Run** Run 5.5 miles @ base pace *or* <u>Nonimpact Cardio Cross-Training Workout</u> 35–45 minutes @ recovery pace	**Resistance Workout** *2 sets each* Single-Leg Squat Oblique Bridge Lying Draw-In w/Hip Flexion Quadruped *1 set each* Lying Hip Abduction Cook Hip Lift Kneeling Overhead Draw-In Knee Fall-Out Single-Leg Squat Jump

FRIDAY	**Fartlek Run** Dynamic stretching warm-up Run 5.5 miles @ base pace w/6 × 90-second intervals @ 3,000m pace "sprinkled in"

SATURDAY	**Base Run** Run 5.5 miles @ base pace	**Resistance Workout** *2 sets each* Single-Leg Squat Oblique Bridge Lying Draw-In w/Hip Flexion Quadruped

SATURDAY (continued)	Base Run	Resistance Workout *1 set each* Lying Hip Abduction Cook Hip Lift Kneeling Overhead Draw-In Knee Fall-Out Wall Jump
SUNDAY	Base Run Run 9 miles @ base pace	

WEEK 6 ◆ Proprioceptive Cue: Pounding the Ground

MONDAY	Off	
TUESDAY	**Base Run + Drills** Run 6 miles @ base pace Stiff-Legged Run 2 × 20 seconds Running No Arms 2 × 20 seconds	
WEDNESDAY	**Hill Repetitions** Dynamic stretching warm-up 1.5-mile warm-up @ recovery pace 8 × 90-second hill repetitions @ 1-mile pace w/2-minute active recoveries 1.5-mile cool-down @ recovery pace	
THURSDAY	**Base Run** Run 6 miles @ base pace *or* Nonimpact Cardio Cross-Training Workout 40–50 minutes @ recovery pace	**Resistance Workout** *3 sets each* Single-Leg Squat Oblique Bridge Lying Draw-In w/Hip Flexion Quadruped *2 sets* Squat Jump
FRIDAY	**Fartlek Run** Dynamic stretching warm-up Run 6 miles @ base pace w/8 × 90-second intervals @ 3,000m pace "sprinkled in"	
SATURDAY	**Base Run** Run 6 miles @ base pace	**Resistance Workout** *3 sets each* Single-Leg Squat Oblique Bridge Lying Draw-In w/Hip Flexion Quadruped *2 sets* Single-Leg Squat Jump
SUNDAY	**Endurance Run** Run 10 miles @ base pace	

Build 1 Phase

Training objectives: Continue to increase aerobic capacity and endurance; increase fatigue resistance at 3,000m pace and 10K pace

WEEK 7 ◆ Proprioceptive Cue: Driving the Thigh

MONDAY	Off	
TUESDAY	**Base Run + Drills** Run 6 miles @ base pace Steep Hill Sprints 2×20 seconds One-Leg Hop 2×20 seconds	
WEDNESDAY	**400m Intervals @ 3,000m Pace** Dynamic stretching warm-up 1-mile warm-up @ recovery pace 8×400m @ 3,000m pace w/3-minute active recoveries 1-mile cool-down @ recovery pace	
THURSDAY	**Recovery Run** 2–6 miles @ recovery pace *or* Nonimpact Cardio Cross-Training Workout 20–45 minutes @ recovery pace	**Resistance Workout** *2 sets each* Single-Leg Squat Oblique Bridge Lying Draw-In w/Hip Flexion Quadruped Split Squat Jump *1 set each* Box Lunge Stability Ball Leg Curl Forearms to Palms Bridge Dead Bug
FRIDAY	**1-Mile Intervals @ 10K Pace** Dynamic stretching warm-up 1.5-mile warm-up @ recovery pace 2×1 mile @ 10K pace w/2-minute active recoveries 1.5-mile recovery-pace-cool-down	

(continued)

WEEK 7 ◆ Proprioceptive Cue: Driving the Thigh
(continued)

SATURDAY	Recovery Run 2–6 miles @ recovery pace	Resistance Workout *2 sets each* Single-Leg Squat Oblique Bridge Lying Draw-In w/Hip Flexion Quadruped Single-Leg Box Jump *1 set each* Box Lunge Stability Ball Leg Curl Forearms to Palms Bridge Dead Bug
SUNDAY	**Base Run** Run 12 miles @ base pace	

WEEK 8 (Recovery) ♦ Proprioceptive Cue: Floppy Feet

MONDAY	Off	
TUESDAY	**Base Run + Drills** Run 5 miles @ base pace High Knees 20 seconds Bounding 20 seconds	
WEDNESDAY	**400m Intervals @ 3,000m Pace** Dynamic stretching warm-up 1-mile warm-up @ recovery pace 8 × 400m @ 3,000m pace w/3-minute active recoveries 1-mile cool-down @ recovery pace	
THURSDAY	**Recovery Run** 2–6 miles @ recovery pace *or* <u>Nonimpact Cardio Cross-Training Workout</u> 20–45 minutes @ recovery pace	**Resistance Workout** *1 set each* Single-Leg Squat Oblique Bridge Lying Draw-In w/Hip Flexion Quadruped *2 sets each* Box Lunge Stability Ball Leg Curl Forearms to Palms Bridge Dead Bug Broad Jump
FRIDAY	**1-Mile Intervals @ 10K Pace** Dynamic stretching warm-up 1.5-mile warm-up @ recovery pace 2 × 1 mile @ 10K pace w/2-minute active recoveries 1.5-mile recovery-pace-cool-down	
SATURDAY	**Recovery Run** 2–6 miles @ recovery pace	**Resistance Workout** *1 set each* Single-Leg Squat Oblique Bridge Lying Draw-In w/Hip Flexion Quadruped

(continued)

WEEK 8 (Recovery) ◆ Proprioceptive Cue: Floppy Feet
(continued)

SATURDAY (continued)	Recovery Run	Resistance Workout 2 sets each Box Lunge Stability Ball Leg Curl Forearms to Palms Bridge Dead Bug Wall Jump
SUNDAY	**Base Run** Run 8 miles @ base pace	

WEEK 9 ◆ Proprioceptive Cue: Butt Squeeze

MONDAY	Off	
TUESDAY	**Base Run + Drills** Run 6 miles @ base pace Stiff-Legged Run 2 × 20 seconds Running No Arms 2 × 20 seconds	
WEDNESDAY	**400m Intervals @ 3,000m Pace** Dynamic stretching warm-up 1-mile warm-up @ recovery pace 10 × 400m @ 3,000m pace w/3-minute active recoveries 1-mile cool-down @ recovery pace	
THURSDAY	**Recovery Run** 2–6 miles @ recovery pace *or* Nonimpact Cardio Cross-Training Workout 20–45 minutes @ recovery pace	**Resistance Workout** *3 sets each* Box Lunge Stability Ball Leg Curl Forearms to Palms Bridge Dead Bug Wall Jump
FRIDAY	**1-Mile Intervals @ 10K Pace** Dynamic stretching warm-up 1-mile warm-up @ recovery pace 3 × 1 mile @ 10K pace w/2-minute active recoveries 1-mile cool-down @ recovery pace	
SATURDAY	**Recovery Run** 2–6 miles @ recovery pace	**Resistance Workout** *3 sets each* Box Lunge Stability Ball Leg Curl Forearms to Palms Bridge Dead Bug Single-Leg Box Jump
SUNDAY	**Base Run** Run 13 miles @ base pace	

WEEK 10 ♦ Proprioceptive Cue: Feeling Symmetry

MONDAY	Off	
TUESDAY	**Base Run + Drills** Run 6.5 miles @ base pace Stiff-Legged Run 2×20 seconds Running No Arms 2×20 seconds	
WEDNESDAY	**400m Intervals @ 3,000m Pace** Dynamic stretching warm-up 1-mile warm-up @ recovery pace 12×400m @ 3,000m pace w/3-minute active recoveries 1-mile cool-down @ recovery pace	
THURSDAY	**Recovery Run** 2–6 miles @ recovery pace *or* Nonimpact Cardio Cross-Training Workout 20–45 minutes @ recovery pace	**Resistance Workout** *2 sets each* Lying Hip Abduction Single-Leg Squat Box Lunge Stability Ball Leg Curl Squat Jump
FRIDAY	**1-Mile Intervals @ 10K Pace** Dynamic stretching warm-up 1-mile warm-up @ recovery pace 4×1 mile @ 10K pace w/2-minute active recoveries 1-mile cool-down @ recovery pace	
SATURDAY	**Recovery Run** 2–6 miles @ recovery pace	**Resistance Workout** *2 sets each* Cook Hip Lift Oblique Bridge Forearms to Palms Bridge Stability Ball Leg Curl Split Squat Jump
SUNDAY	**Base Run** Run 14 miles @ base pace	

Build 2

Training objectives: Increase fatigue resistance at 5K pace and 10K pace; build efficiency at half-marathon pace

WEEK 11 ◆ Proprioceptive Cue: Axle Between the Knees

MONDAY	Off	
TUESDAY	**Base Run + Drills** Run 6.5 miles @ base pace Steep Hill Sprints 2 × 20 seconds One-Leg Hop 2 × 20 seconds	
WEDNESDAY	**1K Intervals @ 5K Pace** Dynamic stretching warm-up 1.5-mile warm-up @ recovery pace 3 × 1K @ 5K pace w/3-minute active recoveries 1.5-mile recovery-pace cool-down	
THURSDAY	**Recovery Run** 2–6 miles @ recovery pace *or* Nonimpact Cardio Cross-Training Workout 20–45 minutes @ recovery pace	**Resistance Workout** *2 sets each* Lying Hip Abduction Single-Leg Squat Box Lunge Stability Ball Leg Curl Single-Leg Squat Jump
FRIDAY	**Tempo Run @ 10K Pace** Dynamic stretching warm-up 2-mile warm-up @ recovery pace 3 miles @ 10K pace 2-mile cool-down @ recovery pace	
SATURDAY	**Recovery Run** 2–6 miles @ recovery pace	**Resistance Workout** *2 sets each* Cook Hip Lift Oblique Bridge Forearms to Palms Bridge Stability Ball Leg Curl Broad Jump

(continued)

WEEK 11 ◆ Proprioceptive Cue: Axle Between the Knees
(continued)

SUNDAY	**Progression Run**
	Run 11 miles
	Start @ recovery pace; gradually increase pace every other mile
	Run last mile @ half-marathon pace

WEEK 12 (Recovery) ◆ Proprioceptive Cue: Running Against a Wall

MONDAY	Off	
TUESDAY	**Base Run + Drills** Run 5 miles @ base pace High Knees 20 seconds Bounding 20 seconds	
WEDNESDAY	**1K Intervals @ 5K Pace** Dynamic stretching warm-up 1.5-mile warm-up @ recovery pace 3 × 1K @ 5K pace w/3-minute active recoveries 1.5-mile recovery-pace cool-down	
THURSDAY	**Recovery Run** 2–6 miles @ recovery pace or Nonimpact Cardio Cross-Training Workout 20–45 minutes @ recovery pace	**Resistance Workout** *2 sets each* Lying Hip Abduction Single-Leg Squat Box Lunge Stability Ball Leg Curl Wall Jump
FRIDAY	**Tempo Run @ 10K Pace** Dynamic stretching warm-up 2-mile warm-up @ recovery pace 2.5 miles @ 10K pace 2-mile cool-down @ recovery pace	
SATURDAY	**Recovery Run** 2 miles @ recovery pace	**Resistance Workout** *2 sets each* Cook Hip Lift Oblique Bridge Forearms to Palms Bridge Stability Ball Leg Curl
SUNDAY	**5K Tune-up Race or Time Trial** Dynamic stretching warm-up 1.5-mile warm-up @ recovery pace 5K tune-up race or time trial 1.5-mile recovery-pace cool-down	

WEEK 13 ◆ Proprioceptive Cue: Falling Forward

MONDAY	Off
TUESDAY	**Base Run + Drills** Run 6 miles @ base pace High Knees 2×20 seconds Bounding 2×20 seconds
WEDNESDAY	**1K Intervals @ 5K Pace** Dynamic stretching warm-up 1.5-mile warm-up @ recovery pace 4×1K intervals @ 5K pace w/3-minute active recoveries 1.5-mile cool-down @ recovery pace

THURSDAY	**Recovery Run** 2–6 miles @ recovery pace *or* Nonimpact Cardio Cross-Training Workout 20–45 minutes @ recovery pace	**Resistance Workout** *2 sets each* Lying Hip Abduction Single-Leg Squat Box Lunge Stability Ball Leg Curl Wall Jump

FRIDAY	**Tempo Run @ 10K Pace** Dynamic stretching warm-up 2-mile warm-up @ recovery pace 3.5 miles @ 10K pace 2-mile cool-down @ recovery pace	
SATURDAY	**Recovery Run** 2–6 miles @ recovery pace	**Resistance Workout** *2 sets each* Cook Hip Lift Oblique Bridge Forearms to Palms Bridge Stability Ball Leg Curl Single-Leg Box Jump
SUNDAY	**Progression Run** Run 13 miles Start @ recovery pace; gradually increase pace every other mile Run last 2 miles @ half-marathon pace	

WEEK 14 ♦ Proprioceptive Cue: Navel to Spine

MONDAY	Off	
TUESDAY	**Base Run + Drills** Run 6.5 miles @ base pace Stiff-Legged Run 2 × 20 seconds Running No Arms 2 × 20 seconds	
WEDNESDAY	**1K Intervals @ 5K Pace** Dynamic stretching warm-up 1.5-mile warm-up @ recovery pace 5 × 1K intervals @ 5K pace w/3-minute active recoveries 1.5-mile cool-down @ recovery pace	
THURSDAY	**Recovery Run** 2–6 miles @ recovery pace or Nonimpact Cardio Cross-Training Workout 20–45 minutes @ recovery pace	**Resistance Workout** *2 sets each* Lying Hip Abduction Single-Leg Squat Box Lunge Stability Ball Leg Curl Squat Jump
FRIDAY	**Tempo Run @ 10K Pace** Dynamic stretching warm-up 1-mile warm-up @ recovery pace 4 miles @ 10K pace 1-mile cool-down @ recovery pace	
SATURDAY	**Recovery Run** 2–6 miles @ recovery pace	**Resistance Workout** *2 sets each* Cook Hip Lift Oblique Bridge Forearms to Palms Bridge Stability Ball Leg Curl Split Squat Jump
SUNDAY	**Progression Run** Run 14 miles Start @ recovery pace; gradually increase pace every other mile Run last mile @ half-marathon pace	

Peak Phase

Training objectives: Achieve peak fatigue resistance and efficiency at half-marathon pace; adapt and recover for peak race day

WEEK 15 ◆ Proprioceptive Cue: Running on Water

MONDAY	Off	
TUESDAY	**Base Run + Drills** Run 7 miles @ base pace Steep Hill Sprints 20 seconds One-Leg Hop 20 seconds	
WEDNESDAY	**Mixed Intervals** Dynamic stretching warm-up 1-mile warm-up @ recovery pace 2 × 2K @ half-marathon pace, 3-minute active recoveries 1 × 1 mile @ 10K pace, 3-minute active recovery 1 × 1K @ 5K pace, 3-minute active recovery 1 × 800m @ 3,000m pace 1-mile cool-down @ recovery pace	
THURSDAY	**Recovery Run** 2–6 miles @ recovery pace *or* Nonimpact Cardio Cross-Training Workout 20–45 minutes @ recovery pace	**Resistance Workout** *2 sets each* Lying Hip Abduction Single-Leg Squat Box Lunge Stability Ball Leg Curl Single-Leg Squat Jump
FRIDAY	**Tempo Run @ Half-Marathon Pace** 1.5-mile warm-up @ recovery pace 5 miles @ half-marathon pace 1.5-mile recovery-pace cool-down	
SATURDAY	**Recovery Run** 2–6 miles @ recovery pace	**Resistance Workout** *2 sets each* Cook Hip Lift Oblique Bridge Forearms to Palms Bridge Stability Ball Leg Curl Broad Jump

SUNDAY	**Marathon-Pace Run**
	2-mile warm-up @ recovery pace
	8 miles @ marathon pace
	2-mile cool-down @ recovery pace

WEEK 16 (Recovery) ◆ Proprioceptive Cue: Pulling the Road

MONDAY	Off	
TUESDAY	**Base Run + Drills** Run 6 miles @ base pace Stiff-Legged Run 2 × 20 seconds Running No Arms 2 × 20 seconds	
WEDNESDAY	**Mixed Intervals** Dynamic stretching warm-up 1-mile warm-up @ recovery pace 1 × 2K @ half-marathon pace, 3-minute active recovery 1 × 1 mile @ 10K pace, 3-minute active recovery 1 × 1K @ 5K pace 1 × 800m @ 3,000m pace 1-mile cool-down @ recovery pace	
THURSDAY	**Recovery Run** 2–6 miles @ recovery pace *or* Nonimpact Cardio Cross-Training Workout 20–45 minutes @ recovery pace	**Resistance Workout** *2 sets each* Lying Hip Abduction Single-Leg Squat Box Lunge Stability Ball Leg Curl Squat Jump
FRIDAY	**Tempo Run @ Half-Marathon Pace** 1-mile warm-up @ recovery pace 4 miles @ half-marathon pace 1-mile cool-down @ recovery pace	
SATURDAY	**Recovery Run** 2 miles @ recovery pace	**Resistance Workout** *1 set each* Cook Hip Lift Oblique Bridge Forearms to Palms Bridge Stability Ball Leg Curl Split Squat Jump
SUNDAY	**10K Tune-up Race or Time Trial** Dynamic stretching warm-up 1.5-mile warm-up @ recovery pace 10K tune-up race or time trial 1.5-mile recovery-pace cool-down	

WEEK 17 ◆ Proprioceptive Cue: Scooting

MONDAY	Off
TUESDAY	**Base Run + Drills** Run 7 miles @ base pace Stiff-Legged Run 2 × 20 seconds Running No Arms 2 × 20 seconds
WEDNESDAY	**Mixed Intervals** Dynamic stretching warm-up 1-mile warm-up @ recovery pace 2 × 2K @ half-marathon pace, 2-minute active recoveries 1 × 1 mile @ 10K pace, 2-minute active recovery 1 × 1K @ 5K pace, 2-minute active recovery 1 × 800m @ 3,000m pace 1-mile cool-down @ recovery pace

THURSDAY	**Recovery Run**
	    2–6 miles @ recovery pace
	or
	Nonimpact Cardio Cross-Training Workout
	    20–45 minutes @ recovery pace
		Resistance Workout
		2 sets each
		Lying Hip Abduction
		Single-Leg Squat
		Box Lunge
		Stability Ball Leg Curl
		Squat Jump

FRIDAY	**Tempo Run @ Half-Marathon Pace** 2-mile warm-up @ recovery pace 6 miles @ half-marathon pace 2-mile cool-down @ recovery pace

SATURDAY	**Recovery Run** 2–6 miles @ recovery pace	**Resistance Workout** *2 sets each* Cook Hip Lift Oblique Bridge Forearms to Palms Bridge Stability Ball Leg Curl Split Squat Jump

SUNDAY	**Marathon-Pace Run** 2-mile warm-up @ recovery pace 9 miles @ marathon pace 2-mile cool-down @ recovery pace

WEEK 18 ◆ Proprioceptive Cue: Pounding the Ground

MONDAY	Off
TUESDAY	**Base Run + Drills** Run 7 miles @ base pace Stiff-Legged Run 2 × 20 seconds Running No Arms 2 × 20 seconds
WEDNESDAY	**Mixed Intervals** Dynamic stretching warm-up 1-mile warm-up @ recovery pace 2 × 2K @ half-marathon pace, 90-second active recoveries 1 × 1 mile @ 10K pace, 90-second active recovery 1 × 1K @ 5K pace, 90-second active recovery 1 × 800m @ 3,000m pace 1-mile cool-down @ recovery pace

THURSDAY	**Recovery Run** 2–6 miles @ recovery pace *or* <u>Nonimpact Cardio Cross-Training Workout</u> 20–45 minutes @ recovery pace	**Resistance Workout** *2 sets each* Lying Hip Abduction Single-Leg Squat Box Lunge Stability Ball Leg Curl Squat Jump

FRIDAY	**Tempo Run @ Half-Marathon Pace** 1-mile warm-up @ recovery pace 7 miles @ half-marathon pace 1-mile cool-down @ recovery pace

SATURDAY	**Recovery Run** 2–6 miles @ recovery pace	**Resistance Workout** *2 sets each* Cook Hip Lift Oblique Bridge Quadruped Dead Bug Single-Leg Squat Jump

SUNDAY	**Marathon-Pace Run** 2-mile warm-up @ recovery pace 9 miles @ marathon pace 2-mile cool-down @ recovery pace

WEEK 19 ♦ Proprioceptive Cue: Driving the Thigh

MONDAY	Off	
TUESDAY	**Base Run + Drills** Run 6 miles @ base pace Steep Hill Sprints 2 × 20 seconds One-Leg Hop 2 × 20 seconds	
WEDNESDAY	**Mixed Intervals** Dynamic stretching warm-up 1-mile warm-up @ recovery pace 2 × 2K @ half-marathon pace, 1-minute active recoveries 1 × 1 mile @ 10K pace, 1-minute active recovery 1 × 1K @ 5K pace, 1-minute active recovery 1 × 800m @ 3,000m pace 1-mile cool-down @ recovery pace	
THURSDAY	**Recovery Run** 2–6 miles @ recovery pace *or* Nonimpact Cardio Cross-Training Workout 20–45 minutes @ recovery pace	**Resistance Workout** *2 sets each* Kneeling Overhead Draw-In Lying Draw-In w/Hip Flexion Box Lunge Stability Ball Leg Curl Broad Jump
FRIDAY	**Tempo Run @ Half-Marathon Pace** 2-mile warm-up @ recovery pace 6 miles @ half-marathon pace 2-mile cool-down @ recovery pace	
SATURDAY	**Recovery Run** 2–6 miles @ recovery pace	**Resistance Workout** *2 sets each* Cook Hip Lift Oblique Bridge Quadruped Dead Bug Single-Leg Squat Jump
SUNDAY	**Marathon-Pace Run** 2-mile warm-up @ recovery pace 8 miles @ marathon pace 2-mile cool-down @ recovery pace	

WEEK 20 (Taper) ◆ Proprioceptive Cue: Your Choice

MONDAY	Off
TUESDAY	**Base Run + Drills** Run 5 miles @ base pace High Knees 20 seconds Bounding 20 seconds
WEDNESDAY	**Mixed Intervals** Dynamic stretching warm-up 1-mile warm-up @ recovery pace 1×2K @ half-marathon pace, 2-minute active recovery 1×1 mile @ 10K pace, 2-minute active recovery 1×1K @ 5K pace, 2-minute active recovery 1-mile cool-down @ recovery pace

THURSDAY	**Recovery Run** 2 miles @ recovery pace *or* Nonimpact Cardio Cross-Training Workout 15–20 minutes @ recovery pace	**Resistance Workout** *2 sets each* Kneeling Overhead Draw-In Lying Draw-In w/Hip Flexion Box Lunge Stability Ball Leg Curl

FRIDAY	**Tempo Run @ Half-Marathon Pace** 1-mile warm-up @ recovery pace 2 miles @ half-marathon pace 1-mile cool-down @ recovery pace
SATURDAY	Off
SUNDAY	**Half-Marathon Peak Race** 1-mile warm-up @ recovery pace Half marathon 1-mile cool-down @ recovery pace

LEVEL 3

Use this plan if you are most comfortable with a half-marathon training plan that features six scheduled runs per week plus up to four additional, optional recovery runs or nonimpact cardio cross-training workouts and a maximum run distance of 16 miles. The plan also includes two resistance workouts per week.

Base Phase

Training objectives: Build aerobic capacity and endurance, increase injury resistance, and increase muscle activation capacity

WEEK 1 ♦ Proprioceptive Cue: Falling Forward

MONDAY	Off	
TUESDAY	**Base Run + Drills** Run 6 miles @ base pace Running No Arms 20 seconds One-Leg Hop 20 seconds	Optional Recovery Run or Cardio Cross-Training Workout 20–60 minutes @ recovery pace
WEDNESDAY	**Hill Repetitions** Dynamic stretching warm-up 2-mile warm-up @ recovery pace 2 × 30-second hill repetitions @ relaxed sprint speed 2-mile cool-down @ recovery pace	Optional Recovery Run or Cardio Cross-Training Workout 20–60 minutes @ recovery pace
THURSDAY	**Base Run** Run 6 miles @ base pace	**Resistance Workout** *1 set each* Lying Hip Abduction Cook Hip Lift Kneeling Overhead Draw-In Knee Fall-Out Squat Jump

FRIDAY	**Fartlek Run**
	Dynamic stretching warm-up
	Run 6 miles @ base pace
	   w/2 × 30-second intervals
	   @ 1-mile pace "sprinkled in"
		Optional Recovery Run or Cardio Cross-Training Workout
		20–60 minutes @ recovery pace

(continued)

WEEK 1 ◆ Proprioceptive Cue: Falling Forward
(continued)

SATURDAY	**Base Run** Run 6 miles @ base pace	**Resistance Workout** *1 set each* Lying Hip Abduction Cook Hip Lift Kneeling Overhead Draw-In Knee Fall-Out Broad Jump
SUNDAY	**Base Run** Run 8 miles @ base pace	<u>Optional Recovery Run or Cardio</u> <u>Cross-Training Workout</u> 20–60 minutes @ recovery pace

WEEK 2 ◆ Proprioceptive Cue: Navel to Spine

MONDAY	Off	
TUESDAY	**Base Run + Drills** Run 6 miles @ base pace High Knees 2 × 20 seconds Bounding 2 × 20 seconds	Optional Recovery Run or Cardio Cross-Training Workout 20–60 minutes @ recovery pace
WEDNESDAY	**Hill Repetitions** Dynamic stretching warm-up 2-mile warm-up @ recovery pace 8 × 30-second hill repetitions @ relaxed sprint speed w/2-minute active recoveries 2-mile cool-down @ recovery pace	Optional Recovery Run or Cardio Cross-Training Workout 20–60 minutes @ recovery pace
THURSDAY	**Base Run** Run 6 miles @ base pace	**Resistance Workout** *2 sets each* Lying Hip Abduction Cook Hip Lift Kneeling Overhead Draw-In Knee Fall-Out Split Squat Jump
FRIDAY	**Fartlek Run** Dynamic stretching warm-up Run 6 miles @ base pace w/8 × 30-second intervals @ 1-mile pace "sprinkled in"	Optional Recovery Run or Cardio Cross-Training Workout 20–60 minutes @ recovery pace
SATURDAY	**Base Run** Run 6 miles @ base pace	**Resistance Workout** *2 sets each* Lying Hip Abduction Cook Hip Lift Kneeling Overhead Draw-In Knee Fall-Out Wall Jump
SUNDAY	**Endurance Run** Run 10 miles @ base pace	Optional Recovery Run or Cardio Cross-Training Workout 20–60 minutes @ recovery pace

WEEK 3 ◆ Proprioceptive Cue: Running on Water

MONDAY	Off	
TUESDAY	**Base Run + Drills** Run 6 miles @ base pace Stiff-Legged Run 2 × 20 seconds Running No Arms 2 × 20 seconds	Optional Recovery Run or Cardio Cross-Training Workout 20–60 minutes @ recovery pace

WEDNESDAY	**Hill Repetitions**
	Dynamic stretching warm-up
	2-mile warm-up @ recovery pace
	10 × 45-second hill repetitions
	  @ 1-mile pace w/2-minute
	  active recoveries
	2-mile cool-down @ recovery pace
		Optional Recovery Run or Cardio
		Cross-Training Workout
		20–60 minutes @ recovery pace

THURSDAY	**Base Run** Run 6 miles @ base pace	**Resistance Workout** *3 sets each* Lying Hip Abduction Cook Hip Lift Kneeling Overhead Draw-In Knee Fall-Out Squat Jump

FRIDAY	**Fartlek Run**
	Dynamic stretching warm-up
	Run 4 miles @ base pace
	  w/10 × 45-second intervals
	  @ 1-mile pace "sprinkled in"
		Optional Recovery Run or Cardio
		Cross-Training Workout
		20–60 minutes @ recovery pace

SATURDAY	**Base Run** Run 6 miles @ base pace	**Resistance Workout** *3 sets each* Lying Hip Abduction Cook Hip Lift Kneeling Overhead Draw-In Knee Fall-Out Broad Jump
SUNDAY	**Endurance Run** Run 12 miles @ base pace	Optional Recovery Run or Cardio Cross-Training Workout 20–60 minutes @ recovery pace

WEEK 4 (Recovery) ◆ Proprioceptive Cue: Pulling the Road

MONDAY	Off	
TUESDAY	**Base Run + Drills** Run 5 miles @ base pace One-Leg Hop 20 seconds High Knees 20 seconds	Optional Recovery Run or Cardio Cross-Training Workout 20–60 minutes @ recovery pace
WEDNESDAY	**Hill Repetitions** Dynamic stretching warm-up 2-mile warm-up @ recovery pace 6 × 1-minute hill repetitions 　@ 1-mile pace w/2-minute 　active recoveries 2-mile cool-down @ recovery pace	Optional Recovery Run or Cardio Cross-Training Workout 20–60 minutes @ recovery pace
THURSDAY	**Base Run** Run 5 miles @ base pace	**Resistance Workout** *1 set each* Single-Leg Squat Oblique Bridge Lying Draw-In w/Hip Flexion Quadruped *2 sets each* Lying Hip Abduction Cook Hip Lift Kneeling Overhead Draw-In Knee Fall-Out Single-Leg Squat Jump Broad Jump
FRIDAY	**Fartlek Run** Dynamic stretching warm-up Run 5 miles @ base pace 　w/6 × 1-minute intervals 　@ 1-mile pace "sprinkled in"	Optional Recovery Run or Cardio Cross-Training Workout 20–60 minutes @ recovery pace

(continued)

WEEK 4 (Recovery) ◆ Proprioceptive Cue: Pulling the Road
(continued)

SATURDAY	Base Run Run 5 miles @ base pace	**Resistance Workout** *1 set each* Single-Leg Squat Oblique Bridge Lying Draw-In w/Hip Flexion Quadruped *2 sets each* Lying Hip Abduction Cook Hip Lift Kneeling Overhead Draw-In Knee Fall-Out Wall Jump Single-Leg Box Jump
SUNDAY	**Base Run** Run 8 miles @ base pace	Optional Recovery Run or Cardio Cross-Training Workout 20–60 minutes @ recovery pace

WEEK 5 ◆ Proprioceptive Cue: Scooting

MONDAY	Off	
TUESDAY	**Base Run + Drills** Run 7 miles @ base pace High Knees 2 × 20 seconds Bounding 2 × 20 seconds	<u>Optional Recovery Run or Cardio</u> <u>Cross-Training Workout</u> 20–60 minutes @ recovery pace

WEDNESDAY	**Hill Repetitions**
	Dynamic stretching warm-up
	1.5-mile warm-up @ recovery pace
	8 × 90-second hill repetitions
	   @ 1-mile pace w/2-minute active
	   recoveries
	1.5-mile cool-down @ recovery
	   pace
		<u>Optional Recovery Run or Cardio</u>
		<u>Cross-Training Workout</u>
		20–60 minutes @ recovery pace

THURSDAY	**Base Run** Run 7 miles @ base pace	**Resistance Workout** *2 sets each* Single-Leg Squat Oblique Bridge Lying Draw-In w/Hip Flexion Quadruped *1 set each* Lying Hip Abduction Cook Hip Lift Kneeling Overhead Draw-In Knee Fall-Out Single-Leg Squat Jump Broad Jump

FRIDAY	**Fartlek Run**
	Dynamic stretching warm-up
	Run 7 miles @ base pace
	   w/8 × 90-second intervals
	   @ 3,000m pace "sprinkled in"
		<u>Optional Recovery Run or Cardio</u>
		<u>Cross-Training Workout</u>
		20–60 minutes @ recovery pace

SATURDAY	**Base Run** Run 7 miles @ base pace	**Resistance Workout** *2 sets each* Single-Leg Squat Oblique Bridge

(continued)

WEEK 5 ◆ Proprioceptive Cue: Scooting
(continued)

SATURDAY (continued)	Base Run	Resistance Workout
		2 sets each (cont.)
		Lying Draw-In w/Hip Flexion
		Quadruped
		1 set each
		Lying Hip Abduction
		Cook Hip Lift
		Kneeling Overhead Draw-In
		Knee Fall-Out
		Wall Jump
		Single-Leg Box Jump
SUNDAY	**Endurance Run** Run 12 miles @ base pace	Optional Recovery Run or Cardio Cross-Training Workout 20–60 minutes @ recovery pace

WEEK 6 ◆ Proprioceptive Cue: Pounding the Ground

MONDAY	Off	
TUESDAY	**Base Run + Drills** Run 7 miles @ base pace Stiff-Legged Run 2 × 20 seconds Running No Arms 2 × 20 seconds	<u>Optional Recovery Run or Cardio</u> <u>Cross-Training Workout</u> 20–60 minutes @ recovery pace

WEDNESDAY	**Hill Repetitions**
	Dynamic stretching warm-up
	1.5-mile warm-up @ recovery pace
	10 × 90-second hill repetitions
	    @ 1-mile pace w/2-minute
	    active recoveries
	1.5-mile cool-down @ recovery
	    pace
		<u>Optional Recovery Run or Cardio</u>
		<u>Cross-Training Workout</u>
		20–60 minutes @ recovery pace

THURSDAY	**Base Run** Run 7 miles @ base pace	**Resistance Workout** *3 sets each* Single-Leg Squat Oblique Bridge Lying Draw-In w/Hip Flexion Quadruped *2 sets* Squat Jump

FRIDAY	**Fartlek Run**
	Dynamic stretching warm-up
	Run 7 miles @ base pace
	    w/10 × 90-second intervals
	    @ 3,000m pace "sprinkled in"
		<u>Optional Recovery Run or Cardio</u>
		<u>Cross-Training Workout</u>
		20–60 minutes @ recovery pace

SATURDAY	**Base Run** Run 6 miles @ base pace	**Resistance Workout** *3 sets each* Single-Leg Squat Oblique Bridge Lying Draw-In w/Hip Flexion Quadruped *2 sets* Single-Leg Squat Jump

(continued)

WEEK 6 ◆ Proprioceptive Cue: Pounding the Ground
(continued)

SUNDAY	**Endurance Run** Run 13 miles @ base pace	Optional Recovery Run or Cardio Cross-Training Workout 20–60 minutes @ recovery pace

Build 1 Phase

Training objectives: Continue to increase aerobic capacity and endurance; increase fatigue resistance at 3,000m pace and 10K pace

WEEK 7 ◆ Proprioceptive Cue: Driving the Thigh

MONDAY	Off	
TUESDAY	**Base Run + Drills** Run 7 miles @ base pace Steep Hill Sprints 2 × 20 seconds One-Leg Hop 2 × 20 seconds	<u>Optional Recovery Run or Cardio</u> <u>Cross-Training Workout</u> 20–60 minutes @ recovery pace
WEDNESDAY	**400m Intervals @ 3,000m Pace** Dynamic stretching warm-up 1.5-mile warm-up @ recovery pace 10 × 400m @ 3,000m pace w/3-minute active recoveries 1.5-mile recovery-pace cool-down	<u>Optional Recovery Run or Cardio</u> <u>Cross-Training Workout</u> 20–60 minutes @ recovery pace
THURSDAY	**Recovery/Base Run** 4–8 miles @ recovery/base pace (Do this workout as a recovery run if you did *not* do an afternoon recovery workout following yesterday's interval workout. Otherwise, do this workout as a base workout.)	**Resistance Workout** *2 sets each* Single-Leg Squat Oblique Bridge Lying Draw-In w/Hip Flexion Quadruped Split Squat Jump Single-Leg Squat Jump *1 set each* Box Lunge Stability Ball Leg Curl Forearms to Palms Bridge Dead Bug
FRIDAY	**1-Mile Intervals @ 10K Pace** Dynamic stretching warm-up 2-mile warm-up @ recovery pace 3 × 1 mile @ 10K pace w/2-minute active recoveries 2-mile recovery-pace cool-down	<u>Optional Recovery Run or Cardio</u> <u>Cross-Training Workout</u> 20–60 minutes @ recovery pace

(continued)

WEEK 7 ◆ Proprioceptive Cue: Driving the Thigh
(continued)

SATURDAY	Recovery/Base Run 4–8 miles @ recovery/base pace	Resistance Workout *2 sets each* Single-Leg Squat Oblique Bridge Lying Draw-In w/Hip Flexion Quadruped Single-Leg Box Jump Squat Jump *1 set each* Box Lunge Stability Ball Leg Curl Forearms to Palms Bridge Dead Bug
SUNDAY	**Endurance Run** Run 14 miles @ base pace	<u>Optional Recovery Run or Cardio</u> <u>Cross-Training Workout</u> 20–60 minutes @ recovery pace

WEEK 8 (Recovery) ♦ Proprioceptive Cue: Floppy Feet

MONDAY	Off	
TUESDAY	**Base Run + Drills** Run 6 miles @ base pace High Knees 20 seconds Bounding 20 seconds	Optional Recovery Run or Cardio Cross-Training Workout 20–60 minutes @ recovery pace
WEDNESDAY	**400m Intervals @ 3,000m Pace** Dynamic stretching warm-up 1-mile warm-up @ recovery pace 9 × 400m @ 3,000m pace w/3-minute active recoveries 1-mile cool-down @ recovery pace	Optional Recovery Run or Cardio Cross-Training Workout 20–60 minutes @ recovery pace
THURSDAY	**Recovery/Base Run** 4–8 miles @ recovery/base pace	**Resistance Workout** *1 set each* Single-Leg Squat Oblique Bridge Lying Draw-In w/Hip Flexion Quadruped *2 sets each* Box Lunge Stability Ball Leg Curl Forearms to Palms Bridge Dead Bug Broad Jump Wall Jump
FRIDAY	**1-Mile Intervals @ 10K Pace** Dynamic stretching warm-up 2-mile warm-up @ recovery pace 3 × 1 mile @ 10K pace w/2-minute active recoveries 2-mile recovery-pace cool-down	Optional Recovery Run or Cardio Cross-Training Workout 20–60 minutes @ recovery pace
SATURDAY	**Recovery/Base Run** 4–8 miles @ recovery/base pace	**Resistance Workout** *1 set each* Single-Leg Squat Oblique Bridge

(continued)

WEEK 8 (Recovery) ♦ Proprioceptive Cue: Floppy Feet
(continued)

SATURDAY (continued)	Recovery/Base Run	**Resistance Workout** *1 set each (cont.)* Lying Draw-In w/Hip Flexion Quadruped *2 sets each* Box Lunge Stability Ball Leg Curl Forearms to Palms Bridge Dead Bug Wall Jump Single-Leg Box Jump
SUNDAY	**Endurance Run** Run 10 miles @ base pace	Optional Recovery Run or Cardio Cross-Training Workout 20–60 minutes @ recovery pace

WEEK 9 ♦ Proprioceptive Cue: Butt Squeeze

MONDAY	Off	
TUESDAY	**Base Run + Drills** Run 8 miles @ base pace Stiff-Legged Run 2 × 20 seconds Running No Arms 2 × 20 seconds	Optional Recovery Run or Cardio Cross-Training Workout 20–60 minutes @ recovery pace
WEDNESDAY	**400m Intervals @ 3,000m Pace** Dynamic stretching warm-up 1.5-mile warm-up @ recovery pace 12 × 400m @ 3,000m pace w/3-minute active recoveries 1.5-mile recovery-pace cool-down	Optional Recovery Run or Cardio Cross-Training Workout 20–60 minutes @ recovery pace
THURSDAY	**Recovery/Base Run** 4–8 miles @ recovery/base pace	**Resistance Workout** *3 sets each* Box Lunge Stability Ball Leg Curl Forearms to Palms Bridge Dead Bug Wall Jump Single-Leg Box Jump
FRIDAY	**1-Mile Intervals @ 10K Pace** Dynamic stretching warm-up 2-mile warm-up @ recovery pace 4 × 1 mile @ 10K pace w/2-minute active recoveries 2-mile recovery-pace cool-down	Optional Recovery Run or Cardio Cross-Training Workout 20–60 minutes @ recovery pace
SATURDAY	**Recovery/Base Run** 4–8 miles @ recovery/base pace	**Resistance Workout** *3 sets each* Box Lunge Stability Ball Leg Curl Forearms to Palms Bridge Dead Bug Single-Leg Box Jump Squat Jump
SUNDAY	**Endurance Run** Run 15 miles @ base pace	Optional Recovery Run or Cardio Cross-Training Workout 20–60 minutes @ recovery pace

WEEK 10 ♦ Proprioceptive Cue: Feeling Symmetry

MONDAY	Off	
TUESDAY	**Base Run + Drills** Run 8 miles @ base pace Stiff-Legged Run 2 × 20 seconds Running No Arms 2 × 20 seconds	<u>Optional Recovery Run or Cardio</u> <u>Cross-Training Workout</u> 20–60 minutes @ recovery pace
WEDNESDAY	**400m Intervals @ 3,000m Pace** Dynamic stretching warm-up 1.5-mile warm-up @ recovery pace 14 × 400m @ 3,000m pace w/3-minute active recoveries 1.5-mile recovery-pace cool-down	<u>Optional Recovery Run or Cardio</u> <u>Cross-Training Workout</u> 20–60 minutes @ recovery pace
THURSDAY	**Recovery/Base Run** 4–8 miles @ recovery/base pace	**Resistance Workout** *2 sets each* Lying Hip Abduction Single-Leg Squat Box Lunge Stability Ball Leg Curl Squat Jump Split Squat Jump
FRIDAY	**1-Mile Intervals @ 10K Pace** Dynamic stretching warm-up 2-mile warm-up @ recovery pace 5 × 1 mile @ 10K pace w/2-minute active recoveries 2-mile recovery-pace cool-down	<u>Optional Recovery Run or Cardio</u> <u>Cross-Training Workout</u> 20–60 minutes @ recovery pace
SATURDAY	**Recovery/Base Run** 4–8 miles @ recovery/base pace	**Resistance Workout** *2 sets each* Cook Hip Lift Oblique Bridge Forearms to Palms Bridge Stability Ball Leg Curl Split Squat Jump Single-Leg Squat Jump
SUNDAY	**Endurance Run** Run 16 miles @ base pace	<u>Optional Recovery Run or Cardio</u> <u>Cross-Training Workout</u> 20–60 minutes @ recovery pace

Build 2

Training objectives: Increase fatigue resistance at 5K pace and 10K pace; build efficiency at half-marathon pace

WEEK 11 ♦ Proprioceptive Cue: Axle Between the Knees

MONDAY	Off	
TUESDAY	**Base Run + Drills** Run 8 miles @ base pace Steep Hill Sprints 2 × 20 seconds One-Leg Hop 2 × 20 seconds	<u>Optional Recovery Run or Cardio</u> <u>Cross-Training Workout</u> 20–60 minutes @ recovery pace
WEDNESDAY	**1K Intervals @ 5K Pace** Dynamic stretching warm-up 2-mile warm-up @ recovery pace 4 × 1K @ 5K pace w/3-minute active recoveries 2-mile cool-down @ recovery pace	<u>Optional Recovery Run or Cardio</u> <u>Cross-Training Workout</u> 20–60 minutes @ recovery pace
THURSDAY	**Recovery/Base Run** 4–8 miles @ recovery/base pace	**Resistance Workout** *2 sets each* Lying Hip Abduction Single-Leg Squat Box Lunge Stability Ball Leg Curl Single-Leg Squat Jump Broad Jump
FRIDAY	**Tempo Run @ 10K Pace** Dynamic stretching warm-up 2-mile warm-up @ recovery pace 4 miles @ 10K pace 2-mile cool-down @ recovery pace	<u>Optional Recovery Run or Cardio</u> <u>Cross-Training Workout</u> 20–60 minutes @ recovery pace
SATURDAY	**Recovery/Base Run** 4–8 miles @ recovery/base pace	**Resistance Workout** *2 sets each* Cook Hip Lift Oblique Bridge Forearms to Palms Bridge Stability Ball Leg Curl Broad Jump Wall Jump

(continued)

WEEK 11 ◆ Proprioceptive Cue: Axle Between the Knees
(continued)

SUNDAY	**Progression Run**
	Run 12 miles
	Start @ recovery pace; gradually
	  increase pace every other mile
	Run last 2 miles @ half-marathon
	  pace
		Optional Recovery Run or Cardio
		Cross-Training Workout
		20–60 minutes @ recovery pace

WEEK 12 (Recovery) ◆ Proprioceptive Cue: Running Against a Wall

MONDAY	Off	
TUESDAY	**Base Run + Drills** Run 6 miles @ base pace High Knees 20 seconds Bounding 20 seconds	<u>Optional Recovery Run or Cardio</u> <u>Cross-Training Workout</u> 20–60 minutes @ recovery pace
WEDNESDAY	**1K Intervals @ 5K Pace** Dynamic stretching warm-up 2-mile warm-up @ recovery pace 3 × 1K @ 5K pace w/3-minute active recoveries 2-mile cool-down @ recovery pace	<u>Optional Recovery Run or Cardio</u> <u>Cross-Training Workout</u> 20–60 minutes @ recovery pace
THURSDAY	**Recovery/Base Run** 4–8 miles @ recovery/base pace	**Resistance Workout** *2 sets each* Lying Hip Abduction Single-Leg Squat Box Lunge Stability Ball Leg Curl Wall Jump Single-Leg Box Jump
FRIDAY	**Tempo Run @ 10K Pace** Dynamic stretching warm-up 2-mile warm-up @ recovery pace 2.5 miles @ 10K pace 2-mile cool-down @ recovery pace	
SATURDAY	**Recovery Run** 2 miles @ recovery pace	**Resistance Workout** *2 sets each* Cook Hip Lift Oblique Bridge Forearms to Palms Bridge Stability Ball Leg Curl
SUNDAY	**5K Tune-up Race or Time Trial** Dynamic stretching warm-up 2-mile warm-up @ recovery pace 5K tune-up race or time trial 2-mile cool-down @ recovery pace	

WEEK 13 ◆ Proprioceptive Cue: Falling Forward

MONDAY	Off	
TUESDAY	**Base Run + Drills** Run 9 miles @ base pace High Knees 2×20 seconds Bounding 2×20 seconds	<u>Optional Recovery Run or Cardio</u> <u>Cross-Training Workout</u> 20–60 minutes @ recovery pace
WEDNESDAY	**1K Intervals @ 5K Pace** Dynamic stretching warm-up 2-mile warm-up @ recovery pace 5×1K intervals @ 5K pace w/3-minute active recoveries 2-mile cool-down @ recovery pace	<u>Optional Recovery Run or Cardio</u> <u>Cross-Training Workout</u> 20–60 minutes @ recovery pace
THURSDAY	**Recovery/Base Run** 4–8 miles @ recovery/base pace	**Resistance Workout** *2 sets each* Lying Hip Abduction Single-Leg Squat Box Lunge Stability Ball Leg Curl Wall Jump Single-Leg Box Jump
FRIDAY	**Tempo Run @ 10K Pace** Dynamic stretching warm-up 2-mile warm-up @ recovery pace 4.5 miles @ 10K pace 2-mile cool-down @ recovery pace	<u>Optional Recovery Run or Cardio</u> <u>Cross-Training Workout</u> 20–60 minutes @ recovery pace
SATURDAY	**Recovery/Base Run** 4–8 miles @ recovery/base pace	**Resistance Workout** *2 sets each* Cook Hip Lift Oblique Bridge Forearms to Palms Bridge Stability Ball Leg Curl Single-Leg Box Jump Squat Jump
SUNDAY	**Progression Run** Run 14 miles Start @ recovery pace; gradually increase pace every other mile Run last 2 miles @ half-marathon pace	<u>Optional Recovery Run or Cardio</u> <u>Cross-Training Workout</u> 20–60 minutes @ recovery pace

WEEK 14 ♦ Proprioceptive Cue: Navel to Spine

MONDAY	Off	
TUESDAY	**Base Run + Drills** Run 9 miles @ base pace Stiff-Legged Run 2 × 20 seconds Running No Arms 2 × 20 seconds	Optional Recovery Run or Cardio Cross-Training Workout 20–60 minutes @ recovery pace
WEDNESDAY	**1K Intervals @ 5K Pace** Dynamic stretching warm-up 2-mile warm-up @ recovery pace 6 × 1K intervals @ 5K pace w/3-minute active recoveries 2-mile cool-down @ recovery pace	Optional Recovery Run or Cardio Cross-Training Workout 20–60 minutes @ recovery pace
THURSDAY	**Recovery/Base Run** 4–8 miles @ recovery/base pace	**Resistance Workout** *2 sets each* Lying Hip Abduction Single-Leg Squat Box Lunge Stability Ball Leg Curl Squat Jump Split Squat Jump
FRIDAY	**Tempo Run @ 10K Pace** Dynamic stretching warm-up 1-mile warm-up @ recovery pace 5 miles @ 10K pace 1-mile cool-down @ recovery pace	Optional Recovery Run or Cardio Cross-Training Workout 20–60 minutes @ recovery pace
SATURDAY	**Recovery/Base Run** 4–8 miles @ recovery/base pace	**Resistance Workout** *2 sets each* Cook Hip Lift Oblique Bridge Forearms to Palms Bridge Stability Ball Leg Curl Split Squat Jump Single-Leg Squat Jump
SUNDAY	**Progression Run** Run 16 miles Start @ recovery pace; gradually increase pace every other mile Run last 2 miles @ half-marathon pace	Optional Recovery Run or Cardio Cross-Training Workout 20–60 minutes @ recovery pace

Peak Phase

Training objectives: Achieve peak fatigue resistance and efficiency at half-marathon pace; adapt and recover for peak race day

WEEK 15 ◆ Proprioceptive Cue: Running on Water

MONDAY	Off	
TUESDAY	**Base Run + Drills** Run 9 miles @ base pace Steep Hill Sprint 2 × 20 seconds Single-Leg Hop 2 × 20 seconds	<u>Optional Recovery Run or Cardio Cross-Training Workout</u> 20–60 minutes @ recovery pace
WEDNESDAY	**Mixed Intervals** Dynamic stretching warm-up 1-mile warm-up @ recovery pace 2 × 2K @ half-marathon pace, 3-minute active recoveries 2 × 1 mile @ 10K pace, 3-minute active recoveries 1 × 1K @ 5K pace, 3-minute active recovery 1 × 800m @ 3,000m pace 1-mile cool-down @ recovery pace	<u>Optional Recovery Run or Cardio Cross-Training Workout</u> 20–60 minutes @ recovery pace
THURSDAY	**Recovery/Base Run** 4–8 miles @ recovery/base pace	**Resistance Workout** *2 sets each* Lying Hip Abduction Single-Leg Squat Box Lunge Stability Ball Leg Curl Single-Leg Squat Jump Broad Jump
FRIDAY	**Tempo Run @ Half-Marathon Pace** 2-mile warm-up @ recovery pace 6 miles @ half-marathon pace 2-mile cool-down @ recovery pace	<u>Optional Recovery Run or Cardio Cross-Training Workout</u> 20–60 minutes @ recovery pace

SATURDAY	**Recovery/Base Run** 4–8 miles @ recovery/base pace	**Resistance Workout** *2 sets each* Cook Hip Lift Oblique Bridge Forearms to Palms Bridge Stability Ball Leg Curl Broad Jump Wall Jump
SUNDAY	**Marathon-Pace Run** 2-mile warm-up @ recovery pace 8 miles @ marathon pace 2-mile cool-down @ recovery pace	Optional Recovery Run or Cardio Cross-Training Workout 20–60 minutes @ recovery pace

WEEK 16 (Recovery) ◆ Proprioceptive Cue: Pulling the Road

MONDAY	Off	
TUESDAY	**Base Run + Drills** Run 6 miles @ base pace Stiff-Legged Run 2 × 20 seconds Running No Arms 2 × 20 seconds	<u>Optional Recovery Run or Cardio</u> <u>Cross-Training Workout</u> 20–60 minutes @ recovery pace

WEDNESDAY	**Mixed Intervals**
	Dynamic stretching warm-up
	1-mile warm-up @ recovery pace
	1 × 2K @ half-marathon pace,
	    3-minute active recovery
	1 × 1 mile @ 10K pace, 3-minute
	    active recovery
	1 × 1K @ 5K pace
	1 × 800m @ 3,000m pace
	1-mile cool-down @ recovery pace
		<u>Optional Recovery Run or Cardio</u>
		<u>Cross-Training Workout</u>
		20–60 minutes @ recovery pace

THURSDAY	**Recovery/Base Run** 4–8 miles @ recovery/base pace	**Resistance Workout** *2 sets each* Lying Hip Abduction Single-Leg Squat Box Lunge Stability Ball Leg Curl Squat Jump Split Squat Jump
FRIDAY	**Tempo Run @ Half-Marathon Pace** 1-mile warm-up @ recovery pace 4 miles @ half-marathon pace 1-mile cool-down @ recovery pace	
SATURDAY	**Recovery Run** 2 miles @ recovery pace	**Resistance Workout** *1 set each* Cook Hip Lift Oblique Bridge Forearms to Palms Bridge Stability Ball Leg Curl Split Squat Jump Single-Leg Squat Jump

SUNDAY	**10K Tune-up Race or Time Trial** Dynamic stretching warm-up 2-mile warm-up @ recovery pace 10K tune-up race or time trial 2-mile cool-down @ recovery pace

WEEK 17 ◆ Proprioceptive Cue: Scooting

MONDAY	Off	
TUESDAY	**Base Run + Drills** Run 10 miles @ base pace Stiff-Legged Run 2 × 20 seconds Running No Arms 2 × 20 seconds	Optional Recovery Run or Cardio Cross-Training Workout 20–60 minutes @ recovery pace

WEDNESDAY	**Mixed Intervals**
	Dynamic stretching warm-up
	1-mile warm-up @ recovery pace
	2 × 2K @ half-marathon pace,
	   2-minute active recoveries
	2 × 1 mile @ 10K pace, 2-minute
	   active recoveries
	1 × 1K @ 5K pace, 2-minute active
	   recovery
	1 × 800m @ 3,000m pace
	1-mile cool-down @ recovery pace
		Optional Recovery Run or Cardio Cross-Training Workout
		20–60 minutes @ recovery pace

THURSDAY	**Recovery/Base Run** 4–8 miles @ recovery/base pace	**Resistance Workout** *2 sets each* Lying Hip Abduction Single-Leg Squat Box Lunge Stability Ball Leg Curl Squat Jump Split Squat Jump
FRIDAY	**Tempo Run @ Half-Marathon Pace** 2-mile warm-up @ recovery pace 7 miles @ half-marathon pace 2-mile cool-down @ recovery pace	Optional Recovery Run or Cardio Cross-Training Workout 20–60 minutes @ recovery pace
SATURDAY	**Recovery/Base Run** 4–8 miles @ recovery/base pace	**Resistance Workout** *2 sets each* Cook Hip Lift Oblique Bridge Forearms to Palms Bridge Stability Ball Leg Curl Split Squat Jump Single-Leg Squat Jump

SUNDAY	**Marathon-Pace Run** 2-mile warm-up @ recovery pace 10 miles @ marathon pace 2-mile cool-down @ recovery pace	Optional Recovery Run or Cardio Cross-Training Workout 20–60 minutes @ recovery pace

WEEK 18 ✦ Proprioceptive Cue: Pounding the Ground

MONDAY	Off	
TUESDAY	**Base Run + Drills** Run 10 miles @ base pace Stiff-Legged Run 2 x 20 seconds Running No Arms 2 x 20 seconds	Optional Recovery Run or Cardio Cross-Training Workout 20–60 minutes @ recovery pace

WEDNESDAY	**Mixed Intervals**
	Dynamic stretching warm-up
	1-mile warm-up @ recovery pace
	2 x 2K @ half-marathon pace,
	   90-second active recoveries
	2 x 1 mile @ 10K pace, 90-second
	   active recoveries
	1 x 1K @ 5K pace, 90-second active
	   recovery
	1 x 800m @ 3,000m pace
	1-mile cool-down @ recovery pace
		Optional Recovery Run or Cardio
		Cross-Training Workout
		20–60 minutes @ recovery pace

THURSDAY	**Recovery/Base Run** 4–8 miles @ recovery/base pace	**Resistance Workout** *2 sets each* Lying Hip Abduction Single-Leg Squat Box Lunge Stability Ball Leg Curl Squat Jump Split Squat Jump
FRIDAY	**Tempo Run @ Half-Marathon Pace** 2-mile warm-up @ recovery pace 8 miles @ half-marathon pace 2-mile cool-down @ recovery pace	Optional Recovery Run or Cardio Cross-Training Workout 20–60 minutes @ recovery pace
SATURDAY	**Recovery/Base Run** 4–8 miles @ recovery/base pace	**Resistance Workout** *2 sets each* Cook Hip Lift Oblique Bridge Quadruped Dead Bug Single-Leg Squat Jump Broad Jump

SUNDAY	**Marathon-Pace Run**	Optional Recovery Run or Cardio
	2-mile warm-up @ recovery pace	Cross-Training Workout
	11 miles @ marathon pace	20–60 minutes @ recovery pace
	2-mile cool-down @ recovery pace	

WEEK 19 ♦ Proprioceptive Cue: Driving the Thigh

MONDAY	Off	
TUESDAY	**Base Run + Drills** Run 8 miles @ base pace Steep Hill Sprints 2 x 20 seconds One-Leg Hop 2 x 20 seconds	Optional Recovery Run or Cardio Cross-Training Workout 20–60 minutes @ recovery pace

WEDNESDAY	**Mixed Intervals**
	Dynamic stretching warm-up
	1-mile warm-up @ recovery pace
	2 x 2K @ half-marathon pace,
	    1-minute active recoveries
	2 x 1 mile @ 10K pace, 1-minute
	    active recoveries
	1 x 1K @ 5K pace, 1-minute active
	    recovery
	1 x 800m @ 3,000m pace
	1-mile cool-down @ recovery pace
		Optional Recovery Run or Cardio
		Cross-Training Workout
		20–60 minutes @ recovery pace

THURSDAY	**Recovery/Base Run** 4–8 miles @ recovery/base pace	**Resistance Workout** *2 sets each* Kneeling Overhead Draw-In Lying Draw-In w/Hip Flexion Box Lunge Stability Ball Leg Curl Broad Jump Wall Jump
FRIDAY	**Tempo Run @ Half-Marathon Pace** 2-mile warm-up @ recovery pace 6 miles @ half-marathon pace 2-mile cool-down @ recovery pace	Optional Recovery Run or Cardio Cross-Training Workout 20–60 minutes @ recovery pace
SATURDAY	**Recovery/Base Run** 4–8 miles @ recovery/base pace	**Resistance Workout** *2 sets each* Cook Hip Lift Oblique Bridge Quadruped Dead Bug Single-Leg Squat Jump Broad Jump

| SUNDAY | **Marathon-Pace Run**
2-mile warm-up @ recovery pace
8 miles @ marathon pace
2-mile cool-down @ recovery pace | <u>Optional Recovery Run or Cardio</u>
<u>Cross-Training Workout</u>
20–60 minutes @ recovery pace |

WEEK 20 (Taper) ◆ Proprioceptive Cue: Your Choice

MONDAY	Off
TUESDAY	**Base Run + Drills** 　Run 6 miles @ base pace 　High Knees 20 seconds 　Bounding 20 seconds
WEDNESDAY	**Mixed Intervals** 　Dynamic stretching warm-up 　1-mile warm-up @ recovery pace 　1 x 2K @ half-marathon pace, 2-minute active recovery 　1 x 1 mile @ 10K pace, 2-minute active recovery 　1 x 1K @ 5K pace, 2-minute active recovery 　1 x 800m @ 3,000m pace 　1-mile cool-down @ recovery pace

THURSDAY	**Recovery Run** 　2 miles @ recovery pace	**Resistance Workout** 　*2 sets each* 　Kneeling Overhead Draw-In 　Lying Draw-In w/Hip Flexion 　Box Lunge 　Stability Ball Leg Curl

FRIDAY	**Tempo Run @ Half-Marathon Pace** 　1-mile warm-up @ recovery pace 　2 miles @ half-marathon pace 　1-mile cool-down @ recovery pace
SATURDAY	Off
SUNDAY	**Half-Marathon Peak Race** 　1-mile warm-up @ recovery pace 　Half Marathon 　1-mile cool-down @ recovery pace

CHAPTER ◆ 14

BRAIN TRAINING PLANS: MARATHON

Ah, the marathon! It's the classic challenge of our sport. If you stay involved in running long enough, eventually you have to run at least one marathon. There's no feeling in the world quite like that of crossing a marathon finish line for the first time. That's why most marathon finishers come back for more. For the serious runner, trying to master the marathon becomes the next great challenge. This chapter offers training plans for first-time marathon runners and personal-best seekers alike.

There are three marathon training plans in this chapter: Level 1, Level 2, and Level 3. Each plan is twenty-four weeks long and includes a 5K tune-up race at the end of Week 12, a 10K tune-up race at the end of Week 16, and a half-marathon tune-up race at the end of Week 20, in addition to the marathon peak race at the end of Week 24.

The plans are divided into Base, Build 1, Build 2, and Peak phases. The Base phase is eight weeks long, the Build 1 and 2 phases last four weeks apiece, and the Peak phase lasts eight weeks. Weeks 4, 8, 12, 16, and 20 are reduced-volume recovery weeks, and Weeks 23 and 24 are reduced-volume taper weeks.

There are three key workouts per week in each plan: a speed workout on Wednesdays, an intensive endurance workout on Fridays, and an extensive endurance workout on Sundays. Key workouts are indicated by shaded boxes.

LEVEL 1

Use this plan if you are most comfortable with a marathon training plan that features four runs per week and a maximum run distance of 20 miles. The plan also includes one optional nonimpact cardio cross-training workout and two resistance workouts per week.

Base Phase

Training objectives: Build aerobic capacity and endurance, increase injury resistance, and increase muscle activation capacity

WEEK 1 ♦ Proprioceptive Cue: Falling Forward

MONDAY	Off	
TUESDAY	**Base Run + Drills** Run 3 miles @ base pace Running No Arms 20 seconds One-Leg Hop 20 seconds	
WEDNESDAY	**Hill Repetitions** Dynamic stretching warm-up 1.5-mile warm-up @ recovery pace 1 × 30-second hill repetition @ relaxed sprint speed 1.5-mile cool-down @ recovery pace	
THURSDAY	<u>Optional Nonimpact Cardio Cross-Training Workout</u> 20–30 minutes @ recovery pace (You may break this workout into a 10–15-minute warm-up before and a 10–15-minute cool-down after your resistance workout.)	**Resistance Workout** *1 set each* Lying Hip Abduction Cook Hip Lift Kneeling Overhead Draw-In Knee Fall-Out Squat Jump
FRIDAY	**Fartlek Run** Dynamic stretching warm-up Run 3 miles @ base pace w/2 × 30-second intervals @ 1-mile pace "sprinkled in"	

SATURDAY	**Resistance Workout**
	1 set each
	Lying Hip Abduction
	Cook Hip Lift
	Kneeling Overhead Draw-In
	Knee Fall-Out
	Broad Jump
SUNDAY	**Base Run**
	Run 4 miles @ base pace

WEEK 2 ◆ Proprioceptive Cue: Navel to Spine

MONDAY	Off
TUESDAY	**Base Run + Drills** Run 3.5 miles @ base pace High Knees 2 × 20 seconds Bounding 2 × 20 seconds
WEDNESDAY	**Hill Repetitions** Dynamic stretching warm-up 1.5-mile warm-up @ recovery pace 4 × 30-second hill repetitions @ relaxed sprint speed w/2-minute active recoveries 1.5-mile cool-down @ recovery pace

THURSDAY	Optional Nonimpact Cardio Cross-Training Workout 20–30 minutes @ recovery pace	**Resistance Workout** *2 sets each* Lying Hip Abduction Cook Hip Lift Kneeling Overhead Draw-In Knee Fall-Out Split Squat Jump

FRIDAY	**Fartlek Run** Dynamic stretching warm-up Run 3.5 miles @ base pace w/4 × 30-second intervals @ 1-mile pace "sprinkled in"
SATURDAY	**Resistance Workout** *2 sets each* Lying Hip Abduction Cook Hip Lift Kneeling Overhead Draw-In Knee Fall-Out Wall Jump
SUNDAY	**Base Run** Run 5 miles @ base pace

WEEK 3 ◆ Proprioceptive Cue: Running on Water

MONDAY	Off
TUESDAY	**Base Run + Drills** Run 4 miles @ base pace Stiff-Legged Run 2×20 seconds Running No Arms 2×20 seconds
WEDNESDAY	**Hill Repetitions** Dynamic stretching warm-up 1.5-mile warm-up @ recovery pace 5×45-second hill repetitions @ 1-mile pace w/2-minute active recoveries 1.5-mile cool-down @ recovery pace

THURSDAY	<u>Optional Nonimpact Cardio</u> <u>Cross-Training Workout</u> 20–30 minutes @ recovery pace	**Resistance Workout** *3 sets each* Lying Hip Abduction Cook Hip Lift Kneeling Overhead Draw-In Knee Fall-Out Squat Jump

FRIDAY	**Fartlek Run** Dynamic stretching warm-up Run 4 miles @ base pace w/5×45-second intervals @ 1-mile pace "sprinkled in"
SATURDAY	**Resistance Workout** *3 sets each* Lying Hip Abduction Cook Hip Lift Kneeling Overhead Draw-In Knee Fall-Out Broad Jump
SUNDAY	**Base Run** Run 6 miles @ base pace

WEEK 4 (Recovery) ◆ Proprioceptive Cue: Pulling the Road

MONDAY	Off
TUESDAY	**Base Run + Drills** Run 3 miles @ base pace One-Leg Hop 20 seconds High Knees 20 seconds
WEDNESDAY	**Hill Repetitions** Dynamic stretching warm-up 1.5-mile warm-up @ recovery pace 3 × 1-minute hill repetitions @ 1-mile pace w/2-minute active recoveries 1.5-mile cool-down @ recovery pace

THURSDAY	<u>Optional Nonimpact Cardio</u>
	<u>Cross-Training Workout</u>
	20–30 minutes @ recovery pace **Resistance Workout**
	    1 set each
	    Single-Leg Squat
	    Oblique Bridge
	    Lying Draw-In w/Hip Flexion
	    Quadruped
	
	    2 sets each
	    Lying Hip Abduction
	    Cook Hip Lift
	    Kneeling Overhead Draw-In
	    Knee Fall-Out
	    Single-Leg Squat Jump

FRIDAY	**Fartlek Run** Dynamic stretching warm-up Run 3 miles @ base pace w/3 × 1-minute intervals @ 1-mile pace "sprinkled in"
SATURDAY	**Resistance Workout** *1 set each* Single-Leg Squat Oblique Bridge Lying Draw-In w/Hip Flexion Quadruped

SATURDAY (continued)	**Resistance Workout** *2 sets each* Lying Hip Abduction Cook Hip Lift Kneeling Overhead Draw-In Knee Fall-Out Wall Jump
SUNDAY	**Base Run** Run 4 miles @ base pace

WEEK 5 ◆ Proprioceptive Cue: Scooting

MONDAY	Off
TUESDAY	**Base Run + Drills** Run 4.5 miles @ base pace High Knees 2×20 seconds Bounding 2×20 seconds
WEDNESDAY	**Hill Repetitions** Dynamic stretching warm-up 1-mile warm-up @ recovery pace 4×75-second hill repetitions @ 1-mile pace w/2-minute active recoveries 1-mile cool-down @ recovery pace

THURSDAY	<u>Optional Nonimpact Cardio</u> <u>Cross-Training Workout</u> 20–30 minutes @ recovery pace	**Resistance Workout** *2 sets each* Single-Leg Squat Oblique Bridge Lying Draw-In w/Hip Flexion Quadruped *1 set each* Lying Hip Abduction Cook Hip Lift Kneeling Overhead Draw-In Knee Fall-Out Single-Leg Squat Jump

FRIDAY	**Fartlek Run** Dynamic stretching warm-up Run 4.5 miles @ base pace w/4×75-second intervals @ 3,000m pace "sprinkled in"
SATURDAY	**Resistance Workout** *2 sets each* Single-Leg Squat Oblique Bridge Lying Draw-In w/Hip Flexion Quadruped

SATURDAY (continued)	**Resistance Workout** *1 set each* Lying Hip Abduction Cook Hip Lift Kneeling Overhead Draw-In Knee Fall-Out Wall Jump
SUNDAY	**Base Run** Run 7 miles @ base pace

WEEK 6 ♦ Proprioceptive Cue: Pounding the Ground

MONDAY	Off
TUESDAY	**Base Run + Drills** Run 5 miles @ base pace Stiff-Legged Run 2 × 20 seconds Running No Arms 2 × 20 seconds
WEDNESDAY	**Hill Repetitions** Dynamic stretching warm-up 1-mile warm-up @ recovery pace 5 × 90-second hill repetitions @ 1-mile pace w/2-minute active recoveries 1-mile cool-down @ recovery pace
THURSDAY	<u>Optional Nonimpact Cardio</u> <u>Cross-Training Workout</u> 20–30 minutes @ recovery pace	**Resistance Workout** *3 sets each* Single-Leg Squat Oblique Bridge Lying Draw-In w/Hip Flexion Quadruped *2 sets* Squat Jump
FRIDAY	**Fartlek Run** Dynamic stretching warm-up Run 4.5 miles @ base pace w/4 × 90-second intervals @ 3,000m pace "sprinkled in"
SATURDAY	**Resistance Workout** *3 sets each* Single-Leg Squat Oblique Bridge Lying Draw-In w/Hip Flexion Quadruped *2 sets* Single-Leg Squat Jump
SUNDAY	**Base Run** Run 8 miles @ base pace

WEEK 7 ◆ Proprioceptive Cue: Driving the Thigh

MONDAY	Off
TUESDAY	**Base Run + Drills** Run 6 miles @ base pace Steep Hill Sprints 2 × 20 seconds One-Leg Hop 2 × 20 seconds
WEDNESDAY	**Hill Repetitions** Dynamic stretching warm-up 1-mile warm-up @ recovery pace 4 × 2-minute hill repetitions @ 3,000m pace w/2-minute active recoveries 1-mile cool-down @ recovery pace
THURSDAY	<u>Optional Nonimpact Cardio</u> <u>Cross-Training Workout</u> 20–30 minutes @ recovery pace	**Resistance Workout** *2 sets each* Single-Leg Squat Oblique Bridge Lying Draw-In w/Hip Flexion Quadruped Split Squat Jump *1 set each* Box Lunge Stability Ball Leg Curl Forearms to Palms Bridge Dead Bug
FRIDAY	**Fartlek Run** Dynamic stretching warm-up Run 5 miles @ base pace w/4 × 2-minute intervals @ 3,000m pace "sprinkled in"
SATURDAY	**Resistance Workout** *2 sets each* Single-Leg Squat Oblique Bridge Lying Draw-In w/Hip Flexion Quadruped Single-Leg Box Jump

(continued)

WEEK 7 ◆ Proprioceptive Cue: Driving the Thigh
(continued)

SATURDAY (continued)	**Resistance Workout** *1 set each* Box Lunge Stability Ball Leg Curl Forearms to Palms Bridge Dead Bug
SUNDAY	**Base Run** Run 9 miles @ base pace

WEEK 8 (Recovery) ◆ Proprioceptive Cue: Floppy Feet

MONDAY	Off
TUESDAY	**Base Run + Drills** Run 4 miles @ base pace High Knees 20 seconds Bounding 20 seconds
WEDNESDAY	**Hill Repetitions** Dynamic stretching warm-up 1-mile warm-up @ recovery pace 3 × 2-minute hill repetitions @ 3,000m pace w/2-minute active recoveries 1-mile cool-down @ recovery pace
THURSDAY	<u>Optional Nonimpact Cardio</u> <u>Cross-Training Workout</u> 20–30 minutes @ recovery pace	**Resistance Workout** *1 set each* Single-Leg Squat Oblique Bridge Lying Draw-In w/Hip Flexion Quadruped *2 sets each* Box Lunge Stability Ball Leg Curl Forearms to Palms Bridge Dead Bug Broad Jump
FRIDAY	**Fartlek Run** Dynamic stretching warm-up Run 4 miles @ base pace w/4 × 2-minute intervals @ 3,000m pace "sprinkled in"
SATURDAY	**Resistance Workout** *1 set each* Single-Leg Squat Oblique Bridge Lying Draw-In w/Hip Flexion Quadruped

(continued)

WEEK 8 (Recovery) ◆ Proprioceptive Cue: Floppy Feet
(continued)

SATURDAY (continued)	**Resistance Workout** *2 sets each* Box Lunge Stability Ball Leg Curl Forearms to Palms Bridge Dead Bug Wall Jump
SUNDAY	**Base Run** Run 6 miles @ base pace

Build 1 Phase

Training objectives: Continue to increase aerobic capacity and endurance; increase fatigue resistance at 3,000m pace and 10K pace

WEEK 9 ◆ Proprioceptive Cue: Butt Squeeze

MONDAY	Off
TUESDAY	**Base Run + Drills** Run 6 miles @ base pace Stiff-Legged Run 2×20 seconds Running No Arms 2×20 seconds
WEDNESDAY	**400m Intervals @ 3,000m Pace** Dynamic stretching warm-up 1-mile warm-up @ recovery pace 6×400m @ 3,000m pace w/3-minute active recoveries 1-mile cool-down @ recovery pace

THURSDAY	Optional Nonimpact Cardio Cross-Training Workout 20–30 minutes @ recovery pace	**Resistance Workout** *3 sets each* Box Lunge Stability Ball Leg Curl Forearms to Palms Bridge Dead Bug Wall Jump

FRIDAY	**1-Mile Intervals @ 10K Pace** Dynamic stretching warm-up 1-mile warm-up @ recovery pace 2×1 mile @ 10K pace w/2-minute active recovery 1-mile cool-down @ recovery pace
SATURDAY	**Resistance Workout** *3 sets each* Box Lunge Stability Ball Leg Curl

(continued)

WEEK 9 ◆ Proprioceptive Cue: Butt Squeeze
(continued)

SATURDAY (continued)	**Resistance Workout** *3 sets each (cont.)* Forearms to Palms Bridge Dead Bug Single-Leg Box Jump
SUNDAY	**Endurance Run** Run 10 miles @ base pace

WEEK 10 ◆ Proprioceptive Cue: Feeling Symmetry

MONDAY	Off
TUESDAY	**Base Run + Drills** Run 6 miles @ base pace Stiff-Legged Run 2×20 seconds Running No Arms 2×20 seconds
WEDNESDAY	**400m Intervals @ 3,000m Pace** Dynamic stretching warm-up 1-mile warm-up @ recovery pace 7×400m @ 3,000m pace w/3-minute active recoveries 1-mile cool-down @ recovery pace

THURSDAY	Optional Nonimpact Cardio Cross-Training Workout 20–30 minutes @ recovery pace	**Resistance Workout** *1 set each* Lying Hip Abduction Single-Leg Squat Box Lunge Stability Ball Leg Curl Squat Jump

FRIDAY	**1-Mile Intervals @ 10K Pace** Dynamic stretching warm-up 1-mile warm-up @ recovery pace 3×1 mile @ 10K pace w/2-minute active recoveries 1-mile cool-down @ recovery pace
SATURDAY	**Resistance Workout** *1 set each* Cook Hip Lift Oblique Bridge Forearms to Palms Bridge Stability Ball Leg Curl Split Squat Jump
SUNDAY	**Endurance Run** Run 11 miles @ base pace

WEEK 11 ◆ Proprioceptive Cue: Axle Between the Knees

MONDAY	Off
TUESDAY	**Base Run + Drills** Run 6 miles @ base pace Steep Hill Sprints 2 × 20 seconds One-Leg Hop 2 × 20 seconds
WEDNESDAY	**400m Intervals @ 3,000m Pace** Dynamic stretching warm-up 1-mile warm-up @ recovery pace 8 × 400m @ 3,000m pace w/3-minute active recoveries 1-mile cool-down @ recovery pace

THURSDAY	<u>Optional Nonimpact Cardio</u>
	<u>Cross-Training Workout</u>
	20–30 minutes @ recovery pace **Resistance Workout**
	   1 set each
	   Lying Hip Abduction
	   Single-Leg Squat
	   Box Lunge
	   Stability Ball Leg Curl
	   Single-Leg Squat Jump

FRIDAY	**1-Mile Intervals @ 10K Pace** Dynamic stretching warm-up 1-mile warm-up @ recovery pace 4 × 1 mile @ 10K pace w/2-minute active recoveries 1-mile cool-down @ recovery pace
SATURDAY	**Resistance Workout** *1 set each* Cook Hip Lift Oblique Bridge Forearms to Palms Bridge Stability Ball Leg Curl Broad Jump
SUNDAY	**Endurance Run** Run 12 miles @ base pace

WEEK 12 (Recovery) ◆ Proprioceptive Cue: Running Against a Wall

MONDAY	Off

TUESDAY	**Base Run + Drills**
	    Run 4.5 miles @ base pace
	    High Knees 20 seconds
	    Bounding 20 seconds

WEDNESDAY	**400m Intervals @ 3,000m Pace**
	    Dynamic stretching warm-up
	    1-mile warm-up @ recovery pace
	    6 × 400m @ 3,000m pace w/3-minute active recoveries
	    1-mile cool-down @ recovery pace

THURSDAY	<u>Optional Nonimpact Cardio</u>
	<u>Cross-Training Workout</u>
	20–30 minutes @ recovery pace **Resistance Workout**
	    1 set each
	    Lying Hip Abduction
	    Single-Leg Squat
	    Box Lunge
	    Stability Ball Leg Curl
	    Wall Jump

FRIDAY	**1-Mile Intervals @ 10K Pace**
	    Dynamic stretching warm-up
	    1-mile warm-up @ recovery pace
	    3 × 1 mile @ 10K pace w/2-minute active recoveries
	    1-mile cool-down @ recovery pace

SATURDAY	**Resistance Workout**
	    1 set each
	    Cook Hip Lift
	    Oblique Bridge
	    Forearms to Palms Bridge
	    Stability Ball Leg Curl

SUNDAY	**5K Tune-up Race or Time Trial**
	    Dynamic stretching warm-up
	    1-mile warm-up @ recovery pace
	    5K tune-up race or time trial
	    1-mile cool-down @ recovery pace

Build 2

Training objectives: Continue to build endurance; increase fatigue resistance at 5K pace and 10K pace; build efficiency at half-marathon pace and marathon pace

WEEK 13 ◆ Proprioceptive Cue: Falling Forward

MONDAY	Off	
TUESDAY	**Base Run + Drills** Run 7 miles @ base pace High Knees 2×20 seconds Bounding 2×20 seconds	
WEDNESDAY	**1K Intervals @ 5K Pace** Dynamic stretching warm-up 1-mile warm-up @ recovery pace 3×1K @ 5K pace w/3-minute active recoveries 1-mile cool-down @ recovery pace	
THURSDAY	Optional Nonimpact Cardio Cross-Training Workout 20–30 minutes @ recovery pace	**Resistance Workout** *1 set each* Lying Hip Abduction Single-Leg Squat Box Lunge Stability Ball Leg Curl Wall Jump
FRIDAY	**Tempo Run @ 10K Pace** 1-mile warm-up @ recovery pace 3 miles @ 10K pace 1-mile cool-down @ recovery pace	
SATURDAY	**Resistance Workout** *1 set each* Cook Hip Lift Oblique Bridge Forearms to Palms Bridge Stability Ball Leg Curl Single-Leg Box Jump	

SUNDAY	**Progression Run**
	Run 12 miles
	Run first 6 miles @ base pace, then gradually increase pace every mile; run last mile @ half-marathon pace

WEEK 14 ◆ Proprioceptive Cue: Navel to Spine

MONDAY	Off
TUESDAY	**Base Run + Drills** Run 7 miles @ base pace Stiff-Legged Run 2×20 seconds Running No Arms 2×20 seconds
WEDNESDAY	**1K Intervals @ 5K Pace** Dynamic stretching warm-up 1-mile warm-up @ recovery pace 4×1K intervals @ 5K pace w/3-minute active recoveries 1-mile cool-down @ recovery pace
THURSDAY	Optional Nonimpact Cardio Cross-Training Workout 20–30 minutes @ recovery pace	**Resistance Workout** *1 set each* Lying Hip Abduction Single-Leg Squat Box Lunge Stability Ball Leg Curl Squat Jump
FRIDAY	**Tempo Run @ 10K Pace** Dynamic stretching warm-up 1-mile warm-up @ recovery pace 4 miles @ 10K pace 1-mile cool-down @ recovery pace
SATURDAY	**Resistance Workout** *1 set each* Cook Hip Lift Oblique Bridge Forearms to Palms Bridge Stability Ball Leg Curl Split Squat Jump
SUNDAY	**Endurance Run** Run 14 miles @ base pace

WEEK 15 ◆ Proprioceptive Cue: Running on Water

MONDAY	Off
TUESDAY	**Base Run + Drills** Run 7 miles @ base pace Steep Hill Sprints 20 seconds One-Leg Hop 20 seconds
WEDNESDAY	**1K Intervals @ 5K Pace** Dynamic stretching warm-up 1-mile warm-up @ recovery pace 4 × 1K intervals @ 5K pace w/3-minute active recoveries 1-mile cool-down @ recovery pace
THURSDAY	Optional Nonimpact Cardio Cross-Training Workout 20–30 minutes @ recovery pace **Resistance Workout** *1 set each* Lying Hip Abduction Single-Leg Squat Box Lunge Stability Ball Leg Curl Single-Leg Squat Jump
FRIDAY	**Tempo Run @ 10K Pace** Dynamic stretching warm-up 1-mile warm-up @ recovery pace 4.5 miles @ 10K pace 1-mile cool-down @ recovery pace
SATURDAY	**Resistance Workout** *1 set each* Cook Hip Lift Oblique Bridge Forearms to Palms Bridge Stability Ball Leg Curl Broad Jump
SUNDAY	**Progression Run** Run 13 miles Run first 7 miles @ base pace, then gradually increase pace every mile; run last mile @ half-marathon pace

WEEK 16 (Recovery) ◆ Proprioceptive Cue: Pulling the Road

MONDAY	Off
TUESDAY	**Base Run + Drills** 　Run 5 miles @ base pace 　Stiff-Legged Run 2×20 seconds 　Running No Arms 2×20 seconds
WEDNESDAY	**1K Intervals @ 5K Pace** 　Dynamic stretching warm-up 　1-mile warm-up @ recovery pace 　3×1K intervals @ 5K pace w/3-minute active recoveries 　1-mile cool-down @ recovery pace

THURSDAY	<u>Optional Nonimpact Cardio</u> <u>Cross-Training Workout</u> 20–30 minutes @ recovery pace	**Resistance Workout** *1 set each* Lying Hip Abduction Single-Leg Squat Box Lunge Stability Ball Leg Curl Squat Jump

FRIDAY	**Tempo Run @ 10K Pace** 　Dynamic stretching warm-up 　1-mile warm-up @ recovery pace 　3.5 miles @ 10K pace 　1-mile cool-down @ recovery pace
SATURDAY	**Resistance Workout** 　*1 set each* 　Cook Hip Lift 　Oblique Bridge 　Forearms to Palms Bridge 　Stability Ball Leg Curl 　Split Squat Jump
SUNDAY	**10K Tune-up Race or Time Trial** 　Dynamic stretching warm-up 　1-mile warm-up @ recovery pace 　10K tune-up race or time trial 　1-mile cool-down @ recovery pace

Peak Phase

Training objectives: Achieve peak fatigue resistance and efficiency at marathon pace; adapt and recover for peak race day

WEEK 17 ◆ Proprioceptive Cue: Scooting

MONDAY	Off
TUESDAY	**Base Run + Drills** Run 8 miles @ base pace Stiff-Legged Run 2 × 20 seconds Running No Arms 2 × 20 seconds
WEDNESDAY	**Mixed Intervals** Dynamic stretching warm-up 1-mile warm-up @ recovery pace 1 × 2K @ half-marathon pace, 2-minute active recovery 1 × 1 mile @ 10K pace, 2-minute active recovery 1 × 1K @ 5K pace, 2-minute active recovery 1 × 800m @ 3,000m pace 1-mile cool-down @ recovery pace
THURSDAY	Optional Nonimpact Cardio Cross-Training Workout 20–30 minutes @ recovery pace || **Resistance Workout** *1 set each* Lying Hip Abduction Single-Leg Squat Box Lunge Stability Ball Leg Curl Squat Jump
FRIDAY	**Tempo Run @ Half-Marathon Pace** 1-mile warm-up @ recovery pace 5 miles @ half-marathon pace 1-mile cool-down @ recovery pace

(continued)

WEEK 17 ◆ Proprioceptive Cue: Scooting
(continued)

SATURDAY	**Resistance Workout** *1 set each* Cook Hip Lift Oblique Bridge Forearms to Palms Bridge Stability Ball Leg Curl Split Squat Jump
SUNDAY	**Endurance Run** Run 16 miles @ base pace

WEEK 18 ◆ Proprioceptive Cue: Pounding the Ground

MONDAY	Off
TUESDAY	**Base Run + Drills** Run 8 miles @ base pace Stiff-Legged Run 2×20 seconds Running No Arms 2×20 seconds
WEDNESDAY	**Mixed Intervals** Dynamic stretching warm-up 1-mile warm-up @ recovery pace 1×3K @ half-marathon pace, 2-minute active recovery 1×1 mile @ 10K pace, 2-minute active recovery 1×1K @ 5K pace, 2-minute active recovery 1×800m @ 3,000m pace 1-mile cool-down @ recovery pace

THURSDAY	Optional Nonimpact Cardio Cross-Training Workout 20–30 minutes @ recovery pace	**Resistance Workout** *1 set each* Lying Hip Abduction Single-Leg Squat Box Lunge Stability Ball Leg Curl Squat Jump

FRIDAY	**Tempo Run @ Half-Marathon Pace** 1-mile warm-up @ recovery pace 6 miles @ half-marathon pace 1-mile cool-down @ recovery pace
SATURDAY	**Resistance Workout** *1 set each* Cook Hip Lift Oblique Bridge Quadruped Dead Bug Single-Leg Squat Jump
SUNDAY	**Marathon-Pace Run** 1-mile warm-up @ recovery pace 8 miles @ marathon pace 1-mile cool-down @ recovery pace

WEEK 19 ◆ Proprioceptive Cue: Driving the Thigh

MONDAY	Off
TUESDAY	**Base Run + Drills** Run 8 miles @ base pace Steep Hill Sprints 2 × 20 seconds One-Leg Hop 2 × 20 seconds
WEDNESDAY	**Mixed Intervals** Dynamic stretching warm-up 1-mile warm-up @ recovery pace 1 × 3K @ half-marathon pace, 2-minute active recovery 1 × 2K @ 10K pace, 2-minute active recovery 1 × 1K @ 5K pace, 2-minute active recovery 1 × 800m @ 3,000m pace 1-mile cool-down @ recovery pace

THURSDAY	Optional Nonimpact Cardio Cross-Training Workout 20–30 minutes @ recovery pace	**Resistance Workout** *1 set each* Kneeling Overhead Draw-In Lying Draw-In w/Hip Flexion Box Lunge Stability Ball Leg Curl Broad Jump

FRIDAY	**Tempo Run @ Half-Marathon Pace** 1-mile warm-up @ recovery pace 7 miles @ half-marathon pace 1-mile cool-down @ recovery pace
SATURDAY	**Resistance Workout** *1 set each* Cook Hip Lift Oblique Bridge Quadruped Dead Bug Single-Leg Squat Jump
SUNDAY	**Endurance Run** Run 18 miles @ base pace

WEEK 20 (Recovery) ◆ Proprioceptive Cue: Floppy Feet

MONDAY	Off
TUESDAY	**Base Run + Drills** Run 6 miles @ base pace High Knees 20 seconds Bounding 20 seconds
WEDNESDAY	**Mixed Intervals** Dynamic stretching warm-up 1-mile warm-up @ recovery pace 1×2K @ half-marathon pace, 2-minute active recovery 1×1 mile @ 10K pace, 2-minute active recovery 1×1K @ 5K pace, 2-minute active recovery 1×800m @ 3,000m pace 1-mile cool-down @ recovery pace

THURSDAY	<u>Optional Nonimpact Cardio</u>
	<u>Cross-Training Workout</u>
	20–30 minutes @ recovery pace **Resistance Workout**
	   1 set each
	   Kneeling Overhead Draw-In
	   Lying Draw-In w/Hip Flexion
	   Box Lunge
	   Stability Ball Leg Curl
	   Squat Jump

FRIDAY	**Tempo Run @ Half-Marathon Pace** 1-mile warm-up @ recovery pace 5 miles @ half-marathon pace 1-mile cool-down @ recovery pace
SATURDAY	**Resistance Workout** *1 set each* Knee Fall-Out Oblique Bridge Quadruped Dead Bug Split Squat Jump
SUNDAY	**Half-Marathon Tune-up Race or Time Trial** 1-mile warm-up @ recovery pace Half-marathon tune-up race or time trial 1-mile cool-down @ recovery pace

WEEK 21   ◆   Proprioceptive Cue: Butt Squeeze

MONDAY	Off
TUESDAY	**Base Run + Drills** Run 9 miles @ base pace Stiff-Legged Run 2 × 20 seconds Running No Arms 2 × 20 seconds
WEDNESDAY	**Mixed Intervals** Dynamic stretching warm-up 1-mile warm-up @ recovery pace 1 × 3K @ half-marathon pace, 2-minute active recovery 1 × 2K @ 10K pace, 2-minute active recovery 1 × 1K @ 5K pace, 2-minute active recovery 1 × 800m @ 3,000m pace 1-mile cool-down @ recovery pace

THURSDAY	<u>Optional Nonimpact Cardio</u> <u>Cross-Training Workout</u> 20–30 minutes @ recovery pace	**Resistance Workout** *1 set each* Lying Hip Abduction Single-Leg Squat Box Lunge Stability Ball Leg Curl Single-Leg Squat Jump

FRIDAY	**Tempo Run @ Half-Marathon Pace** 2-mile warm-up @ recovery pace 7 miles @ half-marathon pace 2-mile cool-down @ recovery pace
SATURDAY	**Resistance Workout** *1 set each* Cook Hip Lift Oblique Bridge Quadruped Dead Bug Broad Jump
SUNDAY	**Endurance Run** Run 20 miles @ base pace

WEEK 22 ◆ Proprioceptive Cue: Feeling Symmetry

MONDAY	Off
TUESDAY	**Base Run + Drills** Run 9 miles @ base pace Steep Hill Sprints 2 × 20 seconds One-Leg Hop 2 × 20 seconds
WEDNESDAY	**Mixed Intervals** Dynamic stretching warm-up 1-mile warm-up @ recovery pace 1 × 3K @ half-marathon pace, 90-second active recovery 1 × 2K @ 10K pace, 90-second active recovery 1 × 1K @ 5K pace, 90-second active recovery 1 × 800 m @ 3,000m pace 1-mile cool-down @ recovery pace

THURSDAY	<u>Optional Nonimpact Cardio</u> <u>Cross-Training Workout</u> 20–30 minutes @ recovery pace	**Resistance Workout** *1 set each* Kneeling Overhead Draw-In Lying Draw-In w/Hip Flexion Box Lunge Stability Ball Leg Curl Wall Jump

FRIDAY	**Tempo Run @ Half-Marathon Pace** 2-mile warm-up @ recovery pace 8 miles @ half-marathon pace 2-mile cool-down @ recovery pace
SATURDAY	**Resistance Workout** *1 set each* Knee Fall-Out Oblique Bridge Quadruped Dead Bug Single-Leg Box Jump
SUNDAY	**Marathon-Pace Run** 2-mile warm-up @ recovery pace 10 miles @ marathon pace 2-mile cool-down @ recovery pace

WEEK 23 (Taper) ◆ Proprioceptive Cue: Axle Between the Knees

MONDAY	Off	
TUESDAY	**Base Run + Drills** Run 7 miles @ base pace High Knees 2 × 20 seconds Bounding 2 × 20 seconds	
WEDNESDAY	**Mixed Intervals** Dynamic stretching warm-up 1-mile warm-up @ recovery pace 1 × 2K @ half-marathon pace, 90-second active recovery 1 × 1 mile @ 10K pace, 90-second active recovery 1 × 1K @ 5K pace, 90-second active recovery 1 × 800 m @ 3,000m pace 1-mile cool-down @ recovery pace	
THURSDAY	Optional Nonimpact Cardio Cross-Training Workout 20–30 minutes @ recovery pace	**Resistance Workout** *1 set each* Lying Hip Abduction Single-Leg Squat Box Lunge Stability Ball Leg Curl Squat Jump
FRIDAY	**Tempo Run @ Half-Marathon Pace** 1-mile warm-up @ recovery pace 7 miles @ half-marathon pace 1-mile cool-down @ recovery pace	
SATURDAY	**Resistance Workout** *1 set each* Cook Hip Lift Oblique Bridge Quadruped Dead Bug Split Squat Jump	
SUNDAY	**Endurance Run** Run 12 miles @ base pace	

WEEK 24 (Taper) ◆ Proprioceptive Cue: Your Choice

MONDAY	Off
TUESDAY	**Base Run + Drills** Run 6 miles @ base pace Stiff-Legged Run 20 seconds Running No Arms 20 seconds
WEDNESDAY	**Mixed Intervals** Dynamic stretching warm-up 1-mile warm-up @ recovery pace 1×2K @ half-marathon pace, 90-second active recovery 1×1 mile @ 10K pace, 90-second active recovery 1×1K @ 5K pace, 90-second active recovery 1-mile cool-down @ recovery pace
THURSDAY	**Resistance Workout** *1 set each* Kneeling Overhead Draw-In Lying Draw-In w/Hip Flexion Box Lunge Stability Ball Leg Curl
FRIDAY	**Tempo Run @ Half-Marathon Pace** 1-mile warm-up @ recovery pace 2 miles @ half-marathon pace 1-mile cool-down @ recovery pace
SATURDAY	Off
SUNDAY	**Marathon Peak Race** Marathon

LEVEL 2

Use this plan if you are most comfortable with a marathon training plan that features six runs per week and a maximum run distance of 22 miles. The plan also contains one optional nonimpact cardio cross-training workout and two resistance workouts per week.

Base Phase

Training objectives: Build aerobic capacity and endurance, increase injury resistance, and increase muscle activation capacity

WEEK 1 ♦ Proprioceptive Cue: Falling Forward

MONDAY	Off	
TUESDAY	**Base Run + Drills** Run 4 miles @ base pace Running No Arms 20 seconds One-Leg Hop 20 seconds	
WEDNESDAY	**Hill Repetitions** Dynamic stretching warm-up 2-mile warm-up @ recovery pace 2 × 30-second hill repetitions @ relaxed sprint speed w/2-minute active recoveries 2-mile cool-down @ recovery pace	
THURSDAY	**Base Run** Run 4 miles @ base pace *or* Nonimpact Cardio Cross-Training Workout 20–30 minutes @ recovery pace	**Resistance Workout** *1 set each* Lying Hip Abduction Cook Hip Lift Kneeling Overhead Draw-In Knee Fall-Out Squat Jump
FRIDAY	**Fartlek Run** Dynamic stretching warm-up Run 4 miles @ base pace w/2 × 30-second intervals @ 1-mile pace "sprinkled in"	

SATURDAY	**Base Run** Run 4 miles @ base pace	**Resistance Workout** *1 set each* Lying Hip Abduction Cook Hip Lift Kneeling Overhead Draw-In Knee Fall-Out Broad Jump
SUNDAY	**Base Run** Run 5 miles @ base pace	

WEEK 2 ♦ Proprioceptive Cue: Navel to Spine

MONDAY	Off	
TUESDAY	**Base Run + Drills** Run 4.5 miles @ base pace High Knees 2 × 20 seconds Bounding 2 × 20 seconds	
WEDNESDAY	**Hill Repetitions** Dynamic stretching warm-up 2-mile warm-up @ recovery pace 4 × 30-second hill repetitions @ relaxed sprint speed w/2-minute active recoveries 2-mile cool-down @ recovery pace	
THURSDAY	**Base Run** Run 4.5 miles @ base pace *or* <u>Nonimpact Cardio Cross-Training</u> <u>Workout</u> 25–35 minutes @ recovery pace	**Resistance Workout** *2 sets each* Lying Hip Abduction Cook Hip Lift Kneeling Overhead Draw-In Knee Fall-Out Split Squat Jump
FRIDAY	**Fartlek Run** Dynamic stretching warm-up Run 4.5 miles @ base pace w/4 × 30-second intervals @ 1-mile pace "sprinkled in"	
SATURDAY	**Base Run** Run 4.5 miles @ base pace	**Resistance Workout** *2 sets each* Lying Hip Abduction Cook Hip Lift Kneeling Overhead Draw-In Knee Fall-Out Wall Jump
SUNDAY	**Base Run** Run 6 miles @ base pace	

WEEK 3 ♦ Proprioceptive Cue: Running on Water

MONDAY	Off
TUESDAY	**Base Run + Drills** Run 5 miles @ base pace Stiff-Legged Run 2 × 20 seconds Running No Arms 2 × 20 seconds
WEDNESDAY	**Hill Repetitions** Dynamic stretching warm-up 2-mile warm-up @ recovery pace 6 × 45-second hill repetitions @ 1-mile pace w/2-minute active recoveries 2-mile cool-down @ recovery pace

THURSDAY	**Base Run** Run 5 miles @ base pace *or* <u>Nonimpact Cardio Cross-Training Workout</u> 30–40 minutes @ recovery pace	**Resistance Workout** *3 sets each* Lying Hip Abduction Cook Hip Lift Kneeling Overhead Draw-In Knee Fall-Out Squat Jump

FRIDAY	**Fartlek Run** Dynamic stretching warm-up Run 5 miles @ base pace w/6 × 45-second intervals @ 1-mile pace "sprinkled in"

SATURDAY	**Base Run** Run 5 miles @ base pace	**Resistance Workout** *3 sets each* Lying Hip Abduction Cook Hip Lift Kneeling Overhead Draw-In Knee Fall-Out Broad Jump

SUNDAY	**Base Run** Run 8 miles @ base pace

WEEK 4 (Recovery) ◆ Proprioceptive Cue: Pulling the Road

MONDAY	Off	
TUESDAY	**Base Run + Drills** Run 4 miles @ base pace One-Leg Hop 20 seconds High Knees 20 seconds	
WEDNESDAY	**Hill Repetitions** Dynamic stretching warm-up 2-mile warm-up @ recovery pace 4 × 1-minute hill repetitions @ 1-mile pace w/2-minute active recoveries 2-mile cool-down @ recovery pace	
THURSDAY	**Base Run** Run 4 miles @ base pace *or* <u>Nonimpact Cardio Cross-Training Workout</u> 25–35 minutes @ recovery pace	**Resistance Workout** *1 set each* Single-Leg Squat Oblique Bridge Lying Draw-In w/Hip Flexion Quadruped *2 sets each* Lying Hip Abduction Cook Hip Lift Kneeling Overhead Draw-In Knee Fall-Out Single-Leg Squat Jump
FRIDAY	**Fartlek Run** Dynamic stretching warm-up Run 4 miles @ base pace w/4 × 1-minute intervals @ 1-mile pace "sprinkled in"	
SATURDAY	**Base Run** Run 4 miles @ base pace	**Resistance Workout** *1 set each* Single-Leg Squat Oblique Bridge Lying Draw-In w/Hip Flexion Quadruped

SATURDAY (continued)	Base Run	Resistance Workout *2 sets each* Lying Hip Abduction Cook Hip Lift Kneeling Overhead Draw-In Knee Fall-Out Wall Jump
SUNDAY	**Base Run** Run 6 miles @ base pace	

WEEK 5 ◆ Proprioceptive Cue: Scooting

MONDAY	Off	
TUESDAY	**Base Run + Drills** Run 5.5 miles @ base pace High Knees 2×20 seconds Bounding 2×20 seconds	
WEDNESDAY	**Hill Repetitions** Dynamic stretching warm-up 1.5-mile warm-up @ recovery pace 6×75-second hill repetitions @ 1-mile pace w/2-minute active recoveries 1.5-mile cool-down @ recovery pace	
THURSDAY	**Base Run** Run 5.5 miles @ base pace *or* Nonimpact Cardio Cross-Training Workout 35–45 minutes @ recovery pace	**Resistance Workout** *2 sets each* Single-Leg Squat Oblique Bridge Lying Draw-In w/Hip Flexion Quadruped *1 set each* Lying Hip Abduction Cook Hip Lift Kneeling Overhead Draw-In Knee Fall-Out Single-Leg Squat Jump
FRIDAY	**Fartlek Run** Dynamic stretching warm-up Run 5.5 miles @ base pace w/6×75-second intervals @ 3,000m pace "sprinkled in"	
SATURDAY	**Base Run** Run 5.5 miles @ base pace	**Resistance Workout** *2 sets each* Single-Leg Squat Oblique Bridge Lying Draw-In w/Hip Flexion Quadruped

SATURDAY (continued)	**Base Run**	**Resistance Workout** *1 set each* Lying Hip Abduction Cook Hip Lift Kneeling Overhead Draw-In Knee Fall-Out Wall Jump
SUNDAY	**Base Run** Run 9 miles @ base pace	

WEEK 6 ◆ Proprioceptive Cue: Pounding the Ground

MONDAY	Off
TUESDAY	**Base Run + Drills** Run 6 miles @ base pace Stiff-Legged Run 2×20 seconds Running No Arms 2×20 seconds
WEDNESDAY	**Hill Repetitions** Dynamic stretching warm-up 1.5-mile warm-up @ recovery pace 6×90-second hill repetitions @ 1-mile pace w/2-minute active recoveries 1.5-mile cool-down @ recovery pace

THURSDAY	**Base Run** Run 6 miles @ base pace *or* <u>Nonimpact Cardio Cross-Training Workout</u> 40–50 minutes @ recovery pace	**Resistance Workout** *3 sets each* Single-Leg Squat Oblique Bridge Lying Draw-In w/Hip Flexion Quadruped *2 sets* Squat Jump

FRIDAY	**Fartlek Run** Dynamic stretching warm-up Run 6 miles @ base pace w/6×90-second intervals @ 3,000m pace "sprinkled in"

SATURDAY	**Base Run** Run 6 miles @ base pace	**Resistance Workout** *3 sets each* Single-Leg Squat Oblique Bridge Lying Draw-In w/Hip Flexion Quadruped *2 sets* Single-Leg Squat Jump

SUNDAY	**Endurance Run** Run 10 miles @ base pace

WEEK 7 ◆ Proprioceptive Cue: Driving the Thigh

MONDAY	Off
TUESDAY	**Base Run + Drills** Run 6 miles @ base pace Steep Hill Sprints 2×20 seconds One-Leg Hop 2×20 seconds
WEDNESDAY	**Hill Repetitions** Dynamic stretching warm-up 1.5-mile warm-up @ recovery pace 6×2-minute hill repetitions @ 3,000m pace w/2-minute active recoveries 1.5-mile cool-down @ recovery pace

THURSDAY	**Base Run** Run 6 miles @ base pace *or* <u>Nonimpact Cardio Cross-Training</u> <u>Workout</u> 40–50 minutes @ recovery pace	**Resistance Workout** *2 sets each* Single-Leg Squat Oblique Bridge Lying Draw-In w/Hip Flexion Quadruped Split Squat Jump *1 set each* Box Lunge Stability Ball Leg Curl Forearms to Palms Bridge Dead Bug

FRIDAY	**Fartlek Run** Dynamic stretching warm-up Run 6 miles @ base pace w/6×2-minute intervals @ 3,000m pace "sprinkled in"

SATURDAY	**Base Run** Run 6 miles @ base pace	**Resistance Workout** *2 sets each* Single-Leg Squat Oblique Bridge Lying Draw-In w/Hip Flexion Quadruped Single-Leg Box Jump

(continued)

WEEK 7 ♦ Proprioceptive Cue: Driving the Thigh
(continued)

SATURDAY (continued)	Base Run	Resistance Workout *1 set each* Box Lunge Stability Ball Leg Curl Forearms to Palms Bridge Dead Bug
SUNDAY	**Endurance Run** Run 11 miles @ base pace	

WEEK 8 (Recovery) ♦ Proprioceptive Cue: Floppy Feet

MONDAY	Off
TUESDAY	**Base Run + Drills** Run 5 miles @ base pace High Knees 20 seconds Bounding 20 seconds
WEDNESDAY	**Hill Repetitions** Dynamic stretching warm-up 1.5-mile warm-up @ recovery pace 4 × 2-minute hill repetitions @ 3,000 m pace w/2-minute active recoveries 1.5-mile cool-down @ recovery pace

THURSDAY	**Base Run** Run 6 miles @ base pace *or* <u>Nonimpact Cardio Cross-Training</u> <u>Workout</u> 40–50 minutes @ recovery pace	**Resistance Workout** *1 set each* Single-Leg Squat Oblique Bridge Lying Draw-In w/Hip Flexion Quadruped *2 sets each* Box Lunge Stability Ball Leg Curl Forearms to Palms Bridge Dead Bug Broad Jump
FRIDAY	**Fartlek Run** Dynamic stretching warm-up Run 5 miles @ base pace w/4 × 2-minute intervals @ 3,000m pace "sprinkled in"	
SATURDAY	**Base Run** Run 6 miles @ base pace	**Resistance Workout** *1 set each* Single-Leg Squat Oblique Bridge Lying Draw-In w/Hip Flexion Quadruped

(continued)

WEEK 8 (Recovery) ◆ Proprioceptive Cue: Floppy Feet
(continued)

SATURDAY (continued)	Base Run	Resistance Workout *2 sets each* Box Lunge Stability Ball Leg Curl Forearms to Palms Bridge Dead Bug Wall Jump
SUNDAY	**Base Run** Run 8 miles @ base pace	

Build 1 Phase

Training objectives: Continue to increase aerobic capacity and endurance; increase fatigue resistance at 3,000m pace and 10K pace

WEEK 9 ◆ Proprioceptive Cue: Butt Squeeze

MONDAY	Off	
TUESDAY	**Base Run + Drills** Run 7 miles @ base pace Stiff-Legged Run 2 × 20 seconds Running No Arms 2 × 20 seconds	
WEDNESDAY	**400m Intervals @ 3,000m Pace** Dynamic stretching warm-up 1.5-mile warm-up @ recovery pace 8 × 400 m @ 3,000m pace w/3-minute active recoveries 1.5-mile cool-down @ recovery pace	
THURSDAY	**Recovery Run** 2–6 miles @ recovery pace *or* <u>Nonimpact Cardio Cross-Training Workout</u> 20–50 minutes @ recovery pace	**Resistance Workout** *3 sets each* Box Lunge Stability Ball Leg Curl Forearms to Palms Bridge Dead Bug Wall Jump
FRIDAY	**1-Mile Intervals @ 10K Pace** Dynamic stretching warm-up 1.5-mile warm-up @ recovery pace 2 × 1 mile @ 10K pace w/2-minute active recoveries 1.5-mile recovery-pace cool-down	
SATURDAY	**Recovery Run** 2–6 miles @ recovery pace	**Resistance Workout** *3 sets each* Box Lunge Stability Ball Leg Curl Forearms to Palms Bridge Dead Bug Single-Leg Box Jump
SUNDAY	**Endurance Run** Run 12 miles @ base pace	

WEEK 10 ♦ Proprioceptive Cue: Feeling Symmetry

MONDAY	Off
TUESDAY	**Base Run + Drills** Run 7 miles @ base pace Stiff-Legged Run 2 × 20 seconds Running No Arms 2 × 20 seconds
WEDNESDAY	**400m Intervals @ 3,000m Pace** Dynamic stretching warm-up 1.5-mile warm-up @ recovery pace 10 × 400m @ 3,000m pace w/3-minute active recoveries 1.5-mile cool-down @ recovery pace

THURSDAY	**Recovery Run** 2–6 miles @ recovery pace *or* Nonimpact Cardio Cross-Training Workout 20–50 minutes @ recovery pace	**Resistance Workout** *2 sets each* Lying Hip Abduction Single-Leg Squat Box Lunge Stability Ball Leg Curl Squat Jump

FRIDAY	**1-Mile Intervals @ 10K Pace** Dynamic stretching warm-up 1.5-mile warm-up @ recovery pace 3 × 1 mile @ 10K pace w/2-minute active recoveries 1.5-mile recovery-pace cool-down

SATURDAY	**Recovery Run** 2–6 miles @ recovery pace	**Resistance Workout** *2 sets each* Cook Hip Lift Oblique Bridge Forearms to Palms Bridge Stability Ball Leg Curl Split Squat Jump

SUNDAY	**Endurance Run** Run 13 miles @ base pace

WEEK 11 ◆ Proprioceptive Cue: Axle Between the Knees

MONDAY	Off
TUESDAY	**Base Run + Drills** Run 7 miles @ base pace Steep Hill Sprints 2 × 20 seconds One-Leg Hop 2 × 20 seconds
WEDNESDAY	**400m Intervals @ 3,000m Pace** Dynamic stretching warm-up 1.5-mile warm-up @ recovery pace 12 × 400 m @ 3,000m pace w/3-minute active recoveries 1.5-mile cool-down @ recovery pace

THURSDAY	**Recovery Run** 2–6 miles @ recovery pace *or* Nonimpact Cardio Cross-Training Workout 20–50 minutes @ recovery pace	**Resistance Workout** *2 sets each* Lying Hip Abduction Single-Leg Squat Box Lunge Stability Ball Leg Curl Single-Leg Squat Jump

FRIDAY	**1-Mile Intervals @ 10K Pace** Dynamic stretching warm-up 1.5-mile warm-up @ recovery pace 4 × 1 mile @ 10K pace w/2-minute active recoveries 1.5-mile recovery-pace cool-down

SATURDAY	**Recovery Run** 2–6 miles @ recovery pace	**Resistance Workout** *2 sets each* Cook Hip Lift Oblique Bridge Forearms to Palms Bridge Stability Ball Leg Curl Broad Jump

SUNDAY	**Endurance Run** Run 14 miles @ base pace

WEEK 12 (Recovery) ♦ Proprioceptive Cue: Running Against a Wall

MONDAY	Off
TUESDAY	**Base Run + Drills** Run 5 miles @ base pace High Knees 20 seconds Bounding 20 seconds
WEDNESDAY	**400m Intervals @ 3,000m Pace** Dynamic stretching warm-up 1.5-mile warm-up @ recovery pace 8 × 400m @ 3,000m pace w/3-minute active recoveries 1.5-mile cool-down @ recovery pace

THURSDAY	**Recovery Run** 2–6 miles @ recovery pace *or* <u>Nonimpact Cardio Cross-Training Workout</u> 20–50 minutes @ recovery pace	**Resistance Workout** *2 sets each* Lying Hip Abduction Single-Leg Squat Box Lunge Stability Ball Leg Curl Wall Jump

FRIDAY	**1-Mile Intervals @ 10K Pace** Dynamic stretching warm-up 1.5-mile warm-up @ recovery pace 3 × 1 mile @ 10K pace w/2-minute active recoveries 1.5-mile recovery-pace cool-down

SATURDAY	**Recovery Run** 2 miles @ recovery pace	**Resistance Workout** *2 sets each* Cook Hip Lift Oblique Bridge Forearms to Palms Bridge Stability Ball Leg Curl

SUNDAY	**5 K Tune-up Race or Time Trial** Dynamic stretching warm-up 1.5-mile warm-up @ recovery pace 5K tune-up race or time trial 1.5-mile cool-down @ recovery pace

Build 2

Training objectives: Continue to build endurance; increase fatigue resistance at 5K pace and 10K pace; build efficiency at half-marathon pace and marathon pace

WEEK 13 ◆ Proprioceptive Cue: Falling Forward

MONDAY	Off	
TUESDAY	**Base Run + Drills** Run 8 miles @ base pace High Knees 2 × 20 seconds Bounding 2 × 20 seconds	
WEDNESDAY	**1K Intervals @ 5K Pace** Dynamic stretching warm-up 1.5-mile warm-up @ recovery pace 3 × 1K @ 5K pace w/3-minute active recoveries 1.5-mile cool-down @ recovery pace	
THURSDAY	**Recovery Run** 2–6 miles @ recovery pace *or* Nonimpact Cardio Cross-Training Workout 20–50 minutes @ recovery pace	**Resistance Workout** *2 sets each* Lying Hip Abduction Single-Leg Squat Box Lunge Stability Ball Leg Curl Wall Jump
FRIDAY	**Tempo Run @ 10K Pace** Dynamic stretching warm-up 1.5-mile warm-up @ recovery pace 4 miles @ 10K pace 1.5-mile cool-down @ recovery pace	
SATURDAY	**Recovery Run** 2–6 miles @ recovery pace	**Resistance Workout** *2 sets each* Cook Hip Lift Oblique Bridge Forearms to Palms Bridge Stability Ball Leg Curl Single-Leg Box Jump
SUNDAY	**Progression Run** Run 14 miles Run first 7 miles @ base pace, then gradually increase pace every mile; run last mile @ half-marathon pace	

WEEK 14 ◆ Proprioceptive Cue: Navel to Spine

MONDAY	Off	
TUESDAY	**Base Run + Drills** Run 8 miles @ base pace Stiff-Legged Run 2 × 20 seconds Running No Arms 2 × 20 seconds	
WEDNESDAY	**1K Intervals @ 5K Pace** Dynamic stretching warm-up 1.5-mile warm-up @ recovery pace 4 × 1K intervals @ 5K pace w/3-minute active recoveries 1.5-mile cool-down @ recovery pace	
THURSDAY	**Recovery Run** 2–6 miles @ recovery pace *or* Nonimpact Cardio Cross-Training Workout 20–50 minutes @ recovery pace	**Resistance Workout** *2 sets each* Lying Hip Abduction Single-Leg Squat Box Lunge Stability Ball Leg Curl Squat Jump
FRIDAY	**Tempo Run @ 10K Pace** Dynamic stretching warm-up 1.5-mile warm-up @ recovery pace 4.5 miles @ 10K pace 1.5-mile cool-down @ recovery pace	
SATURDAY	**Recovery Run** 2–6 miles @ recovery pace	**Resistance Workout** *2 sets each* Cook Hip Lift Oblique Bridge Forearms to Palms Bridge Stability Ball Leg Curl Split Squat Jump
SUNDAY	**Endurance Run** Run 16 miles @ base pace	

WEEK 15 ◆ Proprioceptive Cue: Running on Water

MONDAY	Off
TUESDAY	**Base Run + Drills** Run 8 miles @ base pace Steep Hill Sprints 20 seconds One-Leg Hop 20 seconds
WEDNESDAY	**1K Intervals @ 5K Pace** Dynamic stretching warm-up 1.5-mile warm-up @ recovery pace 5 × 1K intervals @ 5K pace w/3-minute active recoveries 1.5-mile cool-down @ recovery pace

THURSDAY	**Recovery Run** 2–6 miles @ recovery pace or Nonimpact Cardio Cross-Training Workout 20–50 minutes @ recovery pace	**Resistance Workout** *2 sets each* Lying Hip Abduction Single-Leg Squat Box Lunge Stability Ball Leg Curl Single-Leg Squat Jump

FRIDAY	**Tempo Run @ 10K Pace** Dynamic stretching warm-up 1.5-mile warm-up @ recovery pace 5 miles @ 10K pace 1.5-mile cool-down @ recovery pace

SATURDAY	**Recovery Run** 2–6 miles @ recovery pace	**Resistance Workout** *2 sets each* Cook Hip Lift Oblique Bridge Forearms to Palms Bridge Stability Ball Leg Curl Broad Jump

SUNDAY	**Progression Run** Run 15 miles Run first 8 miles @ base pace, then gradually increase pace every mile; run last mile @ half-marathon pace

WEEK 16 (Recovery) ◆ Proprioceptive Cue: Pulling the Road

MONDAY	Off	
TUESDAY	**Base Run + Drills** Run 6 miles @ base pace Stiff-Legged Run 2 × 20 seconds Running No Arms 2 × 20 seconds	
WEDNESDAY	**1K Intervals @ 5K Pace** Dynamic stretching warm-up 1.5-mile warm-up @ recovery pace 3 × 1K intervals @ 5K pace w/3-minute active recoveries 1.5-mile cool-down @ recovery pace	
THURSDAY	**Recovery Run** 2–6 miles @ recovery pace *or* Nonimpact Cardio Cross-Training Workout 20–50 minutes @ recovery pace	**Resistance Workout** *2 sets each* Lying Hip Abduction Single-Leg Squat Box Lunge Stability Ball Leg Curl Squat Jump
FRIDAY	**Tempo Run @ 10K Pace** Dynamic stretching warm-up 1.5-mile warm-up @ recovery pace 3.5 miles @ 10K pace 1.5-mile cool-down @ recovery pace	
SATURDAY	**Recovery Run** 2 miles @ recovery pace	**Resistance Workout** *1 set each* Cook Hip Lift Oblique Bridge Forearms to Palms Bridge Stability Ball Leg Curl Split Squat Jump
SUNDAY	**10 K Tune-up Race or Time Trial** Dynamic stretching warm-up 1.5-mile warm-up @ recovery pace 10K tune-up race or time trial 1.5-mile cool-down @ recovery pace	

Peak Phase

Training objectives: Achieve peak fatigue resistance and efficiency at marathon pace; adapt and recover for peak race day

WEEK 17 ◆ Proprioceptive Cue: Scooting

MONDAY	Off	
TUESDAY	**Base Run + Drills** Run 9 miles @ base pace Stiff-Legged Run 2×20 seconds Running No Arms 2×20 seconds	
WEDNESDAY	**Mixed Intervals** Dynamic stretching warm-up 1-mile warm-up @ recovery pace 1×2K @ half-marathon pace, 2-minute active recovery 1×1 mile @ 10K pace, 2-minute active recovery 1×1K @ 5K pace, 2-minute active recovery 1×800m @ 3,000m pace 1-mile cool-down @ recovery pace	
THURSDAY	**Recovery Run** 2–6 miles @ recovery pace or Nonimpact Cardio Cross-Training Workout 20–50 minutes @ recovery pace	**Resistance Workout** *2 sets each* Lying Hip Abduction Single-Leg Squat Box Lunge Stability Ball Leg Curl Squat Jump
FRIDAY	**Tempo Run @ Half-Marathon Pace** 1.5-mile warm-up @ recovery pace 5.5 miles @ half-marathon pace 1.5-mile cool-down @ recovery pace	

(continued)

WEEK 17 ◆ Proprioceptive Cue: Scooting
(continued)

SATURDAY	Recovery Run	Resistance Workout
	2–6 miles @ recovery pace	*2 sets each*
		Cook Hip Lift
		Oblique Bridge
		Forearms to Palms Bridge
		Stability Ball Leg Curl
		Split Squat Jump
SUNDAY	Endurance Run	
	Run 18 miles @ base pace	

WEEK 18 ♦ Proprioceptive Cue: Pounding the Ground

MONDAY	Off
TUESDAY	**Base Run + Drills** Run 9 miles @ base pace Stiff-Legged Run 2 × 20 seconds Running No Arms 2 × 20 seconds
WEDNESDAY	**Mixed Intervals** Dynamic stretching warm-up 1-mile warm-up @ recovery pace 1 × 3K @ half-marathon pace, 2-minute active recovery 1 × 1 mile @ 10K pace, 2-minute active recovery 1 × 1K @ 5K pace, 2-minute active recovery 1 × 800m @ 3,000m pace 1-mile cool-down @ recovery pace

THURSDAY	**Recovery Run** 2–6 miles @ recovery pace *or* <u>Nonimpact Cardio Cross-Training Workout</u> 20–50 minutes @ recovery pace	**Resistance Workout** *2 sets each* Lying Hip Abduction Single-Leg Squat Box Lunge Stability Ball Leg Curl Squat Jump

FRIDAY	**Tempo Run @ Half-Marathon Pace** 1.5-mile warm-up @ recovery pace 6.5 miles @ half-marathon pace 1.5-mile cool-down @ recovery pace

SATURDAY	**Recovery Run** 2–6 miles @ recovery pace	**Resistance Workout** *2 sets each* Cook Hip Lift Oblique Bridge Quadruped Dead Bug Single-Leg Squat Jump

SUNDAY	**Marathon-Pace Run** 2-mile warm-up @ recovery pace 8 miles @ marathon pace 2-mile cool-down @ recovery pace

WEEK 19 ◆ Proprioceptive Cue: Butt Squeeze

MONDAY	Off	
TUESDAY	**Base Run + Drills** Run 9 miles @ base pace Steep Hill Sprints 2 × 20 seconds One-Leg Hop 2 × 20 seconds	
WEDNESDAY	**Mixed Intervals** Dynamic stretching warm-up 1-mile warm-up @ recovery pace 1 × 3K @ half-marathon pace, 2-minute active recovery 1 × 2K @ 10K pace, 2-minute active recovery 1 × 1K @ 5K pace, 2-minute active recovery 1 × 800m @ 3,000m pace 1-mile cool-down @ recovery pace	
THURSDAY	**Recovery Run** 2–6 miles @ recovery pace *or* <u>Nonimpact Cardio Cross-Training Workout</u> 20–50 minutes @ recovery pace	**Resistance Workout** *2 sets each* Kneeling Overhead Draw-In Lying Draw-In w/Hip Flexion Box Lunge Stability Ball Leg Curl Broad Jump
FRIDAY	**Tempo Run @ Half-Marathon Pace** 1.5-mile warm-up @ recovery pace 7.5 miles @ half-marathon pace 1.5-mile cool-down @ recovery pace	
SATURDAY	**Recovery Run** 2–6 miles @ recovery pace	**Resistance Workout** *2 sets each* Cook Hip Lift Oblique Bridge Quadruped Dead Bug Single-Leg Squat Jump
SUNDAY	**Endurance Run** Run 20 miles @ base pace	

WEEK 20 (Recovery) ◆ Proprioceptive Cue: Floppy Feet

MONDAY	Off	
TUESDAY	**Base Run + Drills** Run 6 miles @ base pace High Knees 20 seconds Bounding 20 seconds	
WEDNESDAY	**Mixed Intervals** Dynamic stretching warm-up 1-mile warm-up @ recovery pace 1 × 2K @ half-marathon pace, 2-minute active recovery 1 × 1 mile @ 10K pace, 2-minute active recovery 1 × 1K @ 5K pace, 2-minute active recovery 1 × 800m @ 3,000m pace 1-mile cool-down @ recovery pace	
THURSDAY	**Recovery Run** 2–6 miles @ recovery pace *or* Nonimpact Cardio Cross-Training Workout 20–50 minutes @ recovery pace	**Resistance Workout** *2 sets each* Kneeling Overhead Draw-In Lying Draw-In w/Hip Flexion Box Lunge Stability Ball Leg Curl Squat Jump
FRIDAY	**Tempo Run @ Half-Marathon Pace** 1.5-mile warm-up @ recovery pace 5.5 miles @ half-marathon pace 1.5-mile cool-down @ recovery pace	
SATURDAY	**Recovery Run** 2 miles @ recovery pace	**Resistance Workout** *1 set each* Knee Fall-Out Oblique Bridge Quadruped Dead Bug Split Squat Jump
SUNDAY	**Half-Marathon Tune-up Race or Time Trial** 1.5-mile warm-up @ recovery pace Half-marathon tune-up race or time trial 1.5-mile cool-down @ recovery pace	

WEEK 21 ◆ Proprioceptive Cue: Butt Squeeze

MONDAY	Off	
TUESDAY	**Base Run + Drills** Run 10 miles @ base pace Stiff-Legged Run 2×20 seconds Running No Arms 2×20 seconds	
WEDNESDAY	**Mixed Intervals** Dynamic stretching warm-up 1-mile warm-up @ recovery pace 1×3K @ half-marathon pace, 2-minute active recovery 1×2K @ 10K pace, 2-minute active recovery 1×1K @ 5K pace, 2-minute active recovery 1×800m @ 3,000m pace 1-mile cool-down @ recovery pace	
THURSDAY	**Recovery Run** 2–6 miles @ recovery pace *or* Non-impact Cardio Cross-Training Workout 20–50 minutes @ recovery pace	**Resistance Workout** *2 sets each* Lying Hip Abduction Single-Leg Squat Box Lunge Stability Ball Leg Curl Single-Leg Squat Jump
FRIDAY	**Tempo Run @ Half-Marathon Pace** 2-mile warm-up @ recovery pace 8 miles @ half-marathon pace 2-mile cool-down @ recovery pace	
SATURDAY	**Recovery Run** 2–6 miles @ recovery pace	**Resistance Workout** *2 sets each* Cook Hip Lift Oblique Bridge Quadruped Dead Bug Broad Jump
SUNDAY	**Endurance Run** Run 22 miles @ base pace	

WEEK 22 ◆ Proprioceptive Cue: Feeling Symmetry

MONDAY	Off
TUESDAY	**Base Run + Drills** Run 10 miles @ base pace Steep Hill Sprints 2 × 20 seconds One-Leg Hop 2 × 20 seconds
WEDNESDAY	**Mixed Intervals** Dynamic stretching warm-up 1-mile warm-up @ recovery pace 1 × 3K @ half-marathon pace, 90-second active recovery 1 × 2K @ 10K pace, 90-second active recovery 1 × 1K @ 5K pace, 90-second active recovery 1 × 800m @ 3,000m pace 1-mile cool-down @ recovery pace

THURSDAY	**Recovery Run** 2–6 miles @ recovery pace *or* Nonimpact Cardio Cross-Training Workout 20–50 minutes @ recovery pace	**Resistance Workout** *2 sets each* Kneeling Overhead Draw-In Lying Draw-In w/Hip Flexion Box Lunge Stability Ball Leg Curl Wall Jump

FRIDAY	**Tempo Run @ Half-Marathon Pace** 2-mile warm-up @ recovery pace 8.5 miles @ half-marathon pace 2-mile cool-down @ recovery pace	
SATURDAY	**Recovery Run** 2–6 miles @ recovery pace	**Resistance Workout** *2 sets each* Knee Fall-Out Oblique Bridge Quadruped Dead Bug Single-Leg Box Jump

SUNDAY	**Marathon-Pace Run** 2-mile warm-up @ recovery pace 12 miles @ marathon pace 2-mile cool-down @ recovery pace

WEEK 23 (Taper) ◆ Proprioceptive Cue: Axle Between the Knees

MONDAY	Off
TUESDAY	**Base Run + Drills** Run 8 miles @ base pace High Knees 2×20 seconds Bounding 2×20 seconds
WEDNESDAY	**Mixed Intervals** Dynamic stretching warm-up 1-mile warm-up @ recovery pace 1×2K @ half-marathon pace, 90-second active recovery 1×1 mile @ 10K pace, 90-second active recovery 1×1K @ 5K pace, 90-second active recovery 1×800m @ 3,000m pace 1-mile cool-down @ recovery pace

THURSDAY	**Recovery Run** 2–6 miles @ recovery pace *or* Nonimpact Cardio Cross-Training Workout 20–50 minutes @ recovery pace	**Resistance Workout** *2 sets each* Lying Hip Abduction Single-Leg Squat Box Lunge Stability Ball Leg Curl Squat Jump

FRIDAY	**Tempo Run @ Half-Marathon Pace** 1-mile warm-up @ recovery pace 7 miles @ half-marathon pace 1-mile cool-down @ recovery pace

SATURDAY	**Recovery Run** 2–6 miles @ recovery pace	**Resistance Workout** *2 sets each* Cook Hip Lift Oblique Bridge Quadruped Dead Bug Split Squat Jump

SUNDAY	**Endurance Run** Run 13 miles @ base pace

WEEK 24 (Taper) ◆ Proprioceptive Cue: Your Choice

MONDAY	Off
TUESDAY	**Base Run + Drills** Run 6 miles @ base pace Stiff-Legged Run 20 seconds Running No Arms 20 seconds
WEDNESDAY	**Mixed Intervals** Dynamic stretching warm-up 1-mile warm-up @ recovery pace 1×2K @ half-marathon pace, 90-second active recovery 1×1 mile @ 10K pace, 90-second active recovery 1×1K @ 5K pace, 90-second active recovery 1-mile cool-down @ recovery pace
THURSDAY	**Resistance Workout** *1 set each* Kneeling Overhead Draw-In Lying Draw-In w/Hip Flexion Box Lunge Stability Ball Leg Curl
FRIDAY	**Tempo Run @ Half-Marathon Pace** 1-mile warm-up @ recovery pace 2 miles @ half-marathon pace 1-mile cool-down @ recovery pace
SATURDAY	Off
SUNDAY	**Marathon Peak Race** Marathon

LEVEL 3

Use this plan if you are most comfortable with a marathon training plan that features six scheduled runs per week plus up to four additional, optional recovery runs or nonimpact cardio cross-training workouts and a maximum run distance of 24 miles. The plan also contains two resistance workouts per week.

Base Phase

Training Objectives: Build aerobic capacity and endurance, increase injury resistance, and increase muscle activation capacity

WEEK 1 ◆ Proprioceptive Cue: Falling Forward

MONDAY	Off	
TUESDAY	**Base Run + Drills** Run 6 miles @ base pace Running No Arms 20 seconds One-Leg Hop 20 seconds	<u>Optional Recovery Run or Cardio</u> <u>Cross-Training Workout</u> 20–60 minutes @ recovery pace
WEDNESDAY	**Hill Repetitions** Dynamic stretching warm-up 2-mile warm-up @ recovery pace 2 × 30-second hill repetitions @ relaxed sprint speed 2-mile cool-down @ recovery pace	<u>Optional Recovery Run or Cardio</u> <u>Cross-Training Workout</u> 20–60 minutes @ recovery pace
THURSDAY	**Base Run** Run 6 miles @ base pace	**Resistance Workout** *1 set each* Lying Hip Abduction Cook Hip Lift Kneeling Overhead Draw-In Knee Fall-Out Squat Jump

FRIDAY	**Fartlek Run**
	Dynamic stretching warm-up
	Run 6 miles @ base pace
	  w/2 × 30-second intervals
	  @ 1-mile pace "sprinkled in"
		<u>Optional Recovery Run or Cardio</u>
		<u>Cross-Training Workout</u>
		20–60 minutes @ recovery pace

SATURDAY	**Base Run** Run 6 miles @ base pace	**Resistance Workout** *1 set each* Lying Hip Abduction Cook Hip Lift Kneeling Overhead Draw-In Knee Fall-Out Broad Jump
SUNDAY	**Base Run** Run 7 miles @ base pace	<u>Optional Recovery Run or Cardio</u> <u>Cross-Training Workout</u> 20–60 minutes @ recovery pace

WEEK 2 ♦ Proprioceptive Cue: Navel to Spine

MONDAY	Off	
TUESDAY	**Base Run + Drills** Run 6 miles @ base pace High Knees 2 × 20 seconds Bounding 2 × 20 seconds	Optional Recovery Run or Cardio Cross-Training Workout 20–60 minutes @ recovery pace

WEDNESDAY	**Hill Repetitions**
	Dynamic stretching warm-up
	2-mile warm-up @ recovery pace
	6 × 30-second hill repetitions
	  @ relaxed sprint speed
	  w/2-minute active recoveries
	2-mile cool-down @ recovery
	  pace
		Optional Recovery Run or Cardio Cross-Training Workout
		20–60 minutes @ recovery pace

THURSDAY	**Base Run** Run 6 miles @ base pace	**Resistance Workout** *2 sets each* Lying Hip Abduction Cook Hip Lift Kneeling Overhead Draw-In Knee Fall-Out Split Squat Jump

FRIDAY	**Fartlek Run**
	Dynamic stretching warm-up
	Run 6 miles @ base pace
	  w/6 × 30-second intervals
	  @ 1-mile pace "sprinkled in"
		Optional Recovery Run or Cardio Cross-Training Workout
		20–60 minutes @ recovery pace

SATURDAY	**Base Run** Run 6 miles @ base pace	**Resistance Workout** *2 sets each* Lying Hip Abduction Cook Hip Lift Kneeling Overhead Draw-In Knee Fall-Out Wall Jump
SUNDAY	**Base Run** Run 8 miles @ base pace	Optional Recovery Run or Cardio Cross-Training Workout 20–60 minutes @ recovery pace

WEEK 3 ◆ Proprioceptive Cue: Running on Water

MONDAY	Off	
TUESDAY	**Base Run + Drills** Run 6 miles @ base pace Stiff-Legged Run 2 × 20 seconds Running No Arms 2 × 20 seconds	<u>Optional Recovery Run or Cardio</u> <u>Cross-Training Workout</u> 20–60 minutes @ recovery pace

WEDNESDAY	**Hill Repetitions**
	Dynamic stretching warm-up
	2-mile warm-up @ recovery pace
	8 × 45-second hill repetitions
	   @ 1-mile pace w/2-minute
	   active recoveries
	2-mile cool-down @ recovery pace
		<u>Optional Recovery Run or Cardio</u>
		<u>Cross-Training Workout</u>
		20–60 minutes @ recovery pace

THURSDAY	**Base Run** Run 6 miles @ base pace	**Resistance Workout** *3 sets each* Lying Hip Abduction Cook Hip Lift Kneeling Overhead Draw-In Knee Fall-Out Squat Jump

FRIDAY	**Fartlek Run**
	Dynamic stretching warm-up
	Run 6 miles @ base pace
	   w/8 × 45-second intervals
	   @ 1-mile pace "sprinkled in"
		<u>Optional Recovery Run or Cardio</u>
		<u>Cross-Training Workout</u>
		20–60 minutes @ recovery pace

SATURDAY	**Base Run** Run 6 miles @ base pace	**Resistance Workout** *3 sets each* Lying Hip Abduction Cook Hip Lift Kneeling Overhead Draw-In Knee Fall-Out Broad Jump
SUNDAY	**Base Run** Run 9 miles @ base pace	<u>Optional Recovery Run or Cardio</u> <u>Cross-Training Workout</u> 20–60 minutes @ recovery pace

WEEK 4 (Recovery) ◆ Proprioceptive Cue: Pulling the Road

MONDAY	Off	
TUESDAY	**Base Run + Drills** Run 5 miles @ base pace One-Leg Hop 20 seconds High Knees 20 seconds	<u>Optional Recovery Run or Cardio</u> <u>Cross-Training Workout</u> 20–60 minutes @ recovery pace
WEDNESDAY	**Hill Repetitions** Dynamic stretching warm-up 2-mile warm-up @ recovery pace 5×1-minute hill repetitions @ 1-mile pace w/2-minute active recoveries 2-mile cool-down @ recovery pace	<u>Optional Recovery Run or Cardio</u> <u>Cross-Training Workout</u> 20–60 minutes @ recovery pace
THURSDAY	**Base Run** Run 5 miles @ base pace	**Resistance Workout** *1 set each* Single-Leg Squat Oblique Bridge Lying Draw-In w/Hip Flexion Quadruped *2 sets each* Lying Hip Abduction Cook Hip Lift Kneeling Overhead Draw-In Knee Fall-Out Single-Leg Squat Jump Broad Jump
FRIDAY	**Fartlek Run** Dynamic stretching warm-up Run 5 miles @ base pace w/5×1-minute intervals @ 1-mile pace "sprinkled in"	<u>Optional Recovery Run or Cardio</u> <u>Cross-Training Workout</u> 20–60 minutes @ recovery pace
SATURDAY	**Base Run** Run 5 miles @ base pace	**Resistance Workout** *1 set each* Single-Leg Squat Oblique Bridge Lying Draw-In w/Hip Flexion Quadruped

SATURDAY (continued)	**Base Run**	**Resistance Workout** *2 sets each* Lying Hip Abduction Cook Hip Lift Kneeling Overhead Draw-In Knee Fall-Out Wall Jump Single-Leg Box Jump
SUNDAY	**Base Run** Run 7 miles @ base pace	Optional Recovery Run or Cardio Cross-Training Workout 20–60 minutes @ recovery pace

WEEK 5 ♦ Proprioceptive Cue: Scooting

MONDAY	Off	
TUESDAY	**Base Run + Drills** Run 7 miles @ base pace High Knees 2×20 seconds Bounding 2×20 seconds	Optional Recovery Run or Cardio Cross-Training Workout 20–60 minutes @ recovery pace
WEDNESDAY	**Hill Repetitions** Dynamic stretching warm-up 2-mile warm-up @ recovery pace 8×75-second hill repetitions @ 1-mile pace w/2.5-minute active recoveries 2-mile cool-down @ recovery pace	Optional Recovery Run or Cardio Cross-Training Workout 20–60 minutes @ recovery pace
THURSDAY	**Base Run** Run 7 miles @ base pace	**Resistance Workout** *2 sets each* Single-Leg Squat Oblique Bridge Lying Draw-In w/Hip Flexion Quadruped *1 set each* Lying Hip Abduction Cook Hip Lift Kneeling Overhead Draw-In Knee Fall-Out Single-Leg Squat Jump Wall Jump
FRIDAY	**Fartlek Run** Dynamic stretching warm-up Run 7 miles @ base pace w/8×75-second intervals @ 3,000m pace "sprinkled in"	Optional Recovery Run or Cardio Cross-Training Workout 20–60 minutes @ recovery pace
SATURDAY	**Base Run** Run 7 miles @ base pace	**Resistance Workout** *2 sets each* Single-Leg Squat Oblique Bridge

SATURDAY (continued)	**Base Run**	**Resistance Workout** *2 sets each (cont.)* Lying Draw-In w/Hip Flexion Quadruped *1 set each* Lying Hip Abduction Cook Hip Lift Kneeling Overhead Draw-In Knee Fall-Out Wall Jump Broad Jump
SUNDAY	**Endurance Run** Run 11 miles @ base pace	Optional Recovery Run or Cardio Cross-Training Workout 20–60 minutes @ recovery pace

WEEK 6 ◆ Proprioceptive Cue: Pounding the Ground

MONDAY	Off	
TUESDAY	**Base Run + Drills** Run 7 miles @ base pace Stiff-Legged Run 2 × 20 seconds Running No Arms 2 × 20 seconds	Optional Recovery Run or Cardio Cross-Training Workout 20–60 minutes @ recovery pace
WEDNESDAY	**Hill Repetitions** Dynamic stretching warm-up 2-mile warm-up @ recovery pace 8 × 90-second hill repetitions @ 1-mile pace w/2-minute active recoveries 2-mile cool-down @ recovery pace	Optional Recovery Run or Cardio Cross-Training Workout 20–60 minutes @ recovery pace
THURSDAY	**Base Run** Run 7 miles @ base pace	**Resistance Workout** *3 sets each* Single-Leg Squat Oblique Bridge Lying Draw-In w/Hip Flexion Quadruped *2 sets* Squat Jump Single-Leg Box Jump
FRIDAY	**Fartlek Run** Dynamic stretching warm-up Run 7 miles @ base pace w/8 × 90-second intervals @ 3,000m pace "sprinkled in"	Optional Recovery Run or Cardio Cross-Training Workout 20–60 minutes @ recovery pace
SATURDAY	**Base Run** Run 7 miles @ base pace	**Resistance Workout** *3 sets each* Single-Leg Squat Oblique Bridge Lying Draw-In w/Hip Flexion Quadruped *2 sets* Single-Leg Squat Jump Broad Jump
SUNDAY	**Endurance Run** Run 12 miles @ base pace	Optional Recovery Run or Cardio Cross-Training Workout 20–60 minutes @ recovery pace

WEEK 7 ◆ Proprioceptive Cue: Driving the Thigh

MONDAY	Off	
TUESDAY	**Base Run + Drills** Run 7 miles @ base pace Steep Hill Sprints 2 × 20 seconds One-Leg Hop 2 × 20 seconds	<u>Optional Recovery Run or Cardio</u> <u>Cross-Training Workout</u> 20–60 minutes @ recovery pace

WEDNESDAY	**Hill Repetitions**
	Dynamic stretching warm-up
	2-mile warm-up @ recovery pace
	8 × 2-minute hill repetitions
	   @ 3,000m pace w/3-minute
	   active recoveries
	2-mile cool-down @ recovery pace
		<u>Optional Recovery Run or Cardio</u>
		<u>Cross-Training Workout</u>
		20–60 minutes @ recovery pace

THURSDAY	**Base Run** Run 7 miles @ base pace	**Resistance Workout** *2 sets each* Single-Leg Squat Oblique Bridge Lying Draw-In w/Hip Flexion Quadruped Split Squat Jump *1 set each* Box Lunge Stability Ball Leg Curl Forearms to Palms Bridge Dead Bug

FRIDAY	**Fartlek Run**
	Dynamic stretching warm-up
	Run 7 miles @ base pace
	   w/8 × 2-minute intervals
	   @ 3,000m pace "sprinkled in"
		<u>Optional Recovery Run or Cardio</u>
		<u>Cross-Training Workout</u>
		20–60 minutes @ recovery pace

SATURDAY	**Base Run** Run 7 miles @ base pace	**Resistance Workout** *2 sets each* Single-Leg Squat Oblique Bridge Lying Draw-In w/Hip Flexion

(continued)

WEEK 7 ◆ Proprioceptive Cue: Driving the Thigh
(continued)

SATURDAY (continued)	Base Run	Resistance Workout
		2 sets each (cont.) Quadruped Single-Leg Box Jump
		1 set each Box Lunge Stability Ball Leg Curl Forearms to Palms Bridge Dead Bug
SUNDAY	**Endurance Run** Run 14 miles @ base pace	Optional Recovery Run or Cardio Cross-Training Workout 20–60 minutes @ recovery pace

WEEK 8 (Recovery) ◆ Proprioceptive Cue: Floppy Feet

MONDAY	Off	
TUESDAY	**Base Run + Drills** Run 5 miles @ base pace High Knees 20 seconds Bounding 20 seconds	Optional Recovery Run or Cardio Cross-Training Workout 20–60 minutes @ recovery pace

WEDNESDAY	**Hill Repetitions**
	Dynamic stretching warm-up
	2-mile warm-up @ recovery pace
	5 × 2-minute hill repetitions
	  @ 3,000m pace w/2-minute
	  active recoveries
	2-mile cool-down @ recovery pace
		Optional Recovery Run or Cardio
		Cross-Training Workout
		20–60 minutes @ recovery pace

THURSDAY	**Base Run** Run 6 miles @ base pace	**Resistance Workout** *1 set each* Single-Leg Squat Oblique Bridge Lying Draw-In w/Hip Flexion Quadruped *2 sets each* Box Lunge Stability Ball Leg Curl Forearms to Palms Bridge Dead Bug Broad Jump Single-Leg Box Jump

FRIDAY	**Fartlek Run**
	Dynamic stretching warm-up
	Run 5 miles @ base pace
	  w/4 × 2-minute intervals
	  @ 3,000m pace "sprinkled in"
		Optional Recovery Run or Cardio
		Cross-Training Workout
		20–60 minutes @ recovery pace

SATURDAY	**Base Run** Run 6 miles @ base pace	**Resistance Workout** *1 set each* Single-Leg Squat Oblique Bridge Lying Draw-In w/Hip Flexion

(continued)

WEEK 8 (Recovery) ◆ Proprioceptive Cue: Floppy Feet
(continued)

SATURDAY (continued)	**Base Run**	**Resistance Workout** *1 set each (cont.)* Quadruped *2 sets each* Box Lunge Stability Ball Leg Curl Forearms to Palms Bridge Dead Bug Wall Jump Squat Jump
SUNDAY	**Base Run** Run 8 miles @ base pace	Optional Recovery Run or Cardio Cross-Training Workout 20–60 minutes @ recovery pace

Build 1 Phase

Training objectives: Continue to increase aerobic capacity and endurance; increase fatigue resistance at 3,000m pace and 10K pace

WEEK 9 ◆ Proprioceptive Cue: Butt Squeeze

MONDAY	Off	
TUESDAY	**Base Run + Drills** Run 8 miles @ base pace Stiff-Legged Run 2 × 20 seconds Running No Arms 2 × 20 seconds	Optional Recovery Run or Cardio Cross-Training Workout 20–60 minutes @ recovery pace
WEDNESDAY	**400m Intervals @ 3,000m Pace** Dynamic stretching warm-up 1.5-mile warm-up @ recovery pace 10 × 400m @ 3,000m pace w/3-minute active recoveries 1.5-mile cool-down @ recovery pace	Optional Recovery Run or Cardio Cross-Training Workout 20–60 minutes @ recovery pace
THURSDAY	**Recovery/Base Run** 4–8 miles @ recovery/base pace (Do this workout as a recovery run if you did *not* do an afternoon recovery workout following yesterday's interval workout. Otherwise, do this workout as a base workout.)	**Resistance Workout** *3 sets each* Box Lunge Stability Ball Leg Curl Forearms to Palms Bridge Dead Bug Wall Jump Squat Jump
FRIDAY	**1-Mile Intervals @ 10K Pace** Dynamic stretching warm-up 2-mile warm-up @ recovery pace 3 × 1 mile @ 10K pace w/2-minute active recoveries 2-mile recovery-pace cool-down	Optional Recovery Run or Cardio Cross-Training Workout 20–60 minutes @ recovery pace

(continued)

WEEK 9 ◆ Proprioceptive Cue: Butt Squeeze
(continued)

SATURDAY	Recovery/Base Run 4–8 miles @ recovery/base pace	Resistance Workout *3 sets each* Box Lunge Stability Ball Leg Curl Forearms to Palms Bridge Dead Bug Single-Leg Box Jump Split Squat Jump
SUNDAY	Endurance Run Run 14 miles @ base pace	Optional Recovery Run or Cardio Cross-Training Workout 20–60 minutes @ recovery pace

WEEK 10 ◆ Proprioceptive Cue: Feeling Symmetry

MONDAY	Off	
TUESDAY	**Base Run + Drills** Run 8 miles @ base pace Stiff-Legged Run 2 × 20 seconds Running No Arms 2 × 20 seconds	Optional Recovery Run or Cardio Cross-Training Workout 20–60 minutes @ recovery pace
WEDNESDAY	**400m Intervals @ 3,000m Pace** Dynamic stretching warm-up 1.5-mile warm-up @ recovery pace 12 × 400m @ 3,000m pace w/3-minute active recoveries 1.5-mile cool-down @ recovery pace	Optional Recovery Run or Cardio Cross-Training Workout 20–60 minutes @ recovery pace
THURSDAY	**Recovery/Base Run** 4–8 miles @ recovery/base pace	**Resistance Workout** *2 sets each* Lying Hip Abduction Single-Leg Squat Box Lunge Stability Ball Leg Curl Squat Jump Single-Leg Squat Jump
FRIDAY	**1-Mile Intervals @ 10K Pace** Dynamic stretching warm-up 2-mile warm-up @ recovery pace 4 × 1 mile @ 10K pace w/2-minute active recoveries 2-mile recovery-pace cool-down	Optional Recovery Run or Cardio Cross-Training Workout 20–60 minutes @ recovery pace
SATURDAY	**Recovery/Base Run** 4–8 miles @ recovery/base pace	**Resistance Workout** *2 sets each* Cook Hip Lift Oblique Bridge Forearms to Palms Bridge Stability Ball Leg Curl Split Squat Jump Broad Jump
SUNDAY	**Endurance Run** Run 15 miles @ base pace	Optional Recovery Run or Cardio Cross-Training Workout 20–60 minutes @ recovery pace

WEEK 11 ◆ Proprioceptive Cue: Axle Between the Knees

MONDAY	Off	
TUESDAY	**Base Run + Drills** Run 8 miles @ base pace Steep Hill Sprints 2 × 20 seconds One-Leg Hop 2 × 20 seconds	<u>Optional Recovery Run or Cardio</u> <u>Cross-Training Workout</u> 20–60 minutes @ recovery pace

WEDNESDAY	**400m Intervals @ 3,000m Pace**
	Dynamic stretching warm-up
	1.5-mile warm-up @ recovery pace
	14 × 400m @ 3,000m pace
	   w/ 3-minute active recoveries
	1.5-mile cool-down @ recovery
	   pace
		<u>Optional Recovery Run or Cardio</u>
		<u>Cross-Training Workout</u>
		20–60 minutes @ recovery pace

THURSDAY	**Recovery/Base Run** 4–8 miles @ recovery/base pace	**Resistance Workout** *2 sets each* Lying Hip Abduction Single-Leg Squat Box Lunge Stability Ball Leg Curl Single-Leg Squat Jump Wall Jump
FRIDAY	**1-Mile Intervals @ 10K Pace** Dynamic stretching warm-up 2-mile warm-up @ recovery pace 5 × 1 mile @ 10K pace w/ 2-minute active recoveries 2-mile recovery-pace cool-down	<u>Optional Recovery Run or Cardio</u> <u>Cross-Training Workout</u> 20–60 minutes @ recovery pace
SATURDAY	**Recovery/Base Run** 4–8 miles @ recovery/base pace	**Resistance Workout** *2 sets each* Cook Hip Lift Oblique Bridge Forearms to Palms Bridge Stability Ball Leg Curl Broad Jump Single-Leg Box Jump
SUNDAY	**Endurance Run** Run 16 miles @ base pace	<u>Optional Recovery Run or Cardio</u> <u>Cross-Training Workout</u> 20–60 minutes @ recovery pace

WEEK 12 (Recovery) ◆ Proprioceptive Cue: Running Against a Wall

MONDAY	Off	
TUESDAY	**Base Run + Drills** Run 5 miles @ base pace High Knees 20 seconds Bounding 20 seconds	Optional Recovery Run or Cardio Cross-Training Workout 20–60 minutes @ recovery pace
WEDNESDAY	**400m Intervals @ 3,000m Pace** Dynamic stretching warm-up 1.5-mile warm-up @ recovery pace 9 × 400m @ 3,000m pace w/3-minute active recoveries 1.5-mile cool-down @ recovery pace	Optional Recovery Run or Cardio Cross-Training Workout 20–60 minutes @ recovery pace
THURSDAY	**Recovery/Base Run** 4–8 miles @ recovery/base pace	**Resistance Workout** *2 sets each* Lying Hip Abduction Single-Leg Squat Box Lunge Stability Ball Leg Curl Wall Jump Squat Jump
FRIDAY	**1-Mile Intervals @ 10K Pace** Dynamic stretching warm-up 2-mile warm-up @ recovery pace 3 × 1 mile @ 10K pace w/2-minute active recoveries 2-mile recovery-pace cool-down	Optional Recovery Run or Cardio Cross-Training Workout 20–60 minutes @ recovery pace
SATURDAY	**Recovery Run** 2 miles @ recovery pace	**Resistance Workout** *2 sets each* Cook Hip Lift Oblique Bridge Forearms to Palms Bridge Stability Ball Leg Curl

(continued)

WEEK 12 (Recovery) ◆ Proprioceptive Cue: Running Against a Wall

(continued)

SUNDAY	**5K Tune-up Race or Time Trial** Dynamic stretching warm-up 2-mile warm-up @ recovery pace 5K tune-up race or time trial 2-mile cool-down @ recovery pace

Build 2 Phase

Training objectives: Continue to build endurance; increase fatigue resistance at 5K pace and 10K pace; build efficiency at half-marathon pace and marathon pace

WEEK 13 ◆ Proprioceptive Cue: Falling Forward

MONDAY	Off	
TUESDAY	**Base Run + Drills** Run 9 miles @ base pace High Knees 2 × 20 seconds Bounding 2 × 20 seconds	<u>Optional Recovery Run or Cardio</u> <u>Cross-Training Workout</u> 20–60 minutes @ recovery pace
WEDNESDAY	**1K Intervals @ 5K Pace** Dynamic stretching warm-up 1.5-mile warm-up @ recovery pace 4 × 1K @ 5K pace w/3-minute active recoveries 1.5-mile cool-down @ recovery pace	<u>Optional Recovery Run or Cardio</u> <u>Cross-Training Workout</u> 20–60 minutes @ recovery pace
THURSDAY	**Recovery/Base Run** 4–8 miles @ recovery/base pace	**Resistance Workout** *2 sets each* Lying Hip Abduction Single-Leg Squat Box Lunge Stability Ball Leg Curl Wall Jump Squat Jump
FRIDAY	**Tempo Run @ 10K Pace** Dynamic stretching warm-up 2-mile warm-up @ recovery pace 4.5 miles @ 10K pace 2-mile cool-down @ recovery pace	<u>Optional Recovery Run or Cardio</u> <u>Cross-Training Workout</u> 20–60 minutes @ recovery pace

(continued)

WEEK 13 ◆ Proprioceptive Cue: Falling Forward
(continued)

SATURDAY	**Recovery/Base Run** 4–8 miles @ recovery/base pace	**Resistance Workout** *2 sets each* Cook Hip Lift Oblique Bridge Forearms to Palms Bridge Stability Ball Leg Curl Single-Leg Box Jump Split Squat Jump
SUNDAY	**Progression Run** Run 16 miles Run first 8 miles @ base pace, then gradually increase pace every mile; run last mile @ half-marathon pace	Optional Recovery Run or Cardio Cross-Training Workout 20–60 minutes @ recovery pace

WEEK 14 ◆ Proprioceptive Cue: Navel to Spine

MONDAY	Off	
TUESDAY	**Base Run + Drills** Run 9 miles @ base pace Stiff-Legged Run 2 × 20 seconds Running No Arms 2 × 20 seconds	<u>Optional Recovery Run or Cardio</u> <u>Cross-Training Workout</u> 20–60 minutes @ recovery pace
WEDNESDAY	**1K Intervals @ 5K Pace** Dynamic stretching warm-up 1.5-mile warm-up @ recovery pace 5 × 1K intervals @ 5K pace w/3-minute active recoveries 1.5-mile cool-down @ recovery pace	<u>Optional Recovery Run or Cardio</u> <u>Cross-Training Workout</u> 20–60 minutes @ recovery pace
THURSDAY	**Recovery/Base Run** 4–8 miles @ recovery/base pace	**Resistance Workout** *2 sets each* Lying Hip Abduction Single-Leg Squat Box Lunge Stability Ball Leg Curl Squat Jump Single-Leg Squat Jump
FRIDAY	**Tempo Run @ 10K Pace** Dynamic stretching warm-up 1.5-mile warm-up @ recovery pace 4.5 miles @ 10K pace 1.5-mile cool-down @ recovery pace	<u>Optional Recovery Run or Cardio</u> <u>Cross-Training Workout</u> 20–60 minutes @ recovery pace
SATURDAY	**Recovery/Base Run** 4–8 miles @ recovery/base pace	**Resistance Workout** *2 sets each* Cook Hip Lift Oblique Bridge Forearms to Palms Bridge Stability Ball Leg Curl Split Squat Jump Broad Jump

(continued)

WEEK 14 ◆ Proprioceptive Cue: Navel to Spine
(continued)

SUNDAY	**Endurance Run** Run 18 miles @ base pace	Optional Recovery Run or Cardio Cross-Training Workout 20–60 minutes @ recovery pace

WEEK 15 ◆ Proprioceptive Cue: Running on Water

MONDAY	Off	
TUESDAY	**Base Run + Drills** Run 9 miles @ base pace Steep Hill Sprints 2×20 seconds One-Leg Hop 2×20 seconds	<u>Optional Recovery Run or Cardio</u> <u>Cross-Training Workout</u> 20–60 minutes @ recovery pace

WEDNESDAY	**1K Intervals @ 5K Pace**
	Dynamic stretching warm-up
	1.5-mile warm-up @ recovery
	  pace
	6×1K intervals @ 5K pace
	  w/3-minute active recoveries
	1.5-mile cool-down @ recovery
	  pace
		<u>Optional Recovery Run or Cardio</u>
		<u>Cross-Training Workout</u>
		20–60 minutes @ recovery pace

THURSDAY	**Recovery/Base Run** 4–8 miles @ recovery/base pace	**Resistance Workout** *2 sets each* Lying Hip Abduction Single-Leg Squat Box Lunge Stability Ball Leg Curl Single-Leg Squat Jump Wall Jump
FRIDAY	**Tempo Run @ 10K Pace** Dynamic stretching warm-up 2-mile warm-up @ recovery pace 5.5 miles @ 10K pace 2-mile cool-down @ recovery pace	<u>Optional Recovery Run or Cardio</u> <u>Cross-Training Workout</u> 20–60 minutes @ recovery pace
SATURDAY	**Recovery/Base Run** 4–8 miles @ recovery/base pace	**Resistance Workout** *2 sets each* Cook Hip Lift Oblique Bridge Forearms to Palms Bridge Stability Ball Leg Curl Broad Jump Single-Leg Box Jump

(continued)

WEEK 15 ♦ Proprioceptive Cue: Running on Water
(continued)

SUNDAY	**Progression Run**	Optional Recovery Run or Cardio Cross-Training Workout
	Run 17 miles	20–60 minutes @ recovery pace
	Run first 9 miles @ base pace, then gradually increase pace every mile; run last mile @ half-marathon pace	

WEEK 16 (Recovery) ◆ Proprioceptive Cue: Pulling the Road

MONDAY	Off	
TUESDAY	**Base Run + Drills** Run 6 miles @ base pace Stiff-Legged Run 2×20 seconds Running No Arms 2×20 seconds	<u>Optional Recovery Run or Cardio</u> <u>Cross-Training Workout</u> 20–60 minutes @ recovery pace
WEDNESDAY	**1K Intervals @ 5K Pace** Dynamic stretching warm-up 1.5-mile warm-up @ recovery pace 4×1K intervals @ 5K pace w/3-minute active recoveries 1.5-mile cool-down @ recovery pace	<u>Optional Recovery Run or Cardio</u> <u>Cross-Training Workout</u> 20–60 minutes @ recovery pace
THURSDAY	**Recovery/Base Run** 4–8 miles @ recovery/base pace	**Resistance Workout** *2 sets each* Lying Hip Abduction Single-Leg Squat Box Lunge Stability Ball Leg Curl Squat Jump Single-Leg Squat Jump
FRIDAY	**Tempo Run @ 10K Pace** 2-mile warm-up @ recovery pace 3.5 miles @ 10K pace 2-mile cool-down @ recovery pace	<u>Optional Recovery Run or Cardio</u> <u>Cross-Training Workout</u> 20–60 minutes @ recovery pace
SATURDAY	**Recovery Run** 2 miles @ recovery pace	**Resistance Workout** *1 set each* Cook Hip Lift Oblique Bridge Forearms to Palms Bridge Stability Ball Leg Curl Split Squat Jump
SUNDAY	**10K Tune-up Race or Time Trial** Dynamic stretching warm-up 2-mile warm-up @ recovery pace 10K race or time trial 2-mile cool-down @ recovery pace	

Peak Phase

Training objectives: Achieve peak fatigue resistance and efficiency at 10K pace; adapt and recover for peak race day

WEEK 17 ◆ Proprioceptive Cue: Scooting

MONDAY	Off	
TUESDAY	**Base Run + Drills** Run 10 miles @ base pace Stiff-Legged Run 2×20 seconds Running No Arms 2×20 seconds	Optional Recovery Run or Cardio Cross-Training Workout 20–60 minutes @ recovery pace
WEDNESDAY	**Mixed Intervals** Dynamic stretching warm-up 1-mile warm-up @ recovery pace 1×3K @ half-marathon pace, 2-minute active recovery 1×1 mile @ 10K pace, 2-minute active recovery 1×1K @ 5K pace, 2-minute active recovery 1×800m @ 3,000m pace 1-mile cool-down @ recovery pace	Optional Recovery Run or Cardio Cross-Training Workout 20–60 minutes @ recovery pace
THURSDAY	**Recovery/Base Run** 4–8 miles @ recovery/base pace	**Resistance Workout** *2 sets each* Lying Hip Abduction Single-Leg Squat Box Lunge Stability Ball Leg Curl Squat Jump Single-Leg Squat Jump
FRIDAY	**Cruise Intervals @ Half-Marathon Pace** 2-mile warm-up @ recovery pace 2×3.5 miles @ half-marathon pace, 0.5-mile active recovery 2-mile cool-down @ recovery pace	Optional Recovery Run or Cardio Cross-Training Workout 20–60 minutes @ recovery pace

SATURDAY	**Recovery/Base Run** 4–8 miles @ recovery/base pace	**Resistance Workout** *2 sets each* Cook Hip Lift Oblique Bridge Forearms to Palms Bridge Stability Ball Leg Curl Split Squat Jump Broad Jump
SUNDAY	**Endurance Run** Run 20 miles @ base pace	Optional Recovery Run or Cardio Cross-Training Workout 20–60 minutes @ recovery pace

WEEK 18 ◆ Proprioceptive Cue: Pounding the Ground

MONDAY	Off	
TUESDAY	**Base Run + Drills** Run 10 miles @ base pace Stiff-Legged Run 2×20 seconds Running No Arms 2×20 seconds	<u>Optional Recovery Run or Cardio Cross-Training Workout</u> 20–60 minutes @ recovery pace
WEDNESDAY	**Mixed Intervals** Dynamic stretching warm-up 1-mile warm-up @ recovery pace 1×3K @ half-marathon pace, 2-minute active recovery 1×2K @ 10K pace, 2-minute active recovery 1×1K @ 5K pace, 2-minute active recovery 1×800m @ 3,000m pace 1-mile cool-down @ recovery pace	<u>Optional Recovery Run or Cardio Cross-Training Workout</u> 20–60 minutes @ recovery pace
THURSDAY	**Recovery/Base Run** 4–8 miles @ recovery/base pace	**Resistance Workout** *2 sets each* Lying Hip Abduction Single-Leg Squat Box Lunge Stability Ball Leg Curl Squat Jump Single-Leg Squat Jump
FRIDAY	**Cruise Intervals @ Half-Marathon Pace** 2-mile warm-up @ recovery pace 2×3.75 miles @ half-marathon pace, 0.5-mile active recovery 2-mile cool-down @ recovery pace	<u>Optional Recovery Run or Cardio Cross-Training Workout</u> 20–60 minutes @ recovery pace
SATURDAY	**Recovery/Base Run** 4–8 miles @ recovery/base pace	**Resistance Workout** *2 sets each* Cook Hip Lift Oblique Bridge

SATURDAY (continued)	**Recovery/Base Run**	**Resistance Workout** *2 sets each (cont.)* Quadruped Dead Bug Single-Leg Squat Jump Wall Jump
SUNDAY	**Marathon-Pace Run** 2-mile warm-up @ recovery pace 9 miles @ marathon pace 2-mile cool-down @ recovery pace	Optional Recovery Run or Cardio Cross-Training Workout 20–60 minutes @ recovery pace

WEEK 19 ◆ Proprioceptive Cue: Driving the Thigh

MONDAY	Off	
TUESDAY	**Base Run + Drills** Run 10 miles @ base pace Stiff Hill Sprints 2 × 20 seconds One-Leg Hop 2 × 20 seconds	Optional Recovery Run or Cardio Cross-Training Workout 20–60 minutes @ recovery pace

WEDNESDAY	**Mixed Intervals**
	Dynamic stretching warm-up
	1-mile warm-up @ recovery pace
	1 × 2 miles @ half-marathon pace,
	   2-minute active recovery
	1 × 2K @ 10K pace, 2-minute active
	   recovery
	1 × 1 mile @ 5K pace, 2-minute
	   active recovery
	1 × 800m @ 3,000m pace
	1-mile cool-down @ recovery
	   pace
		Optional Recovery Run or Cardio
		Cross-Training Workout
		20–60 minutes @ recovery pace

THURSDAY	**Recovery/Base Run** 4–8 miles @ recovery/base pace	**Resistance Workout** *2 sets each* Kneeling Overhead Draw-In Lying Draw-In w/Hip Flexion Box Lunge Stability Ball Leg Curl Squat Jump Single-Leg Squat Jump

FRIDAY	**Cruise Intervals @ Half-Marathon Pace**
	2-mile warm-up @ recovery pace
	2 × 4 miles @ half-marathon pace,
	   0.5-mile active recovery
	2-mile cool-down @ recovery
	   pace
		Optional Recovery Run or Cardio
		Cross-Training Workout
		20–60 minutes @ recovery pace

SATURDAY	**Recovery/Base Run** 4–8 miles @ recovery/base pace	**Resistance Workout** *2 sets each* Cook Hip Lift Oblique Bridge

SATURDAY (continued)	**Recovery/Base Run**	**Resistance Workout** *2 sets each (cont.)* Quadruped Dead Bug Single-Leg Squat Jump Wall Jump
SUNDAY	**Endurance Run** Run 22 miles @ base pace	Optional Recovery Run or Cardio Cross-Training Workout 20–60 minutes @ recovery pace

WEEK 20 (Recovery) ◆ Proprioceptive Cue: Floppy Feet

MONDAY	Off	
TUESDAY	**Base Run + Drills** Run 6 miles @ base pace High Knees 20 seconds Bounding 20 seconds	<u>Optional Recovery Run or Cardio</u> <u>Cross-Training Workout</u> 20–60 minutes @ recovery pace

WEDNESDAY	**Mixed Intervals**
	Dynamic stretching warm-up
	1-mile warm-up @ recovery pace
	1 × 2K @ half-marathon pace,
	    2-minute active recovery
	1 × 1 mile @ 10K pace, 2-minute
	    active recovery
	1 × 1K @ 5K pace, 2-minute active
	    recovery
	1 × 800m @ 3,000m pace
	1-mile cool-down @ recovery
	    pace
		<u>Optional Recovery Run or Cardio</u>
		<u>Cross-Training Workout</u>
		20–60 minutes @ recovery pace

THURSDAY	**Recovery/Base Run** 4–8 miles @ recovery/base pace	**Resistance Workout** *2 sets each* Kneeling Overhead Draw-In Lying Draw-In w/Hip Flexion Box Lunge Stability Ball Leg Curl Squat Jump
FRIDAY	**Cruise Intervals @ Half-Marathon Pace** 2-mile warm-up @ recovery pace 2 × 2 miles @ half-marathon pace, 0.5-mile active recovery 2-mile cool-down @ recovery pace	
SATURDAY	**Recovery Run** 2 miles @ recovery pace	**Resistance Workout** *1 set each* Knee Fall-Out Oblique Bridge Quadruped Dead Bug Split Squat Jump

SUNDAY	**Half-Marathon Tune-up Race or Time Trial**
	2-mile warm-up @ recovery pace
	Half-marathon tune-up race or time trial
	2-mile cool-down @ recovery pace

WEEK 21 ◆ Proprioceptive Cue: Butt Squeeze

MONDAY	Off	
TUESDAY	**Base Run + Drills** Run 11 miles @ base pace Stiff-Legged Run 2×20 seconds Running No Arms 2×20 seconds	<u>Optional Recovery Run or Cardio</u> <u>Cross-Training Workout</u> 20–60 minutes @ recovery pace
WEDNESDAY	**Mixed Intervals** Dynamic stretching warm-up 1-mile warm-up @ recovery pace 1×2 miles @ half-marathon pace, 2-minute active recovery 1×2K @ 10K pace, 2-minute active recovery 1×1 mile @ 5K pace, 2-minute active recovery 1×800m @ 3,000m pace 1-mile cool-down @ recovery pace	<u>Optional Recovery Run or Cardio</u> <u>Cross-Training Workout</u> 20–60 minutes @ recovery pace
THURSDAY	**Recovery/Base Run** 4–8 miles @ recovery/base pace	**Resistance Workout** *2 sets each* Lying Hip Abduction Single-Leg Squat Box Lunge Stability Ball Leg Curl Single-Leg Squat Jump Wall Jump
FRIDAY	**Cruise Intervals @ Half-Marathon Pace** 2-mile warm-up @ recovery pace 2×4.25 miles @ half-marathon pace, 0.5-mile active recovery 2-mile cool-down @ recovery pace	<u>Optional Recovery Run or Cardio</u> <u>Cross-Training Workout</u> 20–60 minutes @ recovery pace
SATURDAY	**Recovery/Base Run** 4–8 miles @ recovery/base pace	**Resistance Workout** *2 sets each* Cook Hip Lift Oblique Bridge

SATURDAY (continued)	**Recovery/Base Run**	**Resistance Workout** *2 sets each (cont.)* Quadruped Dead Bug Squat Jump Single-Leg Box Jump
SUNDAY	**Endurance Run** Run 24 miles @ base pace	Optional Recovery Run or Cardio Cross-Training Workout 20–60 minutes @ recovery pace

WEEK 22 ◆ Proprioceptive Cue: Feeling Symmetry

MONDAY	Off	
TUESDAY	**Base Run + Drills** Run 11 miles @ base pace Steep Hill Sprints 2×20 seconds One-Leg Hop 2×20 seconds	<u>Optional Recovery Run or Cardio Cross-Training Workout</u> 20–60 minutes @ recovery pace
WEDNESDAY	**Mixed Intervals** Dynamic stretching warm-up 1-mile warm-up @ recovery pace 1×2 miles @ half-marathon pace, 90-second active recovery 1×2K @ 10K pace, 90-second active recovery 1×1 mile @ 5K pace, 90-second active recovery 1×800m @ 3,000m pace 1-mile cool-down @ recovery pace	<u>Optional Recovery Run or Cardio Cross-Training Workout</u> 20–60 minutes @ recovery pace
THURSDAY	**Recovery/Base Run** 4–8 miles @ recovery/base pace	**Resistance Workout** *2 sets each* Kneeling Overhead Draw-In Lying Draw-In w/Hip Flexion Box Lunge Stability Ball Leg Curl Wall Jump Squat Jump
FRIDAY	**Cruise Intervals @ Half-Marathon Pace** 2-mile warm-up @ recovery pace 2×4.5 miles @ half-marathon pace, 0.5-mile active recoveries 2-mile cool-down @ recovery pace	<u>Optional Recovery Run or Cardio Cross-Training Workout</u> 20–60 minutes @ recovery pace
SATURDAY	**Recovery/Base Run** 4–8 miles @ recovery/base pace	**Resistance Workout** *2 sets each* Knee Fall-Out Oblique Bridge

SATURDAY (continued)	Recovery/Base Run	**Resistance Workout** *2 sets each (cont.)* Quadruped Dead Bug Single-Leg Box Jump Split Squat Jump
SUNDAY	**Marathon-Pace Run** 2-mile warm-up @ recovery pace 13 miles @ marathon pace 2-mile cool-down @ recovery pace	Optional Recovery Run or Cardio Cross-Training Workout 20–60 minutes @ recovery pace

WEEK 23 (Taper) ◆ Proprioceptive Cue: Axle Between the Knees

MONDAY	Off	
TUESDAY	**Base Run + Drills** Run 8 miles @ base pace High Knees 2×20 seconds Bounding 2×20 seconds	<u>Optional Recovery Run or Cardio Cross-Training Workout</u> 20–60 minutes @ recovery pace

WEDNESDAY	**Mixed Intervals**
	Dynamic stretching warm-up
	1-mile warm-up @ recovery pace
	1×3K @ half-marathon pace,
	   90-second active recovery
	1×2K @ 10K pace, 90-second
	   active recovery
	1×1K @ 5K pace, 90-second
	   active recovery
	1×800m @ 3,000m pace
	1-mile cool-down @ recovery
	   pace
		<u>Optional Recovery Run or Cardio Cross-Training Workout</u>
		20–60 minutes @ recovery pace

THURSDAY	**Recovery/Base Run** 4–8 miles @ recovery/base pace	**Resistance Workout** *2 sets each* Lying Hip Abduction Single-Leg Squat Box Lunge Stability Ball Leg Curl Squat Jump Single-Leg Squat Jump

FRIDAY	**Cruise Intervals @ Half-Marathon Pace**
	2-mile warm-up @ recovery pace
	2×2.5 miles @ half-marathon
	   pace, 0.5-mile active recoveries
	2-mile cool-down @ recovery
	   pace
		<u>Optional Recovery Run or Cardio Cross-Training Workout</u>
		20–60 minutes @ recovery pace

SATURDAY	**Recovery/Base Run** 4–8 miles @ recovery/base pace	**Resistance Workout** *2 sets each* Cook Hip Lift

SATURDAY (continued)	**Recovery/Base Run**	**Resistance Workout** *2 sets each (cont.)* Oblique Bridge Quadruped Dead Bug Split Squat Jump
SUNDAY	**Endurance Run** Run 15 miles @ base pace	Optional Recovery Run or Cardio Cross-Training Workout 20–60 minutes @ recovery pace

WEEK 24 (Taper) ◆ Proprioceptive Cue: Your Choice

MONDAY	Off
TUESDAY	**Base Run + Drills** Run 6 miles @ base pace Stiff-Legged Run 20 seconds Running No Arms 20 seconds
WEDNESDAY	**Mixed Intervals** Dynamic stretching warm-up 1-mile warm-up @ recovery pace 1×2K @ half-marathon pace, 90-second active recovery 1×1 mile @ 10K pace, 90-second active recovery 1×1K @ 5K pace, 90-second active recovery 1-mile cool-down @ recovery pace
THURSDAY	**Resistance Workout** *1 set each* Kneeling Overhead Draw-In Lying Draw-In w/Hip Flexion Box Lunge Stability Ball Leg Curl
FRIDAY	**Tempo Run @ Half-Marathon Pace** 1-mile warm-up @ recovery pace 2 miles @ half-marathon pace 1-mile cool-down @ recovery pace
SATURDAY	Off
SUNDAY	**Marathon Peak Race** Marathon

INDEX

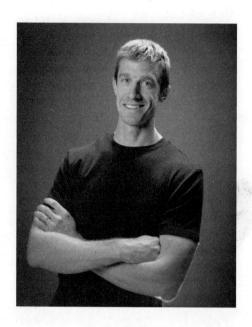

Matt Fitzgerald is a runner, coach, and widely published writer. A frequent contributor to *Runner's World* and *Triathlete,* he has authored five previous books for runners and triathletes. Matt is also a certified sports nutritionist and a TrainingPeaks.com featured coach. He lives in Northern California with his wife, Nataki.